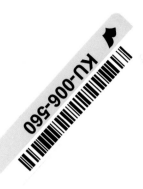

Perspectives in Exercise Science
and Sports Medicine: Volume 10

Optimizing Sport Performance

Edited by

David R. Lamb
The Ohio State University

Robert Murray
The Gatorade Company

Publishing
Group

Library of Congress Cataloging in Publication Data:
LAMB, DAVID R., 1939-
PERSPECTIVES IN EXERCISE SCIENCE AND SPORTS MEDICINE
VOLUME 10: OPTIMIZING SPORT PERFORMANCE

Cover Design: Gary Schmitt

Library of Congress Catalog Card number: 88-70343

ISBN: 1-884125-63-8

Printed in the United States of America by Cooper Publishing Group, 1048 Summit Drive, Carmel, IN 46032
10 9 8 7 6 5 4 3 2 1

Contents

Contributors vii
Acknowledgement xi
Preface xiii

Chapter 1   Mind Games: The Psychology of Sport 1
William P. Morgan

Introduction 1
Historical Anecdotes 3
Applied Sport Psychology 5
Ethical Principles and Training 18
Cognituve Strategies 22
Performance and Mood States 38
Earlier Reviews 41
Practical Implications 44
Directions for Future Practice 46
Directions for Future Research 46
Summary 46
Acknowledgements 50
Bibliography 50
Discussion 54

Chapter 2   Advances in the Evaluation of Sports Training 63
Harm Kuipers

Introduction 64
Sports Training 65
Exercise Testing 67
Indices of Endurance Capacity 70
Measurement of Anaerobic Energy Production 79
Indices of Strength and Speed 80
Field Tests of Sport Performance Capacity 81
Practical Implications 84
Directions for Future Research 85
Summary 86

Bibliography 87
Discussion 90

Chapter 3   Fuels for Sport Performance 95
Edward F. Coyle

Introduction 96
Body Fat Stores 97
Body Carbohydrate Stores 98
Substrate Use During Exercise of Various Intensities 98
Fat Supplementation During Exercise .104
Diets High in Fat and Low in Carbohydrate 105
Endurance Training Increases Fat Oxidation
    During Exercise 107
Dietary Carbohydrate Influences Fat Oxidation
    During Exercise 109
Carbohydratate Feeding During Exercise 110
Metabolic Responses to Various Types of Dietary
    Carbohydrate 115
Muscle Glycogen Resynthesis Following Exercise 116
Maximizing Muscle Glycogen Prior to Competition 119
Preexercise Nutrition 120
Practical Applications for Active People 123
Directions for Future Research 124
Summary 124
Bibliography 125

Chapter 4   Optimizing Hydration for Competitive Sport 139
R.J. Maughan

Introduction 139
Thermoregulation and Fluid Balance .141
Limitations to Fluid Replacement 151
Preexercise Hydration 160
Postexercise Rehydration 161
Formulation of Rehydration Fluids 166
Practical Implications for the Athlete .170
Bibliography 172
Discussion 176

Chapter 5 Erogogenic Aids: Recent Advances and Retreats 185
Lawrence L. Spriet

Introduction 186
Creatine 187
Carnitine 201
Caffeine 210
Erythropoietin 222
Directions for Future Research 227
Summary 228
Bibliography 230
Discussion 234

**Chapter 6 Detection of Cardiovascular and Other
Health Problems in Athletes** 239
E. Randy Eichner

Introduction 240
Sudden Deaths of Athletes: Scope and Impact 240
Epidemiological Information on Sudden Deaths 241
Athlete's Heart 244
Screening Athletes for Cardiovascular Problems 246
Leading Problems: Developments and Implications 251
Conflicts for Team Physicians 258
Practical Implications 258
Directions for Future Research 259
Summary 259
Bibliography 260
Discussion 263

**Chapter 7 The Athlete's Immune System, Intense Exercise,
and Overtraining** 269
J. Mark Davis and Lisa Hertler-Colbert

Introduction 270
Overview of the Immune System 272
Intense Exercise and Immune Function 278
Exercise Training, Competition, and Infection 287
Overtraining, Immune Function, and Infection 290
Potential Mechanisms of Overtraining 297
Practical Implications 303
Summary 305
Bibliography 307
Discussion 311

**Chapter 8   Stay in the Game: Prevention of and Recovery
from Sports Injuries** 317
John R. Perry, Thomas P. Knapp, and Bert R. Mandelbaum

Introduction 318
Injury to the Anterior Cruciate Ligament 319
Osteochondral Knee Injuries 331
Stress Fractures 334
Ankle Impingement Syndromes 344
Summary 350
Bibliography 351
Discussion 353

Index 361

Contributors

Luis Aragon, Ph.D.
c/o Quaker Oats (Guatemala)
Edicifio Topaz Azul, Oficina 801
13 Calle 2-60 Zona 10
Guatemala City, Guatemala C.A.

Francisco Arroyo, M.D.
c/o Beverages Division
Ave. Americas #1600-ler Piso
Col. Providenica - 44620 Guadalajara
Jal., Mexico

Bobby Barton, Ed.D., ATC
Department of Athletics
Eastern Kentucky University
Richmond, KY 40475

Oded Bar-Or, M.D.
Children's Exercise and Nutrition
  Centre
Chedoke Hospital Division
Hamilton, ON L8N 3Z5
CANADA

Ronald Behnke, HSD, ATC
Dept. of Physical Education
Indiana State University
Terre Haute, IN 47809

JiDi Chen, M.D.
Institute of Sports Medicine
Beijing Medican University
Beijing 100083 China

Nancy Clark, M.S., R.D.
830 Boylston St.
Brookline, MA 02167

Priscilla M. Clarkson, Ph.D.
Department of Exercise Science
University of Massachusetts
Amherst, MA 01003

Edward F. Coyle, Ph.D.
Human Performance Lab
University of Texas
Austin, TX 78712

J. Mark Davis, Ph.D.
Department of Exercise Science
University of South Carolina
Columbia, SC 29208

Rod K. Dishman, Ph.D.
University of Georgia
Dept. of Exercise Science
Athens, GA 30602-3654

E. Randy Eichner, M.D.
Section of Hematology (EB-271)
University of Oklahoma
Health Sciences Center
Oklahoma City, OK 73190

Carl V. Gisolfi, Ph.D.
Dept. of Exercise Science
University of Iowa
Iowa City, IA 52242

Consuelo Gonalez-Suarez, M.D.
Sports Medicine Assoc. of the
  Phillipines
Manila, PHILLIPINES

Mark Hargreaves, Ph.D.
School of Human Movement
Deakin University
Burwood 3125
AUSTRALIA

Elizabeth Hernandez, N.D.
Division Beverages
Avenida 4 Norte #6N-67-Oficina 209
Edificio Siglo XXI
Cali, COLUMBIA

Craig A. Horswill, Ph.D.
Gatorade Exercise Physiology
  Laboratory
The Gatorade Company
Barrington, IL 60010

David O. Hough, M.D.
Michigan State University
East Lansing, MI 48824-1315

Carmen S.Y. Jahja, M.D.
National Sports Council of Indonesia
Sports Science Centre
PIO-KONI Pusat Jl. Pintu I Senayan
Jakarta 10270 INDONESIA

Ricardo Javornik, M.D.
c/o Productors Quaker, C.A.
Centro Plaza, Torre C, Piso 16
Avendida Francisco de Miranda
Los Palos Grandes
Caracas, VENEZUELA

Steve Johnsen, B.S.
710 Lancashire Court
Lincoln, NE 68510

Mitchell Kanter, Ph.D.
Gatorade Exercise Physiology
  Laboratory
The Gatorade Company
Barrington, IL 60010

W. Larry Kenney, Ph.D.
Noll Physiological Research Center
The Pennsylvania State University
University Park, PA 16802-6900

Susan Kleiner, Ph.D., R.D., L.D.
2456 63rd Avenue SE
Mercer Island, WA 98040

Howard Knuttgen, Ph.D.
Center for Sports Medicine
Pennsylvania State University
University Park, PA 16082

Tom Koto, ATC
Idaho Sports Medicine Institute
Boise, ID 83706

Harm Kuipers, Ph.D.
University of Limburg
Dept. of Movement Sciences
6229 ER MAASTRICHT
THE NETHERLANDS

David R. Lamb, Ph.D.
508 Greenglade Avenue
Worthington, Ohio 43085

Antonio Lancha, Jr. Ph.D.
4949 W. Pine Blvd., #13K
St. Louis, MO 63108

Bert R. Mandelbaum, M.D.
Santa Monica Sports Medicine,
Suite 150
Santa Monica, CA 90404

Ronald J. Maughan, Ph.D.
University Medical School
Dept. Environmental/Occupational
  Medicine
Foresterhill
Aberdeen AB9 2ZD
SCOTLAND

William P. Morgan, Ed.D.
University of Wisconsin
Sport Psychology Lab
Madison, WI 53706

Robert Murray, Ph.D.
Gatorade Exercise Physiology
  Laboratory
The Gatorade Company
Barrington, IL 60010

Ethan R. Nadel, Ph.D.
John B. Pierce Foundation Laboratory
New Haven, CT 06519

David C. Nieman, Ph.D.
Dept. of Health, Leisure, and
Exercise Science
Applachian State University
Boone, NC 28608

Dennis Passe, Ph.D.
Gatorade Exercise Physiology Laboratory
The Gatorade Company
Barrington, IL 60010

Chris Patrick, M.A., ATC
Department of Athletics
University of Florida
Gainesville, FL 32604

Srimurni P. Prastowo, M.D.
Bagian Ilmu Gixi F.K.U.I.
Jl. Salemba 6
Jakarta Pusal 10450 INDONESIA

Thomas Rowland, M.D.
Department of Pediatric Cardiology
Baystate Medical Center
Children's Hospital
Springfield, MA 01199

Warren Scott, M.D.
7221 Viewpoint Rd.
Aptos, CA 95003

Xiaocai Shi, Ph.D.
Gatorade Exercise Physiology Laboratory
The Gatorade Company
Barrington, IL 60010

Lawrence Spriet, Ph.D.
University of Guelph
Human Biology & Nutritional Sciences
Guelph, Ontario
CANADA N1G 2W1

Ronald L. Terjung, Ph.D.
Dept. of Physiology
SUNY Health Science Center
Syracuse, NY 13210

Janet Walberg-Rankin, Ph.D.
Human Nutrition & Foods Dept.
Virginia Tech
Blacksburg VA 24061-0351

Clyde Williams, Ph.D.
Department of Physical Education,
Sports Science & Recreation
Management
Loughborough University
Loughborough
Leicestershire, LE11 3TU
ENGLAND, UK

Sergio Zucas, Ph.D.
c/o Quaker Alimentos Ltda.
Beverages Division
Rua Alexandre Dumas 2100-16 andar
Chacara Santo Antonio
04717-004 Sao Paulo - SP, BRAZIL

Acknowledgement

For the past decade, The Gatorade Company has been proud to sponsor the textbook series, *Perspectives in Exercise Science and Sports Medicine*. The publication of this tenth volume in the series is part of our continuing commitment in support of research and education programs in sports science. As in previous years, this textbook resulted from a meeting of scientific experts in the areas of sports medicine, exercise science, and sports nutrition. The topics that comprise each of the chapters were presented and enthusiastically discussed and debated. The end result of that writing, presentation, and discussion is captured in this text on *Optimizing Sports Performance*. Once again, the authors, reviewers, and editors are to be commended on a superior result.

James F. Doyle
Executive Vice President
President, Quaker Worldwide Beverages

Preface

The publication of this book marks the tenth anniversary of the Gatorade Sports Science Conference, an annual meeting in which experts from a variety of disciplines meet to present, discuss, and debate topics in sports medicine, exercise science, and sports nutrition. The authors write the chapters months in advance of the meeting, allowing the reviewers an opportunity to provide suggestions and raise questions. Revised versions of the chapters are then compiled in large notebooks that each conference participant receives prior to the meeting. At the meeting, each author has an opportunity to present the highlights of the chapter followed by an extensive discussion session, the highlights of which are published at the end of each chapter.

The meeting that spawned this book was held in June 1996 in Vancouver, British Columbia and its success is attributable to the hard work of a number of people. Barb Jackson and Kathryn Bowling from McCord Travel did a great job juggling the myriad travel arrangements for the conference participants. Joan Seye and Betty Dye of The University of Iowa performed their typically splendid work at transcribing all of the discussion tapes, an enormous job that allowed the participants to make their edits before leaving Vancouver. We greatly appreciate the efforts of Cozette Lamb in her superb job at editing the work of the editors to help ensure that the contents of this text are both readable and accurate. Last, but certainly not least, special recognition is owed to The Gatorade Company whose long-standing commitment to research and education programs in exercise science and sports nutrition has established an impressive standard for cooperation between science and business.

With each volume of the *Perspectives* series, we attempt to include a broad range of information that is of use to scientists and practitioners alike. We hope that we have succeeded in that regard and that you find this book to be a useful addition to your professional library.

David Lamb
Robert Murray

1

Mind Games: The Psychology of Sport

WILLIAM P. MORGAN, ED.D.

INTRODUCTION
HISTORICAL ANECDOTES
APPLIED SPORT PSYCHOLOGY
    Relaxation
    Mental Practice
    Goal-Setting
    Self-Efficacy
    External Validity
    Section Summary
ETHICAL PRINCIPLES AND TRAINING
COGNITIVE STRATEGIES
    Qualitative Survey Data
    Lung-Gom and Tumo
    Evaluation of Lung-Gom
    Elite Distance Runners
    Pre-Elite and Non-Elite Distance Runners
    Section Summary
PERFORMANCE AND MOOD STATES
EARLIER REVIEWS
    Section Summary
PRACTICAL IMPLICATIONS
DIRECTIONS FOR FUTURE PRACTICE
DIRECTIONS FOR FUTURE RESEARCH
SUMMARY
    Consumers
    Conclusion
FOOTNOTE
ACKNOWLEDGEMENTS
BIBLIOGRAPHY
DISCUSSION

INTRODUCTION

> "The mind is its own place,
> and in itself can make a Heaven
> of Hell, a Hell of Heaven."
> —John Milton, *Paradise Lost*

There is always a danger in referring to the "mind" in discussions of psychology because the author and reader alike can be easily deluded into thinking of the mind as not only its own place, but one that is separate from the body. However, there is now an extensive body of literature in the fields of clinical and experimental psychology, neuroscience, and psychosomatic medicine arguing in favor of viewing mind and body as one. While this principle can be thought of as a given, it is both parsimonious and heuristic at times to think of the mind and body as occupying different domains from a conceptual and operational standpoint. Hence, when one speaks of "mind games" in sport settings, this usually implies that cognitive psychology is given primacy, but it does not mean that the mind is independent of the body, nor does it mean that "body games" cannot occur as well.

Early work in sport psychology was devoted primarily to the creation of new knowledge and the elucidation of mechanisms underlying various psychological phenomena, and very little attention was paid to applied issues. However, there was a collective rejection of the natural science models by many writers in this field during the late 1970s and early 1980s when the center of gravity shifted toward applied sport psychology. In other words, the contemporary focus in this field involves issues such as: (1) packaging psychological principles for delivery to athletes and coaches, (2) concerns about whether or not the packages are appreciated or accepted by consumers, and (3) the relative efficacy of various psychological approaches. However, little attention has been paid to the question of whether or not these psychological interventions actually work in settings in which they are used and promoted. An argument has emerged in the field of sport psychology for the adoption of *intuitive* as opposed to *natural science* or *empirical* models, so there are very few new perspectives of a scientific nature in this field. Therefore, this chapter will emphasize some of the older principles that have stood the test of time, as well as what needs to be done if this important area is to move forward.

It should also be noted that the limited research carried out on applied sport psychology topics has been characterized by numerous methodological problems. As a consequence, it is not uncommon for authors to review the published literature in this area and conclude that various psychological interventions are effective. However, this sort of conclusion is not possible if the reviewer employs conventional methodological standards in the process of evaluating the applied research in this field.

In the history and sociology of modern psychological inquiry, the psychoanalytic approach is usually regarded as the "first" force followed by behaviorism as the "second" force. The "inward movement" in contemporary psychology was influenced by many developments.

Members of the humanistic psychology movement, for example, described themselves as the "third" force, and this movement, along with developments within the larger culture, served to emphasize the importance of "consciousness" in academic psychology (Hilgard, 1977). In some respects, developments in sport psychology have paralleled those in cognitive psychology. One of the first examples of the "inward" movement in sport psychology was the appearance of a book by Gallwey (1976) titled *Inner Tennis*. Another was the development of a technique known as visuo-motor behavior rehearsal (VMBR) by Suinn (1972). Suinn made a distinction in his writings between "Self 1" (mind over body), in which the mind directs the body in an instructional or evaluative way, and "Self 2" (body over mind), in which the body takes over its own performance. Suinn has emphasized that Self 1 should be predominant during the precompetitive preparation phase, but as soon as competition is underway, Self 2 should be employed. This performance model seems to imply a clear distinction between the role of mind and body and even the separate nature of mind and body, but Suinn also points out that mind and body should work in harmony as one. Again, it appears that workers in sport psychology sometimes make a distinction between mind and body for the sake of application, but this does not reflect true dualism.

Another recent example taken directly from the field of exercise and sport science is the instructive volume by Newsholme, Leech, and Duester (1994) titled *Keep on Running: The Science of Training and Performance*. These authors devoted an entire chapter to "The Mind and Performance." They opened their discussion of this topic with the statement that ". . . few can doubt the importance of correct mental attitude in any human endeavor taken to its limits" (p. 198), and they concluded this chapter with the rejoinder that "We cannot choose our parents but we can make the best of what they have given us!" (p. 212). These authors suggested that our basic physiological, biochemical, and psychological characteristics are governed by heredity, and they emphasized that psychological training can serve to maximize performance. In other words, the view that "mind games" can enhance performance is held by biochemists and physiologists, as well as by psychologists. The validity of this assumption, as well as its generalizability, will be explored in this chapter.

HISTORICAL ANECDOTES

The role that cognitive psychology plays in endurance performance can be illustrated in the history of record setting in the mile run. Gunder Haegg of Sweden was one of the greatest runners of all times, and he once broke the world records in races over distances of 1,500 m, 2,000 m, 3,000 m, 5,000 m, 2 mi, and 3 mi, all within an 80-d period! While he came very close to breaking the 4-min mile, having run a 4:04.6 in 1942 and a 4:01.4 in 1945, he was unable to break the mythical 4-min barrier. It has been reported by Lars-Eric Unestahl (1982), a Swedish sport psychologist, that Gunder Haegg had read in a book that no man would ever run the mile in less than 4 min because it was thought to be physiologically impossible to achieve this feat; Unestahl speculated that this belief prevented Haegg from breaking the 4-min-mile record. It is also of interest that Haegg's countryman, Arne Anderson, also came close to breaking this record, having run a 4:02.6 in 1943 and a 4:01.6 in 1944. As a matter of fact, the rivalry between Haegg and Anderson brought the 4-min mile within sight, according to Bannister (1981). In discussing the nature of muscular effort in general, Bannister (1956) stated:

> Though physiology may indicate respiratory and circulatory limits to muscular effort, psychological and other factors beyond the ken of physiology set the razor's edge of defeat or victory and determine how close an athlete approaches the absolute limits of performance.

Many dimensions of the assault on the 4-min-mile barrier warrant attention. (The interested reader is referred to the detailed treatment of this topic by Bannister, 1981.) A few of the more salient features of this performance that hold relevance for the present discussion follow. First, it is important to recognize that Roger Bannister was training about 30-min, 5-d/wk when he set the world record, and this certainly falls well below the training volumes pursued by runners in recent years. Second, even with this level of training, Bannister and his teammates experienced what we would label "staleness" by today's standards (Morgan et al., 1987), and following active rest (e.g., hiking and rock climbing) their performances improved. It is clear that Bannister and his teammates were convinced that it was possible to run the mile in less than 4 min (Bannister, 1981), whereas Haegg apparently did not think it was possible. It would seem reasonable to propose that cognitive psychology can explain, in part, Roger Bannister's historic record-shattering performance. Also, it is a matter of record that other runners were soon able to run the mile under 4 min when it was recognized that such a performance was possible. This historical anecdote should not be used to argue that cognitive psychology can be used to facilitate physical performance in the absence of requisite biologic substrate, yet precisely such arguments are being made in the area of applied sport psychology.

Workers in the field of sport psychology often maintain that athletes can achieve essentially any level of performance if they believe it is possible. Indeed, applied sport psychologists often teach athletes to employ "self-talk" monologues designed to enhance performance. Because most of the interventions in applied sport psychology are based upon unverified hypotheses and unsubstantiated pedagogical principles, rather than on scientific evidence, an overview of this area of sport psychology follows.

APPLIED SPORT PSYCHOLOGY

The applied sport psychology movement has been objectively discussed in a series of publications by Dishman (1982, 1983a, 1989, 1991), which should be required reading for anyone contemplating interventions with athletes. Dishman (1991) proposed that applied sport psychology has thrived because of a ". . . bullish consumer market for practical psychology applications in sport and exercise settings." There have been many problems in the area of applied sport psychology, but the most significant has been the apparent lack of concern for scientific verification of the various interventions commonly employed. As a matter of fact, Dishman (1991) pointed out that ". . . it is estimated that the topics of greatest practical concern to coaches are those where applied research with athletes is the most sparse" (p. 156). In many respects this problem is remarkably similar to the state of affairs in the field of psychotherapy when Eysenck (1952) reported that untreated patients recovered as well or better than those treated with eclectic psychotherapy or psychoanalysis. While Eysenck's paper has been subjected to criticism on methodological grounds, it had the effect of stimulating controlled experimental research dealing with the efficacy of psychotherapy.

At the present time there are many applied sport psychologists who employ a variety of procedures with athletes in the hope of enhancing performance. In some cases there is an absence of scientifically acceptable evidence in support of the interventions. In other cases, there is a solid theoretical rationale backed by empirical evidence suggesting that the interventions might actually impair performance. Given this unfortunate state of affairs, the logical question is—"Why do applied sport psychologists employ these procedures?" Dishman (1991) offered three possible explanations. First, he suggested that this error in judgement might be due to primary or secondary ignorance. That is, there is an absence of research evidence (i.e., primary ignorance) or practitioners are unaware (i.e., secondary ignorance) of the absence of supporting evidence or the availability of published research indicating that such interventions are actually contraindicated. Second, the demand by consumers ("bullish market") for services involving practical applications of psychology stimulates sport psychologists to prescribe untested interventions. Third, Dishman pointed out that many sport psychologists believe that an intervention is valid if there is consensus about a given procedure's efficacy among practitioners, coupled with consumer satisfaction. Dishman labels this questionable belief system as "social validity." The history of psychology and medicine instructs us that many procedures (e.g., bloodletting, lobotomy procedure, etc.) were based on similar fallacious thinking (Valenstein, 1986). Several examples of the problem will be presented to further illustrate the point. Additional examples are discussed by Dishman (1991). An effort will be made throughout the chapter to introduce suggestions as to how this situation can be remedied.

Relaxation

The relationship between level of arousal and physical performance has been discussed a great deal in the sport psychology literature (Gould & Udry, 1994; Landers & Boucher, 1993; Weinberg et al.; 1987), but much of this work has been concerned with comparisons of interventions such as "psyching" or "relaxing" individuals prior to the performance of laboratory tasks that have little or no relevance to complex motor behavior in competitive sport situations. The individuals who have taken part in this experimental research have often not been athletes, and when athletes have been employed in such research, the tasks have been of a non-sport nature (e.g., performance on a grip dynamometer, dart throwing, ring tossing, etc.). Sport psychologists have also tended to employ *idiographic* or *nomothetic* research models. In the case of idiographic modeling, emphasis is placed upon the unique nature of the individual, whereas nomothetic approaches emphasize principles of behavior derived from the study of groups. It is difficult to make the case that one approach is superior to the other because the question being asked in the research will ultimately favor one approach over the other. However, when one attempts to predict performance for any given individual in a specific sport setting, a theoretical rationale and compelling empirical research data support the superiority of idiographic modeling and applications. An example of this approach is the recent research involving application of Hanin's "zone of optimal function" (ZOF) model, which maintains that each individual has an optimal zone of function (i.e., IZOF) from an arousal standpoint and that this optimal state of arousal can be low, moderate, or high. The original work by Hanin (1989) has been replicated and extended (Hanin & Syrjä, 1994, 1995; Morgan, 1993; Morgan & Ellickson, 1989; Raglin, 1992; Raglin & Morris, 1994; Raglin & Turner, 1993).

The idea that certain tasks require a high level of arousal, and others a low level, or the view that all tasks require a moderate level of arousal (i.e., inverted U function) is no longer defensible. There is now compelling evidence that each individual has an optimal zone, and this optimal zone might represent low, moderate, or high levels of state anxiety as measured by the state anxiety scale (± 4 units) developed by Spielberger et al. (1983). Research evidence supporting the IZOF model has been presented by Hanin (1989), Morgan et al., (1987, 1988b), Raglin (1992), Raglin & Morris (1994), and Raglin and Turner (1993). In other words, it is now clear that attempting to relax or excite groups of individuals is contraindicated because such attempts have the potential of impairing the performance of approximately two thirds of individuals in most cases.

It is commonly believed by many applied sport psychologists that relaxation procedures will enhance performance. There are several relaxation procedures that are quite effective in reducing anxiety, and there is no question about whether or not an anxious athlete *can be* relaxed. The important question, however, is whether or not an anxious athlete *should be* relaxed. This is a complex question, and it requires a complex answer. A detailed discussion of this matter will be found in the review by Raglin (1992), but for the sake of brevity it can be concluded that the routine use of relaxation procedures with athletes is inappropriate for a number of reasons. First, it is known that some individuals with high anxiety levels actually experience panic attacks when administered standard relaxation procedures (Borkovec, 1985; Borkovec et al., 1987; Heide & Borkovec, 1984). Therefore, it is imperative that sport psychologists not employ relaxation procedures in a laissez-faire manner, and anyone employing this procedure should be familiar with the problem of relaxation-induced panic. Second, there is evidence that some athletes perform optimally when their anxiety is elevated, whereas others tend to perform best when relaxed or moderately anxious (Raglin, 1992). Third, it has been shown by Mittelman et al. (1992) that relaxation and imagery can provoke undesired effects in subjects exposed to a cold stressor.

This instructive investigation demonstrated that Navy divers who could best use relaxation and imagery were the least effective in coping with exposure to cold water. While this finding is counterintuitive at first glance, the authors presented a compelling physiological explanation for the observation. The divers used images of a warm environment during immersion in 25°C water in an effort to increase their abilities to cope with the cold stress. Most of the divers were unable to influence thermoregulation with this hypnotic procedure; furthermore, 3 of 12 divers actually lost heat at a faster rate under hypnosis than under the control condition. The investigators suggested that relaxation and images of warmth reduced shivering, with a concomitant loss of heat production. In other words, using images of a warm day may have produced vasodilation in the skin and muscles, which in turn produced a greater rate of heat loss. This investigation emphasizes the importance of not employing a psychological intervention unless the procedure's efficacy has first been demonstrated. Indeed, in this case it appears that use of hypnosis, imagery, and relaxation not only failed to enhance coping ability but actually placed these divers at an increased risk of hypothermia (Mittleman et al., 1992).

In addition to the potential for decreasing performance in an individual or group by using a relaxation strategy, another reason why such a practice should not be employed is, "relaxation-induced anxiety." The explanation for this paradoxical production of anxiety with relaxation training is complex. Anecdotal reports of relaxation-induced anxiety have been associated with interventions such as autogenic relaxation, biofeedback, progressive muscular relaxation, and transcendental mediation. This paradoxical effect has been most common in chronically anxious individuals (Borkovec, 1985; Borkovec et al., 1987). In addition to anecdotal reports, empirical research supports this phenomenon of relaxation-induced anxiety. For example, Heide and Borkovec (1984) conducted an experiment in which progressive relaxation and mantra meditation were presented in counterbalanced order to seven men and seven women suffering from general tension. During a preliminary practice session, four of these individuals displayed evidence of an anxiety reaction, and another stopped practice prematurely because of an anxiety response. It was later found that 31% of the total group experienced increased tension following progressive relaxation, and 54% had increased tension due to focused relaxation in the meditation condition. These findings are particularly relevant to the field of applied sport psychology because it is probable that individuals with chronic anxiety are the most likely to request relaxation training for the management of this condition. In other words, in addition to theoretically decreasing performance in those athletes who perform best when anxious, it is also probable that use of relaxation procedures with such individuals would produce relaxation-induced anxiety in some of them. It is remarkable that the problem of relaxation-induced anxiety is not even discussed in recent reviews designed to promote the use of applied sport psychology interventions such as relaxation (e.g., Greenspan & Feltz, 1989; Kirschenbaum et al. 1995; Whelan et al., 1991).

Relaxation-induced anxiety has practical and theoretical implications, but the mechanisms responsible for this phenomenon are unclear. However, of the mechanisms proposed to date, the ". . . fear of losing control or exerting undue effort to achieve control" (Heide & Borkovec, 1984) has received the most support. At any rate, individuals who employ various relaxation procedures need to be sensitive to the possibility that the paradoxical response known as relaxation-induced anxiety can and does occur in chronically anxious individuals.

Williamson (1996) reported that it is important for athletes to develop an "awareness" of the factors responsible for distracting them during competition, and this is true regardless of an athlete's level of experience. Furthermore, Williamson advises the athlete:

> If you notice your heart racing, you are breathing too quickly. If your palms are sweating, take a couple of deep breaths and repeat key words, or cues such as "calm," "cool," "focused." Use words that come naturally to you, but be sure that the words can produce a calming affect, not an increase in arousal. (p. 2)

Williamson does not present any research evidence in support of such an intervention, whereas a considerable amount of theoretical and empirical evidence supports the view that some athletes should actually be aroused, not calm, in order to maximize performance in such a setting (Raglin, 1992).

Another example involving a similar approach has been described by Kabat-Zinn and Beall (1985) for the sport of rowing. These authors reported that relaxation is of particular importance immediately before a race and that competitive pressures often lead to elevated arousal, which in turn can reduce an individual's alertness and can adversely affect rowing techniques. In an effort to deal with this arousal, rowers are advised by these investigators to keep their "minds" on their ". . . breathing at the abdomen prior to the start of races" (Kabat-Zinn & Beall, 1985). On the other hand, Ellickson (1986) observed that successful rowing teams reported that they experienced significant elevations in anxiety just prior to their best performances. Furthermore, an increase in body awareness or arousal prior to a runner's personal best has been reported for elite men and women distance runners (Morgan et al., 1987; 1988b). Also, the men's and women's rowing teams studied by Ellickson (1986) went on to win the National Collegiate Athletic Association Championships. Results of this study are summarized in Figure 1-1. It could be argued that these teams would have experienced impairments in performance if a relaxation intervention had been employed with them just prior to the national championship.

Murphy (1988) reported that the psychological support service most frequently requested by athletes competing in the U.S. Olympic Festival was help for "coping with preperformance anxiety." However, the fact that athletes request support for coping with anxiety prior to a competition does not mean that it is necessarily in their best interests to have anxiety reduced with various relaxation strategies. Indeed, if an in-

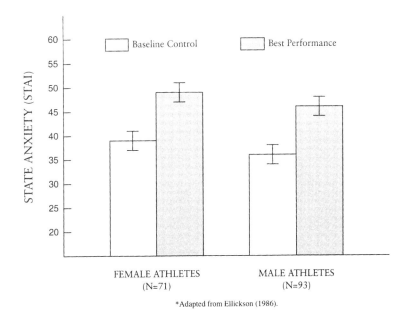

FIGURE 1-1. *Recall of pre-competition state anxiety in collegiate rowers.* Adapted from Ellickson (1986).

dividual performs best when anxious, it might be more appropriate to employ a cognitive strategy designed to help the athlete cope with the anxiety by use of "restructuring," in which the anxiety is perceived as a positive signal. The relative merits of various psychological approaches must be considered on theoretical grounds at this point. There is a need for applied research dealing with questions of whether or not one approach is superior to another. At any rate, it would be inappropriate to imply that a particular approach was superior at this stage if a given intervention is based entirely on an untested model or theory. Also, while there is a popular conception that sport psychologists should be made available on site, an alternative view is that psychologists can be of greatest value preparing athletes for upcoming competitions in advance of, not on the day of, a competition (Desharnais, 1983; Unestahl, 1982).

The question of how a counselor, clinical psychologist, or psychiatrist should proceed when faced with a client who seems to have an anxiety problem can be quite challenging. It is common for such problems to be presented within the context of performance decrements in the athlete. However, it often becomes apparent during the therapeutic intervention that the presenting problem is merely a symptom, and the actual problem can be far more serious and complex at times (e.g., depression of clinical significance). Hence, it is imperative that service providers not only possess appropriate licensure and certification to help insure that serious psychological problems will be recognized, but they should also have the necessary background and training in exercise and sport science in order to have a full appreciation for the nature of the psychological problem in an exercise or sport setting. It should also be understood that excessive anxiety during the precompetitive setting may actually serve an ergogenic function, and elimination of this distress with various procedures such as biofeedback, hypnosis, meditation or relaxation would theoretically impair performance (Hanin, 1989; Raglin, 1992). In such cases, the preferred intervention may be to attempt to *increase* the athlete's perceived anxiety before competition.

Relaxation training represents one of the most frequently employed interventions used by applied sport psychologists, and a review of self-help books in "pop" psychology, as well as a number of books and articles published in the area of applied sport psychology, gives the impression that a number of tried and proven interventions (i.e., "mind games") can be employed as a means of enhancing performance. However, closer inspection of the basis or foundation for various sport psychology interventions, such as relaxation, visualization and imagery, goal setting strategies, and treatment of alleged problems associated with phenomena such as insomnia and jet lag, reveals a striking absence of compelling research evidence for these applications. Indeed, it is fair to say that most of these interventions are based upon a series of *yet-to-be-confirmed* hypotheses. A discussion of several of the most commonly employed interventions, for which there is little or no support and in several cases evidence arguing against their employment, will be discussed.

Mental Practice

Druckman and Swets (1988) reported that mental practice of a motor skill such as dart throwing, basketball foul shooting, or bowling is associated with improved performance, and the effect size across all practice treatments was 0.43 standard deviations. Effect size is sometimes used in place of standard tests of significance between control and experimental conditions. It is computed by subtracting the control mean from the experimental mean and dividing by the pooled standard deviation. Although this effect size was statistically significant, it is noteworthy that the effect size for physical practice (0.79) showed the greatest change effects. Furthermore, the results of Druckman and Swets cannot be generalized to competitive athletic settings. Importantly, there would be no reason to assume that improvement in the *learning* of a motor skill such as throwing darts would have relevance for the *performance* of already well-ingrained sport skills in competition, such as throwing a discus in a track-and-field meet.

In a meta-analysis of 60 studies yielding 146 effect sizes, Feltz and Landers (1983) found an average effect size of 0.48 for mental practice and concluded that ". . . mentally practicing a motor skill influences performance somewhat better than no practice at all" (p.25). This, of course, is the same as saying that mental practice is "better than nothing," and it raises a question about whether or not the effect is merely due to differences between *no* treatment and *any* treatment (i.e., the Hawthorne effect (Morgan, 1997). It has been recognized for many years that muscular performance can be increased significantly with a placebo or inert treatment (Morgan, 1972).

It is remarkable that investigators concerned with the efficacy of "mind games" seldom employ appropriate (i.e., blind) placebo paradigms. There is also a tendency for journals not to publish negative findings. This is especially important in the area of mental practice and motor performance because published studies apparently report larger average effect sizes than unpublished investigations (Feltz & Landers, 1983; p. 25).

In terms of possible mechanisms underlying the alleged effect of mental practice on the learning and performance of motor skills, several authors have proposed that the "effect" is due to neuromuscular facilitation; however, this point of view is not without opposition. Dishman (1991) pointed out that such a position fails to recognize that feedback or some form of feedforward control is included in modern theories of motor skill acquisition. Indeed, Dishman (1991) concludes this critique with the statement that:

No plausible explanation can currently be mustered for enhancing motor control by imaging in the absence of movement and knowledge of results, yet the practice persists in the literatures of applied sport psychology in isolation from the traditions and methods of what is known about motor skill acquisition and retention. (p. 45)

A cardinal principle of research design is to employ a control group, or a control condition in which participants in the study serve as their own controls for comparison purposes. A recent study by Tenenbaum et al. (1995) dealing with the effects of selected psychological interventions on isokinetic leg strength illustrates the importance of employing a control in exercise science research. These investigators randomly assigned 45 men to one of three groups that received (1) a cognitive intervention based on positive statements (self-efficacy), (2) relaxation, visualization, and "autogenic" relaxation training, and (3) control (no treatment). Knee extensor strength was evaluated before and following four sessions of the psychological interventions and the control condition. The self-efficacy condition resulted in an increase of 24.6% in peak force compared with a gain of 9.0% for the relaxation-visualization condition. This difference of 15.6% favoring the self-efficacy group was statistically significant ($P < 0.05$). The most remarkable feature of this study, however, was the observation that the untreated control group improved 39.1%—a gain significantly greater ($P < 0.05$) than both of the psychological interventions. This study has many implications for investigations dealing with the efficacy of any intervention designed to enhance muscular strength. Tenenbaum and colleagues concluded that it is possible that four sessions of mental preparation may actually hinder optimal strength performance ". . . by diverting the individuals' full concentration away from the exercise movement."

If a control group had not been employed by Tenenbaum et al. (1995), it would have been easy to conclude that the two psychological interventions were both effective in producing significant gains in muscular strength. However, because the control also experienced a significant improvement—superior to either of the formal psychological interventions—alternative hypotheses must be considered. For example, it is possible that repeated testing on an isokinetic dynamometer improves strength simply because the subject learns from experience how to better apply force against the resistance supplied by the dynamometer. It is also possible that the gain in strength by the control group was superior to the psychological treatments because those treatments generated some form of interference with the ability to exert force. Although these hypotheses are speculative, it is important to realize that in this study "nothing" (i.e., control) was superior to "something" (i.e., psychological interventions). Furthermore, it has been known for many years that expression of maximal force is regulated by inhibitory mechanisms. The classical work by Ikai and Steinhaus (1961) demonstrated that maximal elbow flexion strength could be enhanced by disinhibition of these inhibitory mechanisms.

Goal-Setting

Weinberg (1994) stated that recent research on goals and performance in exercise and sport settings has been equivocal, but Locke (1991) asserted that the disappointing results from many of these goal-setting studies can be explained by the various methodological flaws in the research. Indeed, Locke devoted his entire article to the shortcomings of goal-setting research in exercise and sport psychology. This position merely serves to reinforce Weinberg's conclusion that research findings in this area are equivocal. The fact remains that goal-setting strategies employed in sport psychology have been derived largely from research and theoretical formulations from industrial and other non-sport settings. There is a good possibility that classical psychological theory involving goal-setting is irrelevant as far as exercise and sport applications are concerned. It is not acceptable from a methodological standpoint to conduct goal-setting research with assembly line workers in a factory or clerical workers in an office setting and proceed to generalize the results to elite athletes performing complex skills at or near maximal levels. However, as pointed out by Weinberg (1994), this is exactly what has occurred in the absence of a scientifically defensible research base and it leads one to question the external validity or generalizability of results in such studies.

If one wishes to perform psychological interventions with elite, pre-elite, or non-elite performers in sport settings, it is imperative that samples of participants be drawn from the appropriate population. This is a fundamental tenet of inferential statistics. A related problem is that the task employed as the dependent variable should possess relevance for the skill to be performed in the sport setting (e.g., $2\frac{1}{2}$ somersault in the tuck position) rather than a clerical skill such as performance on a word processing task.

Nevertheless, there has been widespread adoption of goal-setting theory and principles developed in non-sport settings by workers in applied sport psychology (Gould, 1993). Furthermore, when exercise and sport skills have been employed in goal-setting research, investigators have often used measures that have little if any relevance to performance by skilled athletes in sport settings (Gould, 1993; Weinberg, 1994; Weinberg et al., 1990).

In a seminal paper, Locke and Latham (1985) presented 10 hypotheses derived primarily from research of a non-sport nature, and emphasized the need for these hypotheses to be tested in appropriately designed research. Unfortunately, most of the necessary research prescribed by Locke and Latham remains to be performed. Subsequently, Locke (1991) published a paper summarizing the methodological problems with previous goal-setting research in sports and suggested improvements in future research in this area.

Self-Efficacy

There are other examples of interventions and beliefs in sport psychology that are not universally accepted in the general field of psychology. A fairly extensive literature in sport psychology is based on the assumption that a causal link exists between self-confidence and performance in exercise and sports settings (Feltz, 1988). Other labels such as "self-efficacy," "perceived ability," and "physical competence" are often used as synonyms for "self-confidence." Interventions designed to improve confidence with an aim toward enhancing physical performance are questionable for several reasons. First, the relationships between perceived physical competence and actual measures of physical fitness are quite modest, with correlations ranging from 0.27 to 0.53 (Sonstroem & Morgan, 1989). Second, there is an absence of evidence in support of a causal link between measures of physical fitness or performance and measures of perceived competence or confidence. Also, there is a surprising absence of appreciation for the role of "biological substrate" in such relationships. For example, individuals with high levels of aerobic power would be expected to be more successful in endurance events than individuals with low aerobic power, and the successful individuals in turn might feel more confident. In other words, using a psychological intervention to improve the confidence of an individual with a maximal aerobic power of only 30 $mL \cdot kg^{-1} \cdot min^{-1}$ would probably have little influence on the individual's success in the marathon.

As with other areas in which interventions are routinely performed in sport psychology, the theoretical formulations and empirical data bases for self–efficacy research were often developed in non-sport settings. Applied sport psychologists make the tacit assumption that improving confidence will result in improved physical performance because successful athletes are found to be confident, but there are actually some counterintuitive findings in this area. Dunn & Dishman (1988), for example, reported the converse to be true. Also, where high confidence/competence scores are noted in the successful athlete, it is possible that success breeds confidence, rather than confidence leading to success. The point is academic because there is no substantive research regarding the issue. This is merely another of the many *yet-to-be-confirmed* hypotheses.

There also seems to have been a tendency for workers in exercise and sport psychology to selectively ignore opposing views published in the self-efficacy literature. One of the most critical papers dealing with this issue, "Self-Efficacy: A Predictor But Not a Cause of Behavior," was written by Hawkins (1992), who argued that self-efficacy is a useful hypothetical construct for predicting behavior, but has no valid claim to being a cause of behavior. Furthermore, Hawkins emphasized that proponents of self-efficacy as a causal factor have not ". . . acknowledged that self-efficacy itself is an epiphenomenon of performance" (p. 251). At any rate, given the weak supportive evidence of efficacy, it seems inappropriate to employ psychological interventions designed to enhance confidence in an effort to facilitate physical performance. Rather than employing "mind games" designed to make a weak person feel stronger, for example, it would seem more prudent to improve the individual's muscular strength with a well-designed resistance training program. Of course, psychobiological theory would predict that such a person would also become more confident following the gain in muscular strength. There are no demonstrated "short cuts" or "quick fixes" in the form of "mind games" that will enable one to quickly facilitate performance. In an interview published in the September, 1989, *American Psychological Association Observer*, Strupp quoted Freud as having said:

> What we cannot reach flying we must reach limping—The Book tells us it is no sin to limp (p. 10).

External Validity

One of the major problems in the area of applied sport psychology involves a methodological issue known as *external validity*. This form of validity is defined as the degree to which findings in a given study can be generalized. A fundamental principle in research design is that the sample of individuals evaluated in the study should represent those in the target population. Numerous publications in the lay and quasi-scientific literature have addressed the role of sport psychology in the enhancement of performance in the Olympic athlete. For example, Livermore (1996) pointed out that ". . . the difference between winning and losing can be fractions of a second . . . That's where the most successful athletes bring their mental edge into play" (p. 77). Livermore interviewed a number of sports psychologists who counseled Olympic athletes in an effort to give them the "mental edge" by teaching techniques such as stress control, goal-setting, and basic mental hygiene. However, Livermore presented no evidence that any of the techniques employed by these sport psychologists was effective. There is no question about the widespread use of "mind games" with Olympic athletes, but whether or not these procedures work is unknown.

Greenspan and Feltz (1989) pointed out that ". . . a great deal of the outcome research in sport psychology does not use athletes as research participants or their performance in competitive situations as the dependent variable" (p. 219). Furthermore, only three of the 23 intervention studies reviewed by Greenspan and Feltz were regarded as having used national or elite athletes as participants. In addition, one of the three studies thus categorized employed "semi-pro" baseball players, and it would probably be more appropriate to regard such athletes as non-elite or pre-elite at best. One of the remaining investigations was restricted to a single athlete performing a single gymnastic skill, and there was no control comparisons or manipulation checks. There is not only a remarkable absence of research dealing with the influence of frequently employed interventions on the performance of elite athletes, but there is also a dearth of studies dealing with simple descriptive characterizations of elite athletes. A review of 1,203 sport psychology articles published during a selected five-year period (1980-1984) revealed that only 21 (1.8%) dealt with individuals regarded as possessing above-average fitness levels (Morgan, 1989). In other words, there is not only an absence of intervention research designed to quantify the outcome of various psychological techniques, there is also a deficiency of descriptive or cross-sectional studies. This is an important point because it is much more difficult to conduct intervention research compared with descriptive studies. It seems reasonable to conclude that interventions commonly employed with elite athletes lack external validity. Because a great deal of the research carried out with non-elite performers has relied upon laboratory as opposed to field assessments and on novel motor tasks as opposed to sport tasks, it is unlikely that the results can be generalized even to non-elite athletes.

The caution urged by Greenspan and Feltz (1989) and Morgan (1989) regarding the matter of external validity is not shared by other authors such as Druckman and Bjork (1991). These authors pointed out that whereas only a few studies have dealt with the influence of psychological interventions on performance in elite athletes, 75% of the investigations ". . . show positive effects of cognitive-behavioral interventions on sports performance" (p. 208). However, these authors located only four intervention studies conducted with "elite" athletes, and while it may be mathematically correct to talk in terms of 75% of the studies yielding positive results, this statistic can be misleading. It would be most unfortunate if reports of the type published by Druckman and Bjork (1991) were to be accepted uncritically.

Section Summary

It is possible that "mind games" based upon interventions such as relaxation, mental practice, imagery, hypnosis, and goal-setting will enhance performance in a causal manner, but there is a very limited number of experimental studies demonstrating the efficacy of such procedures. In most of the cases in which efficacy studies have actually been conducted, the research designs have been characterized by methodological shortcomings. The experimental literature in this area of inquiry suffers from numerous problems such as a lack of external validity and inadequate experimental designs, along with a host of behavioral artifacts such as the Halo effect, Hawthorne effect, and demand characteristics to name a few (Morgan, 1972, 1997). In other words, the hypothesis that an intervention such as imagery can improve sport performance has not been refuted at this point, but rather it remains to be confirmed. Second, a number of alternative, and quite plausible, explanations can be offered for the modest effects observed with mental practice (Dishman, 1991). It is difficult to believe that applied sport psychologists would perform interventions with athletes when the limited supportive research is restricted to investigations based on the learning of irrelevant motor skills by non-athletes. In those cases in which sport skills have been tested using athletes, there has been a tendency to evaluate athletes at one level (e.g., non-elite) and to generalize to athletes at another level (e.g., elite). This absence of external validity has been largely ignored in applied sport psychology.

There is evidence that numerous interventions are employed in applied sport psychology. According to Vealey (1994), imagery, goal-setting, and arousal regulation are extremely popular in sport psychology. Vealey's conclusion that ". . . the effectiveness of sport psychology interventions is supported in the literature" (p. 495) should be viewed with caution. First, much of the research cited by Vealey investigated the *learning* of motor skills as opposed to the *performance* of previously learned skills. Second, much of this literature is based upon motor skills that have little relevance to sport settings. Third, participants in many of these studies have been non-athletes, and it would not be appropriate to generalize to athletes. Fourth, control of behavioral artifacts such as the Halo effect and Hawthorne effect has generally been ignored in this literature. Fifth, Vealey selectively ignored opposing views expressed by investigators such as Dishman (1982, 1983a, 1989, 1991).

It is understandable that athletes and coaches might be eager to employ a psychological intervention that is promoted as possessing performance-enhancing properties; small improvements (e.g., hundredths of a second) can represent the difference between a medal in Olympic competition and not placing. It is less obvious why service providers would be willing and eager to employ interventions with individual athletes or teams in the absence of scientific evidence supporting the treatment's efficacy; however, this does not represent a recent development. Coleman Griffith (1925), the "Father of American Sport Psychology," commented over seven decades ago that:

> During the last few years and at the present time, there have been and are (men) short in psychological training and long in the use of the English language, who are doing psychology damage by advertising that they are ready to answer any and every question that comes up in any and every field. No sane psychologist is deceived by these self-styled apostles of a new day. Coaches and athletes have a right to be wary of such stuff. (p. 194)

ETHICAL PRINCIPLES AND TRAINING

A review of the "Ethical Principles of Psychologists and Code of Conduct" published by the American Psychological Association (1992) is an important document to consider when reviewing this overall matter. This document contains a preamble, five general principles, and 102 ethical standards to which it is imperative that applied sport psychologists adhere to. It is stated in the preamble that, "Psychologists work to develop a valid and reliable body of scientific knowledge based on research." This position differs markedly from the commonly employed "intuitive" models employed by applied sport psychologists (Straub & Hinman, 1992). The issue of a research basis for practice is also addressed in Principle A (Competence), which emphasizes that psychologists ". . . maintain knowledge of relevant scientific and professional information related to the services they render." In other words, a case can be made that an applied sport psychologist who elects to use relaxation with an anxious athlete, but who is unaware (i.e., secondary ignorance) of the phenomenon known as relaxation-induced anxiety (Borkovec, 1985) would probably be in violation of this ethical principle. Principle A of this document also emphasizes that psychologists provide only ". . . those services and use only those techniques for which they are qualified by education, training, or experience." In commenting on the issue of competence and ethicality in psychodiagnostic work, Weiner (1989) stated: "Although it is, therefore, possible in psychodiagnostic work to be competent without being ethical, it is not possible to be ethical without being competent" (p. 829). If this point of view were extended to applied sport psychology, it could be argued that a practitioner could not be ethical unless he or she were competent. It is undoubtedly the case that some applied sport psychologists are well trained, licensed, and/or certified in counseling or clinical psychology, but they may have little or no training in exercise and sport science. Conversely, it is readily apparent that some applied sport psychologists are well trained in exercise and sport science but have little or no training in psychology. The basis for this view is the observation that some and perhaps many practices in applied sport psychology are not based upon a sound theoretical rationale and ignore research evidence presently existing in the fields of exercise science and psychology (Dishman, 1991).

The principal reason for the overuse of unproven interventions in applied sport psychology is the tendency to focus on providing "services" rather than on conducting research involving the outcomes or efficacy of various interventions. It is noteworthy that Griffith (1925) made the following observation many years ago:

> Experience is, of course, a good school; but everyone now knows that a sane use of laboratories and of scientific methods will take us in a day to results not gotten in years in other ways. (p. 194)

Consumers should become aware of what proven services can be delivered by a practitioner according to the current state-of-the-art in sport psychology. Needless to say, practitioners should not overstate the efficacy of a given intervention, and in those cases in which a potential for undesired outcomes may exist, it is imperative that these potential risks be communicated to the consumer. Dishman's 1991 position echoes that of Leopold (1938a), who stated in an editorial many years ago that:

> A profession is a body of (men) who voluntarily measure their work by a higher standard than their clients demand. To be professionally acceptable, a policy must be sound as well as salable (p. 3).

This view possesses currency even today, and it has relevance for workers in the field of sport psychology.

According to Kimble (1984), scientific and humanistic cultures exist within psychology, and these cultures have conflicting values. Kimble has identified six value dimensions, which are summarized in Table 1-1.

Kimble (1984) reported that psychologists who are associated with institutions and programs that emphasize the natural science components of psychology usually exhibit the "scientific culture" characteristics shown in the table, whereas other psychologists tend to exhibit the "humanistic culture" characteristics with one exception, the "lawfulness of behavior" item, because, according to Kimble, psychologists are all determinists (but to different degrees). Kimble proposes in this insightful paper that the existence of these two cultures is due to processes of self-selection and the value enhancement that follows. On the basis of empirical data, Kimble reached the conclusion that there is little chance of an epistemic armistice between the two cultures because the value differences are not trivial—they are very basic.

It is often not possible to make generalizations from developments taking place in the field of psychology in general to those occurring in the emerging specialty known as sport psychology, but Straub and Hinman (1992), who interviewed 10 of the leading sport psychologists in North America, suggest some striking parallels with the findings from Kimble's study. These 10 sport psychologists expressed values similar to

TABLE 1-1. *Summary of value dimensions held by psychologists representing scientific and humanistic cultures.* Comparison adapted from Kimble (1984).

Value Dimension	Scientific Culture	Humanistic Culture
Most important scholarly values	Scientific	Humanistic
Lawfulness of behavior	Determinism	Indeterminism
Basic source of knowledge	Observation	Intuition
Appropriate setting for discovery	Laboratory	Field/Case history
Generality of laws	Nomothetic	Idiographic
Appropriate level of analysis	Elementism	Holism

those of the "humanistic culture" in Kimble's taxonomy (1984). Indeed, Straub and Hinman (1992) concluded their reviews of opinions with a quote attributed to a prominent sport psychologist who ". . . voiced concern about the relevance of what he called 'orthodox science' to the enterprise of applied sport psychology." Furthermore, this survey respondent suggested that ". . . applied sport psychologists should abandon the goal of scientific objectivity and rely instead on personal 'experiential knowledge'" (p. 309).

There is a general tendency in applied sport psychology to perform interventions without first establishing the necessary research base called for by Mahoney (1977). The validity of this generalization is corroborated by the survey reported by Straub and Hinman (1992). It has also been stated by Gould (1988) in an editorial published in *The Sport Psychologist*, that:

> No profession, whether it be medicine, education, or engineering, has a complete data base, and to demand such a data base before offering professional services is extreme. It is akin to a physician refusing to treat a patient because the scientific data base on the illness in question is not complete. Does the physician ignore the patient because not all the answers are available? Certainly not! He or she recognizes the limited nature of scientific knowledge and integrates what knowledge exists with accepted professional practices and experience. (p. 96)

The position expressed by Gould (1988) seems reasonable at first glance, but there are potential problems associated with the adoption of such a position. First, although it is true that physicians and others perform interventions without having a "complete" data base, this can be problematic at times. The history of medicine informs us that well-intentioned interventions such as bloodletting, the lobotomy procedure, mammary artery ligation, and the use of various drugs such as thalidomide were ultimately shown to be ineffective, life threatening, and/or associated with various undesired side-effects or after-effects (Valenstein, 1986). Second, while physicians may employ procedures at times for which efficacy remains to be proven, it is customary to present the patient or legal guardian with a consent procedure that spells out the: (1) lack of proven efficacy, (2) the possibility that the intervention will not improve the patient, and (3) the possibility, where appropriate, that the intervention may have undesired after-effects and side-effects. Hence, if the "medical model" were to be employed when performing interventions in sport psychology, it would seem prudent to inform the consumer of whether or not a given intervention possessed proven efficacy, and, if the efficacy is unproven, the possibility that the interventions: (1) might not work, (2) might lead to a decrement in performance, or (3) might possibly place the individual at risk. Furthermore, published articles and books clearly show that applied sport psychologists implicitly or explicitly lead consumers to assume that selected interventions possess efficacy. The application of interventions for which there is no scientific basis raises ethical, moral, and legal concerns.

It was emphasized by Mahoney (1977) almost two decades ago that sport psychologists not only lacked "data-based" answers regarding the parameters of athletic performance, but some of the questions being asked (at the time) were probably characterized by naivete. Mahoney went on to point out that sport psychology could be a fertile area for research, and he then commented on the area's ". . . delinquency in the empirical cultivation of this field" (p. 24). Mahoney also addressed the potential promise of cognitive-skills training, one of the principal directions taken by many applied sport psychologists, but he also cautioned that we would first need experimental scrutiny in order for the promise of this approach to be achieved. Unfortunately, the application has taken place, but the "experimental scrutiny" prescribed by Mahoney has not occurred. This is clearly illustrated in several subsequent reviews (Greenspan & Feltz, 1989; Kirschenbaum, 1995; Whelan et al., 1991).

There are parallels in other areas as well. Dawes (1994) has published a provocative book dealing with the view that some aspects of psychology and psychotherapy have been built on myth. Dawes argued that the professional community has become disconnected from clinical research, and in the process of doing so it has lost its legitimacy. It is Dawes' view that segments of the professional community can be characterized as a culture of professionals concerned with self-preservation and self-aggrandizement—a striking parallel exists in the area of applied sport psychology. It is imperative that applied sport psychologists conduct experimental or quasi-experimental research designed to evaluate the efficacy of interventions designed to enhance athletic performance. It is equally, if not more, important that applied sport psychologists become familiar with the existing research evidence. Because there is a paucity of recent research in this area, a summary of earlier research that has relevance for application with endurance athletes will be reviewed in the next section.

COGNITIVE STRATEGIES

Individuals vary considerably in maximal aerobic power ($\dot{V}O_2max$), which influences endurance performance to a considerable degree, and although it can be modified with training, a substantial portion of the variance in $\dot{V}O_2max$ is influenced by heredity. Investigators often attempt to resolve this problem of individual differences when conducting exercise experiments involving prolonged endurance efforts by having all participants exercise at the same relative intensity. In theory, individuals differing widely in $\dot{V}O_2$max but exercising at the same relative intensity should attain similar scores on time-to-exhaustion in an endurance task. However, experimentation based on the relative exercise intensity (e.g., 80% $\dot{V}O_2$max) is also characterized by considerable variability (Horstman et al., 1979). Efforts to elucidate the principal psychologic mechanisms underlying long-term endurance efforts have yielded several insights into the use of cognitive strategies such as association and dissociation, which are often linked to attempts to minimize perceived exertion (Morgan, 1973, 1984, 1985a, 1994), which will be reviewed in the following section.

Qualitative Survey Data

Morgan and Pollock (1977) interviewed a sample of marathon runners (n = 20) who were living and training in the Boston metropolitan area during the mid 1970s and reported two primary findings. First, all of the runners said they had little difficulty completing the first 18–20 mi of the marathon, at which time a difficult point was reached. They termed this point "the wall" and indicated that negotiating this difficult point in the marathon was a principal challenge. Second, when these taped interviews were studied, it became apparent that each runner employed a cognitive strategy that seemed to involve a dissociative state. In short, these runners attempted to ignore the discomfort and pain experienced during competition by dissociating themselves from the sensory distress. In each case, the runner employed a stereotypical form of dissociative cognitive involvement such as imagining that they were: (1) writing letters to friends and relatives, (2) designing, building, furnishing, and landscaping a house, (3) stepping on the faces of two hostile coworkers with the left and then the right foot for the entire 42.2 km, (4) placing a stack of Beethoven records on the record player and "grooving on Beethoven" for the entire run, (5) age regressing to the first grade classroom and then progressing forward through each successive year of schooling through the postdoctoral period, (6) calculating the volume of an imaginary multi-colored box on the horizon, letting the box drop, and attempting to calculate the new volume in a high-speed, computer-like manner taking into account the influence of changes in temperature and pressure, and (7) staring at the body's shadow on the pavement, and then at a certain point, letting the body "leave" and enter the shadow. Surprisingly, one of the marathoners in this sample reported that "Heartbreak Hill" in the Boston Marathon was the easiest part of the race for him because:

I look over my shoulder at the bottom of "Heartbreak Hill," and I go into a trance. This enables me to negotiate the hill with no pain. My dad was an engineer on the railroad, and I spent a lot of time as a kid riding in the cab of my dad's train on weekends. The thing I remember the most is looking out of the window when we pulled out of a station in one of those little towns. I would see those powerful pistons driving the wheels, and the steam squirting on the tracks and platform as we pulled out. So, when I look over my left shoulder at the bottom of "Heartbreak Hill," I am actually back in the cab, my legs become the powerful pistons, and my exhalation becomes the steam, and I sail right over the top of the hill. It's the easiest part of the race for me—I really don't feel a thing.

The form of dissociation described above represents a form of age regression, and it is important to recognize that the marathon runner had never received any formal training in using this cognitive strategy. When asked to explain when and why he started using this approach, he replied: "I don't recall—it just sort of came to me—it seems like I have always done this—anyway it really works for me."

Lung-Gom and Tumo

At the time we were doing this work, a book titled *Supernature* was published by Watson (1973) in which a description of *lung-gom* or "swiftness of foot" appeared. Tibetan monks trained in the art of *lung-gom* are reported to have traversed a distance of over 300 mi in approximately 30 h. This would have resulted in an average pace of 10 mi/h over rough terrain, with a good portion of these efforts happening at night. It is difficult to imagine an individual running the equivalent of 11.5 marathons at a 2:37 pace, or three 100-mi runs back-to-back at 10 h each. Elite marathon runners today average at least 12 mi/h, but this faster pace is only for 26.2 mi. Also, today's marathon runners have the advantage of good roads and state-of-the-art footwear, and they do not normally race at high altitude with exposure to cold temperatures. According to Watson (1973), the Tibetan monks trained in "swiftness of foot" were known as *Mahetangs*, and their training consisted of ". . . living in complete darkness and seclusion for 39 months of deep-breathing exercises" (p. 225). Also, an anthropological report by David-Neel (1967) described one of these *Mahetangs* running at high altitude and reported that the monk's eyes were wide open and his gaze was fixed on some distant object high up in space.

Most of Tibet is at an altitude greater than 10,000 feet, and the custom known as *tumo* is learned by some of the monk initiates as a means of combating the effects of cold. This custom involves a complex set of breathing exercises and meditation, and the student retires to a remote area for the training. Watson (1973) reported that individuals who learn this custom ". . . bathe in icy streams and sit naked in the snow thinking of internal fires" (p. 226). When the training has been completed, a sheet is dipped in the water of a frozen stream, and the student is wrapped in the sheet. The sheet is expected to be dried by the student's body heat alone, and this is done at least three times during the night. When the training has been completed, the individual is expected to wear nothing more than a cotton garment in all seasons, regardless of the altitude. The members of several Mount Everest expeditions have seen completely naked hermits living at altitudes where there is permanent snow. Given the reported physical performance of the *Mahetangs*, in concert with the clothing worn, the altitude, and the cold, it is reasonable to assume that they were also trained in *tumo* (Watson, 1973).

Evaluation of Lung-Gom

A review of the "cognitive strategy" employed by the *Mahetangs* suggests that the procedure was principally of a dissociative nature. These monks are reported to have fixed their gaze on a distant object and repeated a mantra or phrase in synchrony with their respiration and locomotion. The efficacy of this cognitive strategy has been evaluated under controlled laboratory conditions (Morgan et al., 1983). In the first experiment a pilot study was conducted with 18 adult males. A $\dot{V}O_2$max test was performed, and this was followed by a test of endurance time carried out at 80% of $\dot{V}O_2$max on a motor-driven treadmill. These individuals were randomly assigned to a control (no treatment), placebo (inert capsule), and dissociation group. The dissociative strategy consisted of (1) selecting a spot or stationary object in the lab and staring at this spot/object throughout the treadmill test of endurance time, (2) repeating a "non-cultic mantra" (the word "down") each time the left and right foot was placed on the treadmill belt, and (3) attempting to synchronize breathing and locomotion. To minimize behavioral artifacts, none of the investigators or technicians involved in testing of these individuals was aware of the exerciser's experimental status (Morgan, 1972, 1996). The participants in this study were next evaluated at 90% of $\dot{V}O_2$max with the assumption that a performance decrement would occur, and this did, in fact, take place for each group. However, the decrease in performance was less for the dissociation group compared to both the control and placebo groups, which experienced comparable decreases. In other words, this pilot work suggested that dissociation is effective in minimizing reduced performance with increasing work load, and this ergogenic phenomenon was not merely due to the Hawthorne effect (Morgan, 1972, 1997). These results are summarized in Figure 1-2.

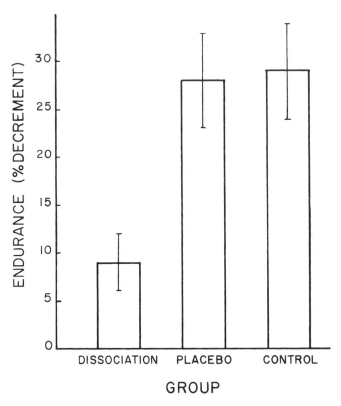

FIGURE 1-2. *Efficacy of a dissociative cognitive strategy compared with control and placebo treatments in minimizing performance decline.* Adapted from Morgan et al. (1983).

A second experiment was conducted with 28 adult males using a design similar to the one described above. Because the previous study suggested the absence of a Hawthorne effect, a placebo group was not involved in this second experiment. Following a test of $\dot{V}O_2$max and a test of endurance time performed at 80% of $\dot{V}O_2$max, the 28 participants were randomly assigned to a dissociation (N = 14) and a control (N = 14) group, and this was followed by a second test of endurance time carried out at 80% of $\dot{V}O_2$max. All of the remaining procedures were identical with those described for the pilot study. Performance for the control group did not change when retested at 80% of $\dot{V}O_2$max, but the dissociation group experienced a gain in endurance performance as hypothesized. These results are summarized in Figure 1-3. Whereas the two groups differed substantially on the measure of endurance time, there were no physiological differences observed between the two groups. Therefore, the enhanced performance that resulted from dissociation was not associated with any of the physiological variables studied (i.e.,

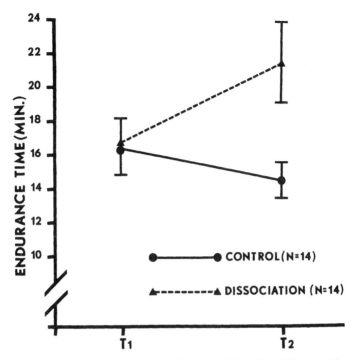

FIGURE 1-3. *Enhancement of endurance performance with a dissociative cognitive strategy.* Adapted from Morgan et al. (1983).

heart rate, oxygen uptake, ventilation, lactate production, and catecholamine levels). However, the fact that the dissociation group exercised for a longer period of time suggests that the individuals in this group were able to better tolerate the distress associated with increased endurance time.

The initial interview data summarized above, along with the anthropological reports of David-Neel (1967) and Watson (1973) in concert with the experimental laboratory research by Morgan et al. (1983), offer convergence from divergent sources regarding the efficacy of dissociation as an ergogenic aid. In other words, the interview data suggested that marathon runners employed a cognitive strategy that could be viewed as dissociative in nature, an older literature based upon anthropological reports provided indirect support for this strategy, and experimental research under controlled laboratory conditions demonstrated that endurance performance could be enhanced with this cognitive strategy. In addition, there are numerous anecdotal reports demonstrating the efficacy of dissociation. One example is that of Rod Dixon, winner of the 1983 New York City Marathon, who reportedly employed a dissociative strategy at the close of the marathon (Olsen, 1984). Having trailed the favorite, Geoff Smith, for most of the marathon, Dixon is quoted as saying that he began thinking about his career as a world-class runner with only a few hundred meters remaining, and he began to recite a sort of mantra over and over as he accelerated and passed the leader with only a few meters remaining. The phrase, "A Miler's Kick Does the Trick," was repeated over and over throughout the remaining few hundred meters. Would this be a desired strategy to employ for an entire marathon, or is such an approach appropriate only if used judiciously and with caution? Would it not seem more prudent to pay attention to distress signals in order to avoid physical problems (e.g., hyperthermia, hypothermia, musculoskeletal discomfort, or cardiovascular dysfunction), as well as fatigue and impairment due to an inappropriate pace? These questions were addressed in a subsequent study involving elite and non-elite distance runners, and the results illustrate the importance of establishing external validity or generalizability of findings (Morgan, 1972, 1997).

Elite Distance Runners

The predominant cognitive strategy employed during competitive distance running was evaluated in a group of 19 elite runners and a group of 8 college runners judged to be non-elite (Morgan & Pollock, 1977). The 19 elite runners included 11 middle- and long-distance runners as well as 8 marathon runners. The elite marathon runners in this investigation did not employ dissociative cognitive strategies during competition. Indeed, these elite runners were found to employ an *associative strategy*. Rather than dissociating and ignoring sensory input, these elite runners paid very close attention to sensations in their feet, calves, and thighs as well as to their respiratory sensations. For example, each of these runners would typically slow his pace when breathing became labored. As one runner in this study stated: "If I am having trouble getting enough air, I know I have to slow the pace." Second, while these runners reported that they paid attention to "the clock," it is clear that pace was governed by how they "felt" rather than the time elapsed. In other words, pace was regulated by "reading their bodies." Third, the elite runners reported there were runners in every race that they would like to maintain contact with; however, these runners preferred to "run their own races" rather than "leech." Fourth, these runners constantly reminded themselves to "stay loose," "relax," "don't get tight," and so on. Fifth, these elite runners did not encounter "pain zones" such as the non-elite runners described earlier, and much to our surprise, these runners dismissed "the wall" as a myth. These runners reported that "pain zones" and "the wall" were easily avoided by simply slowing the pace. As one elite runner stated:

If I am having trouble during a marathon, I know that everyone else is in trouble as well. If others do not slow the pace when I do, they will probably crash at some point down the line. I don't worry about what the other runners are doing in a race. I pay attention to my body. . . I read the signs . . . I sort of have the equivalent of a shopping list that I keep going over . . . I seem to dehydrate very easily, and I know that I have to drink a lot during a marathon so I am constantly reminding myself to drink . . . I pick up the pace, and I slow my pace based on how I feel.

Three additional findings from this investigation of elite runners are relevant to the present discussion. First, the elite runners possessed a higher $\dot{V}O_2$max than did the non-elite runners; therefore, it was expected that the elite runners would have significantly lower values for measures such as heart rate, ventilatory minute volume, and blood lactate when running at absolute paces of 10 mi/h and 12 mi/h. This finding was confirmed as expected, but the perception of effort did not differ significantly for the two groups during a 6-min run at a 10 mi/h pace. Even though the metabolic demand was significantly greater for the non-elite runners at both 10 mi/h and 12 mi/h, it was not perceived as more effortful until treadmill speed was increased to 12 mi/h. This finding provides additional evidence that elite marathon runners are more likely to employ an associative strategy than are non-elite runners. Of course, the dissociative strategy employed by the non-elite runners would theoretically be associated with a greater likelihood of injury, along with performances that would fall below their probable maximum.

A second finding that has considerable practical and theoretical implications was the observation that the elite runners consumed significantly less oxygen at the same treadmill speed despite an absence of biomechanical differences favoring the elite runners (Cavanagh et al., 1977). It is possible that the associative strategy along with the conscious effort to remain relaxed might have been responsible for the small but significant difference in oxygen uptake while running at both 10 and 12 mi/h. Third, these elite runners possessed a stereotypical "iceberg" profile that is characterized by low scores on the tension, depression, anger, fatigue, and confusion scales of the Profile of Mood States (POMS), along with an elevated score on vigor. This profile is summarized in Figure 1-4. The standard instructional set employed with the POMS asks the respondents to indicate how they have been feeling during the past week including today. Hence, the resulting profile reflects more of a state than a trait measure. Nevertheless, there is a trait component to this measure, and it has been shown that the "iceberg" profile observed

The "Iceberg" Profile

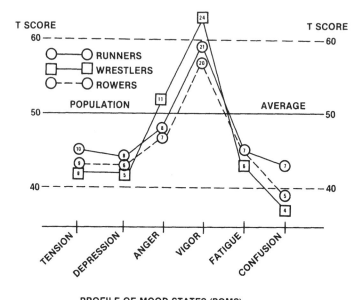

FIGURE 1-4. *The stereotypical "iceberg" profile observed in elite male athletes.* Adapted from Morgan and Pollock (1977).

in elite marathon runners persists across 17–23 y of follow-up (Morgan & Costill, 1996).

The initial report on runners by Morgan and Pollock (1977) has been replicated and extended with independent samples of both elite female and male distance runners. A sample of elite and non-elite female distance runners and marathon runners was evaluated by Morgan et al. (1987). These elite female distance runners were also found to possess the "iceberg" profile reported for the elite male distance runners described above, and these results are summarized in Figure 1-5. This sample of elite female runners was characterized by scores that fell below the population mean for tension, depression, anger, fatigue, and confusion and above the population mean for vigor. Assessment of cognitive strategies and selected variables such as motivation were obtained in the same manner described earlier by Morgan and Pollock (1977), with the exception that the principal cognitive strategy during *training* was quantified in addition to *racing* strategies. The proportion of elite and non-elite runners who were classified as using an associative strategy during training, as well as racing, did not differ significantly (P > .05);

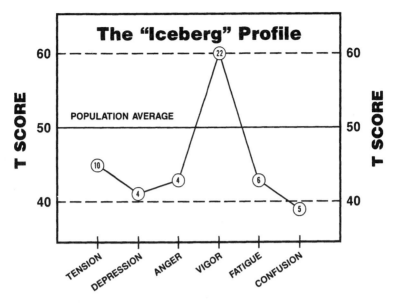

FIGURE 1-5. *The stereotypical "iceberg" profile observed in elite female distance runners.* Adapted from Morgan et al. (1987).

therefore, the data for the two groups were combined for analysis purposes. Some of the runners employed both association and dissociation strategies during races, but the proportion employing association (56%) was significantly (P < .05) higher than the proportion reporting the use of dissociation (22%). However, none of the runners employed association during training runs, and 56% reported the active use of dissociation while training.

The predominant race strategy for these runners consisted of moderating pace in order to maintain "contact" with the lead runners, and they would try to "kick" at a critical point toward the end of a race. In other words, these runners did not typically go out fast and lead a race. The proportion (52%) of runners in this group who would follow the lead group was significantly (P < .05) higher than the proportion who would lead (22%) or use a combination of leading and following (26%).

Two additional findings are worth noting. First, 60% of the elite runners and 33% of the non-elite had experienced "staleness" at some point in their competitive careers. While this difference of 27% was not statistically significant, the elite runners were running significantly more miles per week (65 vs 39). However, training 65 mi/wk on the average did not have an impact on mood state, and these elite runners exhibited the stereotypical "iceberg" profile reported for elite athletes in general. Second, retrospective recall of precompetitive arousal levels was significantly higher than baseline levels for both groups prior to recall of usual, best, and worst performances. Of these runners, 52% reported that they had their best performances when arousal levels were moderate or high.

A second replication of the initial study by Morgan and Pollock (1977) was conducted with male distance runners and marathon runners involved in an elite distance runners project conducted at the U.S. Olympic Training Center (Morgan et al., 1988b). This replication confirmed results of the earlier studies with elite male (Morgan & Pollock, 1977) and female (Morgan et al., 1987) distance runners. The runners in this investigation had the stereotypical "iceberg" profile previously described for elite male and female distance runners. These runners became involved in distance running because of intrinsic reasons, and this also served as the motivation for continued running, as found with earlier samples. The predominant cognitive strategy employed by these runners during competition was association as opposed to dissociation, and this is also in direct agreement with earlier findings for elite female and male distance runners alike. The principal racing strategy (72% of the sample) reported by this group consisted of "laying back" in races but maintaining contact with the front runners throughout a race. They reported attempting to accelerate toward the end of races in an effort to win. Another 14% of these runners indicated that they would typically "set-the-pace" and lead races from the outset, whereas the remaining 14% preferred to use both strategies (i.e., lead or follow), depending on the nature of the race and other runners. The number of male runners in this sample reporting a period of staleness at some point in their careers was 64%, and this is similar to the career prevalence (60%) reported earlier for elite female distance runners. A significant increase in arousal was reported by these runners as a group prior to competition, but as was the case for elite female runners, some runners reported no increase in arousal prior to competition, whereas others reported moderate to large increases in arousal as the usual case. These findings serve to reinforce the individual-zone-of-optimal-function concept described earlier in this chapter. An effort was made in this study to evaluate the relationship between ability ratings for the 10,000-m run and selected psychological measures. A significant multiple R of 0.67 (P < 0.04) was observed between performance on the one hand and trait anxiety and mood state on the other. This observation provides additional support for the mental health model (Morgan, 1985).

Pre-Elite and Non-Elite Distance Runners

There have been several related studies with non-elite or potentially pre-elite distance runners and marathon runners. Although these subsequent studies have been in general agreement with the earlier work of Morgan and Pollock (1977) and Morgan et al. (1987, 1988b), the later studies suffered from a number of design problems. Silva and Appelbaum (1989), for example, reported that the cognitive strategies of marathon runners finishing in the first 50 places in a U.S. Olympic Marathon Trial differed from those finishing at slower paces. The better runners relied on both associative and dissociative techniques, while the slower runners adopted a dissociative strategy early in a competition, which was maintained throughout the run. Although this finding is in general agreement with the earlier work of Morgan and Pollock (1977) and Morgan et al. (1987, 1988b), there is one fundamental difference. Silva and Appelbaum (1989) reported that the top runners in their study actually ". . . shifted their cognitive strategy according to the demands of the race" (p.190). Indeed, they stated that although the top runners " . . . tended to associate more regularly over the course of the race, they also exhibited cognitive flexibility in that during later stages of the race (18–24 miles), when pain was felt, they dissociated more than lower placers" (p. 191). These authors also stated that "Pushing through the pain would be facilitated by dissociation, even though the risk of injury would be increased" (p. 191). The basis for this view was the study by Morgan et al. (1983) reviewed earlier; however, there is an absence of both external and ecological validity for the proposal by Silva and Appelbaum (1989).

It is possible that the earlier research by Morgan and Pollock (1977) and Morgan et al. (1987, 1988b) cannot be compared to the subsequent work by Silva and Appelbaum (1989) for several reasons. First, the elite marathon runners described in the earlier research included individuals who had placed in the top three at Olympic trials, competed in the Olympic Marathon, and in some instances actually earned Olympic medals or placed high in Olympic and World Competition on at least one occasion. The highest place finisher in the Olympic trials competition studied by Silva and Appelbaum (1989) came in at tenth place. Therefore, these investigators were probably working with pre-elite or non-elite marathoners, and it would not be appropriate to generalize these findings to the elite population. Indeed, the marathon runners described in the report by Silva and Appelbaum seem to resemble the non-elite runners described by Morgan and Pollock. That is, rather than paying attention to discomfort and pain in order to avoid injury and maintain a steady state, the "top" runners in the study by Silva and Appelbaum employed dissociative strategies to cope with the pain.

Individuals can be classified as employing a predominant associative (A) or dissociative (D) cognitive strategy during competition, and this results in a nominal score (i.e., A or D). This was the procedure employed in our early research, and it is important to understand that the classification is not only nominal, but it relies on a taxonomy based on the qualification that it is the principal or dominant strategy. In an effort to improve this taxonomy by increasing the classification to an interval scale, Silva and Appelbaum (1989) developed the "Running Style Questionnaire" (RSQ), but there is no evidence presented that the RSQ possesses construct validity. Also, the test-retest reliability between "days" resulted in a modest correlation coefficient of r = 0.73. If a marathon runner reported that he or she usually employed a particular strategy when competing in the marathon on one day, it would be expected that a similar reply would be given a few days later. In other words, the association-dissociation construct has always been conceptualized as a trait. The reported reliability coefficient for the RSQ only accounts for 53% of the variance, and this implies that the scale lacks adequate reliability as well as construct validity. Also, the reliability of the RSQ was evaluated on 43 males who were members of a college cross-country team and students enrolled in a distance-running class. It would be inappropriate to generalize from such a sample to runners competing in the Olympic Marathon Trials. That is, the sample on which the RSQ was developed would most likely have lacked experience in marathon competition at the elite level. Furthermore, the overall prediction accuracy of the discriminant function analysis was 72% in the study reported by Silva and Applebaum (1989), but this was not cross validated on an independent sample. In other words, the group prediction model was based upon data collected from the sample studied. Construct validation of the RSQ would require a major research effort, and there is no evidence that a need exists for such a scale in the first place.

One of the most important findings made in the initial work by Morgan and Pollock (1977) relates to the observation that the elite marathon runners in their sample were rather unique from both a physiological and a psychological perspective. This research has been replicated in studies with other independent samples of marathon runners (Morgan & Costill, 1972, 1996). There has been a general failure for investigators to recognize that elite marathon runners, as opposed to non-elite, may employ an associative strategy during competition because of their unique physiological capacity. In other words, they may be able to rely on an associative strategy because of their high aerobic power, high proportion of slow-twitch muscle fibers, greater anaerobic threshold, and so on. Furthermore, it would be desirable in research of this nature to compare prediction efforts based on psychological parameters (e.g., personality structure, mood profiles, cognitive strategies) with the success of prediction based upon physiological parameters and/or performance histories. Marathon runners with previous performances below

2:15 would probably do better in an Olympic trial than runners with personal best performances above 2:30, regardless of cognitive strategies employed. In other words, the best predictor of performance would likely be a marathon runner's prior performance levels. At any rate, the top marathon runners (i.e., first through fourth place) in the Olympic Marathon Trial studied by Silva and Applebaum (1989) did not participate in their study.[1]

A sharp distinction may not exist between athletes classified as elite and non-elite. Also, some investigators add a third category known as "pre-elite," which falls between the two extremes. Workers at the U.S. Olympic Training Center routinely conduct camps and workshops for "elite," "pre-elite," and "non-elite" athletes. It is possible to classify individuals into one of these three categories with a reasonable degree of objectivity (inter-judge) and reliability (test-retest). And, whereas this construct may exist on a continuum, it is difficult to imagine that one could be much more precise than using a trichotomy of this type. It is probably preferable to focus on the "elite" and "non-elite" in research of this nature in order to avoid the intermediate grey zone when making generalizations. That is, individuals in the "pre-elite" category might easily drift into the "elite" or "non-elite" domains at some point.

The marathon runners classified as elite in work by Morgan and Pollock (1977) and Morgan et al. (1988b) all had personal best marathon times under 2:15, and each had won or placed in the top five of all runners in (1) Olympic Games Competition, (2) U.S. Olympic Marathon Trials, and/or (3) major marathons (e.g., Boston, Grandma's, New York, Pittsburgh).

A case was made earlier in this chapter for the use of psychobiological models in exercise science, and a report by Smith et al. (1995) illustrates the use of such an approach with distance runners. These investigators studied the physiological and psychological effects of attentional strategy use by experienced distance runners. The participants in this study included 27 men and 9 women ranging in age from 18-40 y, and they were running an average of 47 mi/wk at the time of the study. These individuals had a minimum of 12 mo of competitive racing experience, and they were recruited from local road races and collegiate cross-country programs. It would be difficult to classify these runners, but their training status and competitive experience indicates that they were not elite runners. Participants completed a modified version of the Running Styles Questionnaire (RSQ), and a standardized treadmill protocol was employed in order to calculate running economy. The least (n = 12) and most (n = 12) economical runners were compared on the use of attentional strategies, and this analysis revealed that the two groups did not differ in associative style use. However, the most economical runners were characterized by more use of relaxation, and these runners reported less use of dissociation than did the less economical runners. In an effort to evaluate whether or not the least economical runners could improve their running economy, an experiment was conducted in which these 12 runners were tested under three conditions. The conditions were counterbalanced and consisted of (1) control, (2) passive association, and (3) active association. The control condition consisted of viewing a neutral video tape, whereas the passive association involved the focusing of attention on bodily states, and the active association consisted of tensing and then relaxing muscle groups. A modified version of the Profile of Mood States was also employed during the treadmill run. None of the three conditions resulted in physiological or psychological changes.

The study by Smith et al. (1995) is one of the most ambitious to be published in recent years on the topic of distance running and attentional strategies. However, this study cannot be compared to the earlier work by Morgan and Pollock (1977) and Morgan et al. (1987, 1988b) for some of the same reasons already addressed in the review of the paper by Silva and Appelbaum (1989). It should also be noted that the more economical elite runners in the study by Morgan and Pollock (1977) did not differ remarkably from the non-elite on several biomechanical variables included in the overall project (Cavanagh et al., 1977). It would have been useful to know if the most and least economical runners in the study by Smith et al. (1995) differed biomechanically because the use of biomechanical assessments might have been potentially instructive. Also, it would have been equally instructive to have had measures of perceived exertion for the experimental manipulations. It is unclear why the modified POMS was employed during the treadmill runs because this could have had a distracting influence, and it could have resulted in dissociative rumination. Further, it is not clear why the runners were instructed to tense and relax muscle groups during the "active association" condition since tensing of muscles would potentially decrease running economy or neutralize the effects of relaxation.

In the report by Smith et al. (1995) the authors reported that the most and least economical runners differed significantly only on age (27.4 vs 21.8 y, respectively). However, inspection of the tabular data indicates that the most economical runners (1) ran in more races each year, (2) had more total months of running and racing, (3) ran more miles per week, and (4) had a faster mean 10-km time. The reason that none of these variables differed significantly may have been due to the small sample size in concert with variability. In other words, the most economical runners in this study appear to differ from the least economical in a number of ways. Furthermore, the faster mean 10-km time for the most economical runners may not have been significantly faster than that reported for the least economical. It would be expected that younger runners would be faster than older runners, but since this was not the case, the two groups may have differed in other unique ways. There has been a tendency in the field of exercise and sport psychology to ignore the importance of external and ecological validity (Morgan, 1972, 1997). It is important to have a clear understanding about the target population when conducting research of this nature.

A case has been made for employing an associative strategy during endurance competition, and this recommendation is based upon a sound theoretical rationale as well as on survey research involving marathon runners (Morgan & Pollock, 1977; Morgan et al., 1987, 1988b). An excellent example of this cognitive strategy being employed successfully has been presented by O'Connor (1992). This report includes a summary of Greg LeMond's performance in the 1989 Tour de France. The event lasted for 23 d, and it covered a total distance of 3,252 km (2,025 mi), including arduous climbs through the Pyrenees and the Alps. Greg LeMond not only won the event, finishing 8 s in front of Laurent Fignon, a two-time winner of the race, but LeMond's effort was characterized by an incredible performance on the final day of the competition. LeMond trailed Fignon by 50 s going into the final day, and it was generally felt that it would not be possible for him to make this up since the remaining distance was too short (i.e., 24.5 km). It has been reported by O'Connor (1992) that, "Despite the improbability of the task, LeMond won by cycling at an average speed of 54.6 km/h (34 mi/h), the fastest average speed ever recorded during a time trial in the 76-y history of the Tour de France" (p.139). While it has been well established that cyclists of LeMond's caliber possess unique physiological characteristics, it is also clear that elite performers at this level are quite homogeneous. This often leads to the suggestion that factors of a psychological nature play an important role in the final analysis. In commenting on the cognitive-perceptual aspects of LeMond's phenomenal performance, O'Connor (1992) reported that:

> He had already decided he didn't want aides in his support vehicle to tell him his splits or how he was faring in relation to Fignon. That would only detract from his concentration. (p. 139)

This is the type of anecdotal report obtained earlier in qualitative research carried out with elite distance runners. These individuals tend to "read" or monitor their own bodies in making decisions about factors such as pace, and they titrate velocity on the basis of how they feel rather than the position of others in a given race (Morgan & Pollock, 1977). Also, they tend to ignore the "clock" and resulting "splits" because doing so can lead to overshooting or undershooting. In short, they prefer to "run their own race," and the anecdote regarding LeMond's performance suggests that he employed a similar cognitive strategy. There are, of course, both a compelling theoretical rationale and research data favoring such an approach.

Section Summary

This section has focused principally on the cognitive strategies employed by distance runners, and this research has yielded several principles that can be potentially applied by runners and coaches. Elite performers rely principally on an "associative" cognitive strategy during competition. The cardinal principle of association is based upon the monitoring of sensory input and symptoms arising during competition with an aim, for example, toward increasing or decreasing energy expenditure by adjusting pace.

Athletes who employ association make a conscious effort to relax rather than ignoring and working through the development of unnecessary muscle tension. Individuals involved in prolonged endurance events must rehydrate during competition, and those athletes who employ association constantly remind themselves to replace fluids as they proceed in a race. Non-elite athletes, on the other hand, tend to employ a "dissociative" strategy, and they have a tendency to ignore sensory input in order to cope with the pain and discomfort of prolonged muscular activity. This has the potential for provoking performance decrements and medical problems (e.g., heat exhaustion, stress fractures) when prolonged efforts take place under extreme conditions. Despite the recognized efficacy of employing an "associative" strategy, there are both research and anecdotal evidence supporting the judicious use of "dissociation" during competition. Some investigators have assumed that research involving association and dissociation in distance runners can be applied to the management of pain tolerance during injury rehabilitation (Pen et al., 1995), but this assumption is not supported by research data. One important issue that has not received adequate attention involves the question of whether or not the use of various cognitive strategies during exercise has an additive or synergistic effect on psychological outcomes. Research on this subject has been reported by Brown et al. (1995), but the results are equivocal.

PERFORMANCE AND MOOD STATES

Personality theory and the psychological assessments that represent applications or extensions of various theories (e.g., Eysenckian, Freudian, Lewinian, Social Psychological) have been a central focus within academic psychology for many years (Hall & Lindzey, 1965). The history of this area of specialization within sport psychology has been summarized in several earlier reviews (Dishman, 1989; Eysenck et al., 1982; Morgan, 1980; Singer, 1988). Despite the fact that predicting the quality of performance of athletes from personality traits is consistently superior to predictions based solely on probability expectancies, there are many false positives and false negatives in these prediction efforts (e.g., Dishman et al., 1980; Morgan, 1995; Morgan & Raven, 1987). Hence, while psychological assessment of athletes has yielded important information regarding the influence of personality structure on performance in sport settings, and while this information enhances prediction accuracy when used in concert with biomechanical, medical, and physiological variables, the resulting low precision does not warrant the use of such models for selection purposes. However, the use of transitory mood states (e.g., tension, depression) within a dynamic context has considerable utility.

It is conceivable from a theoretical perspective that various psychological interventions might succeed or fail on the basis of an athlete's mood state at any given time. In other words, an intervention based on a cognitive psychology principle might enhance performance at a time when an athlete has a desirable mood state, but the same cognitive strategy might be ineffective when the same individual is characterized by elevated levels of tension, depression, fatigue, and confusion. There is not only a good theoretical rationale for the hypothesis that a depressed and confused athlete would experience impairment of information-processing abilities along with performance decrements, but there is also an emerging research literature supporting this theoretical position. A brief summary of this work will be presented in the next section.

A mental health model has been developed for use in predicting performance in a variety of sport settings, and the model specifies that performance and psychopathology are inversely correlated (Morgan, 1985b). That is, individuals scoring within the normal range on standardized measures of psychological constructs such as anxiety and depression will be more likely to perform well compared with individuals who are characterized by elevated scores on the same measures. The model is *nomothetic* in nature to the extent that it views ". . . behavior in terms of general principles, universal variables, and a large number of subjects" (Hall & Lindzey, 1965). It also includes an *idiographic* component in the sense that it focuses ". . . on the individual case, using methods and variables that are adequate to the individuality of each person" (Hall & Lindzey, 1965). For example, an athlete might score at or near the population mean on a construct such as depression when evaluated with a standardized instrument (e.g., POMS or the Minnesota

Multiphasic Personality Inventory (MMPI)), but this score might reflect a significant elevation (e.g., 1.0–1.5 standard deviations) above the individual's customary level of depression.

The idiographic component of the mental health model is particularly useful when attempting to carry out applied interventions with athletes who train at extreme loads. For example, the stereotypical "iceberg" profile noted in elite athletes tends to disappear with an overtraining stimulus, and this profile can actually regress to the population mean and flatten, or it can even invert during and following a particularly arduous training cycle (Morgan, 1985b; Morgan et al., 1987, 1988a).

Mood disturbances seem to increase as training volumes increase at high levels, so it should be possible to prevent the undesired consequences of overtraining by monitoring mood state and adjusting training loads. There is not only preliminary support for this view, but monitoring of overtraining with a measure of mood turns out to be comparable to using a battery of physiological measures commonly employed to assess the consequences of overtraining (Morgan et al., 1988a). This is probably one of the principal benefits of psychological testing with athletes, and it argues in favor of decreasing training volume when depression and other negative signs appear rather than introducing a psychological intervention such as cognitive therapy that is designed to reduce depression.

Much of the depression that occurs in athletes undergoing overtraining is thought to be caused by the training itself, and rest or reductions in training loads usually have immediate antidepressant effects (Morgan et al., 1987). However, psychological testing is of potential value only when there is an established "template" or "psychogram" that describes the individual athlete when she or he was healthy and performing well. Although the "iceberg" profile is the stereotypical profile of the elite performer, some successful athletes are characterized by "flat" profiles as measured by the POMS instrument (McNair & Lorr, 1992). This observation emphasizes the importance of employing both a nomothetic and idiographic approach, and it is important to have a reference point available when evaluating training status or making decisions about increasing or decreasing training loads. Psychological testing can provide an important source of information to the sports medicine team in such cases, and Raglin (1996) has recently presented a comprehensive update of the mental health model. Raglin's overview includes a discussion of the model's theoretical and empirical underpinnings, summarizes recent research involving the model, and explains why some investigators (e.g., Druckman and Bjork, 1991; and Rowley et al., 1995) have been unable to confirm the model's efficacy.

EARLIER REVIEWS

There have been several earlier reviews dealing with the psychological and psychophysiological mechanisms underlying endurance efforts of a prolonged nature (Dishman & Landy, 1988; Morgan, 1981; O'Connor, 1992). One of the common themes in these earlier reviews is the importance of a holistic mind-body approach when studying endurance performance. Also, as Dishman and Landy (1988) pointed out ". . . increased performance in prolonged exercise requires a training volume that will place many athletes at risk for pathological adaptations" (p. 341). In other words, while it is possible to "play" or employ "mind games" in an effort to cope with the distress of overtraining, this might well be done at the risk of ignoring important pathophysiological and/or psychopathological developments. It has also been noted by Dishman and Landy that ". . . only a single study has demonstrated that an applied cognitive intervention can enhance performance during prolonged exercise . . ." (p. 342). These authors also noted that this area has potential for making practical applications, but there is an absence of scientifically acceptable evidence to justify such interventions. Even though their position was advanced almost a decade ago, it still has currency.

Dishman and Landy (1988) devoted considerable attention to discussion of theoretical views derived from valence-expectancy and goal-setting models to illustrate ways in which cognitive psychology might be used to explain existing research evidence as well as to generate testable hypotheses for use in future research. This was done principally because there has been a lack of theoretical formulations in predicting or explaining outcomes in research or applied interventions. There has been a considerable amount of theory-driven research since that time, but it has generally been found that various theoretical formulations that are effective in non-sport areas (e.g., goal-setting theory) do not necessarily work well when applied in exercise and sport psychology.

Whelan et al. (1991) prepared one of the most ambitious reviews dealing with the influence of interventions such as imagery and mental rehearsal, arousal management, goal-setting, and self instruction and self-monitoring, as well as multi-component treatment programs on performance enhancement. Although this review was generally comprehensive, there appeared to be a selective omission of relevant papers. The classic work by Hanin (1989) involving the zone of optimal function (ZOF) was not even cited, and this is unfortunate because Hanin's ZOF (now labeled IZOF) model contradicts much of the discussion by Whelan et al. (1991) dealing with anxiety and performance.

Whelan et al. (1991) reviewed a considerable amount of research that has been conducted since the time of Mahoney's earlier review in 1977, but the authors concluded that ". . . questions about the efficacy of such interventions (e.g., cognitive behavioral) with athletes remained" (p. 320). This guarded conclusion is warranted for many of the same reasons previously discussed in the section on applied sport psychology, including:

1. The research was limited to samples of non-athletes or non-elite athletes; this is of special concern considering the widespread application of these interventions with elite athletes by sport psychologists involved with the United States Olympic Committee (USOC) and elsewhere (Kirschenbaum et al., 1995).

2. Many of the tasks—dart throwing, maximum sit-ups in a prescribed time, squeezing a grip dynamometer, juggling objects, and tracking a target on the pursuit rotor device—employed in the studies reviewed by Whelan et al. (1991) lacked direct relevance to sport performance.

3. Many of the investigations included in their review, it appears, were based on performance measures obtained during the *learning* of a motor task, as opposed to the study of *performance* in athletes who have already learned the skill in question.

4. Most of the research cited in this review was characterized by one or more fatal methodological flaws. In most cases, for example, investigators failed to employ adequate control and placebo groups or treatments, and the use of experimental "blinds" appears to be non-existent. As a consequence, even when there is a suggestion of possible performance enhancement, it is difficult to attribute such gains to the intervention employed because of the many alternative hypotheses that exist in such studies. That is, it is seldom possible in this field to rule out factors such as the Halo effect, Hawthorne effect, demand characteristics, expectancies of the experimenter and the participant, pre-test sensitization, "pact of ignorance," inappropriate sample size, lack of randomization, statistical regression, and so on (Morgan, 1997). These concerns are compounded when one considers additional problems associated with internal validity in concert with an inability to generalize to the target population (external validity) in many cases.

5. The results of an unpublished meta-analysis dealing with various interventions is summarized by Whelan et al. (1991), and included a quantitative analysis of 56 studies published between 1970 and 1988. It is probable that many of these studies suffered from the same methodological problems outlined above. It is reported, for example, that sample sizes varied from 4 to 70 per group, but the matter of statistical power is not addressed. It was also reported that 48% of the participants

in these studies were non-athletes or judged to be "moderately competent (33%) on the target performance" (p. 320). These investigators reported that the average effect size across the 56 studies was ". . . slightly larger than a half standard deviation" (p.320). However, the authors noted that questions remain about the efficacy of these psychological interventions with athletes and that many of the studies failed to present adequate descriptions of the interventions employed or the context in which the treatments were presented. This is particularly problematic for other investigators who might be interested in replicating the results of a given study as well as for sport psychologists who might wish to employ these interventions at an applied level. Finally, only one of the 56 studies included follow-up evaluations, and a "minority" dealt with athletic competition—the target domain.

Section Summary

There are undoubtedly many reasons why various theoretical formulations from the field of cognitive psychology have not met with success in exercise and sport settings. In the case of goal-setting research and applications, for example, Locke (1991) and Weinberg (1994) have engaged in a sort of point-counterpoint dialogue that explains the failure of classical goal-setting theory to work well in sport psychology. However, there is one point that is often overlooked in these discussions, and the issue actually has relevance for many of the popular interventions employed in applied sport psychology. The problem is that it is often impossible to verify that a change in the independent variable (e.g., mental practice, imagery, or visualization) actually occurred in the intervention group, or, if such a change did occur, that it did not also occur in the control group. Some investigators have been sensitive to this problem, and this has resulted in "debriefing" of participants by using interviews and self-reports. Nevertheless, in the absence of some sort of "brain activity snapshot," it is unlikely that we will ever be able to adequately assess the efficacy of interventions designed to alter the quality or even the presence of the desired brain "images." In other words, the scientific criterion of "falsifiability" does not exist.

Some sport psychologists argue that imagery based upon an "internal" perspective is superior to imagery involving a third-person or "external" perspective. Arguments of this nature are impossible to totally support or refute, owing to the inability to determine whether or not the desired imagery took place. Wang and Morgan (1992) attempted to quantify the effect of imagery perspectives (internal versus external) on the psychophysiological responses to imagined exercise and found during debriefing of participants that some subjects assigned to each condition reported that they employed the opposite perspective at times during the treatment. It is important to realize that the presence or absence of images has never been confirmed in the imagery literature; that is, imagery has only been *inferred*.

A sport psychologist or coach might employ classical goal-setting approaches with an athlete, but the athlete might elect to accept or reject the goal(s). Unestahl (1982) described the case of an elite runner on Sweden's National Team. The coach had worked with the runner in an effort to establish short-term goals that were both proximal and readily achievable, as well as realistic long-term or distal goals. The runner eventually set the world record in his event, and this performance exceeded the established goal. A retrospective analysis revealed that the runner had rejected both the proximal and distal goals, and he had established an "unrealistic" private goal that exceeded the coach's expectation. Furthermore, the runner had written his goal in the soles of all of his running and dress shoes, and he reported looking at this private goal, that no one else was aware of, each time he placed his left and right shoes on his left and right feet! This anecdote is presented in order to emphasize that goal-setting strategies in exercise and sport settings, just like imagery and many other interventions in applied sport psychology, are not verifiable. This may be one of the many reasons why research on these topics tends to be equivocal, and it may be an explanation for why applied sport psychologists favor the use of "intuitive models" over models based upon traditional experimental research designed to quantify the efficacy of a given intervention.

PRACTICAL IMPLICATIONS

The points that follow do not represent a traditional "cookbook" or "how to" list of applications as much as they reflect a cautionary note to consumers about many of the interventions that are used in applied sport psychology without the benefit of either an empirical data base or a sound theoretical rationale. Nevertheless, it is important that practitioners have a sound and critical understanding of exactly which interventions are based on *fact* as opposed to *fiction*. Another way of thinking about this is to make a distinction between myth and reality. Furthermore, it is important for *consumers* (e.g., athletes, coaches) to objectively evaluate the competence of *providers* (e.g., sport psychologists) as well as to critically analyze the basis for interventions offered by providers. It is also important that *observers* (e.g., trainers, team physicians) become sensitive to the issue of competency (e.g., training, licensure) with respect to sport psychology providers as well as to the validity of interventions offered by these providers. Conclusions and recommendations are summarized in the following points.

- There is compelling anecdotal evidence that success in sports, and maximal performance in general, is governed by factors of a psychological nature.
- Various "cognitive strategies" may be useful during endurance competition. Two approaches are known as association and dissociation.
- Association is based upon the monitoring of bodily sensations and symptoms arising during competition with an aim, for example, toward using the best pace. Athletes who employ association make a conscious effort to relax rather than ignoring and working through the development of unnecessary muscle tension.
- Another strategy is known as dissociation, whereby the athlete tends to ignore bodily sensations in order to cope with the pain and discomfort of prolonged muscular activity. Although this can improve performance in some situations, it may also worsen performance and cause medical problems when prolonged efforts take place under extreme conditions.
- Individuals involved in prolonged endurance events must rehydrate during competition, and those athletes who employ association regularly remind themselves to replace fluids during prolonged exercise.
- Despite the recognized advantage of employing an associative strategy, there is both research and anecdotal evidence that also supports the judicious use of dissociation during competition.
- There is little compelling scientific evidence to support the widespread use of uniform interventions such as relaxation, imagery, visualization, goal-setting, or treatment of alleged performance problems associated with various conditions (e.g., insomnia, jet lag).
- Providers of sport psychology services are too often not trained in psychology or exercise/sport science, and very few providers are trained in both psychology and exercise/sport science.
- Much of the limited research dealing with "mind games" and performance enhancement should be viewed with caution for two reasons. First, the research has involved *learning* simple, unfamiliar movement skills rather than *performing* complex skills (such as those used in elite sport) that have already been finely tuned over many years of practice.
- Athletes, coaches, trainers, team physicians, and consumers in general are encouraged to develop a healthy skepticism regarding many of the "services" provided by applied sport psychologists.
- To develop principles and guidelines for sport psychology education and interventions, there needs to be a healthy collaboration between practitioners and the scientific community in sport settings.

DIRECTIONS FOR FUTURE PRACTICE

Theory, research, and practice, in concert with the provider's level of competence, are crucial for the future of applied sport psychology. It is imperative that providers have both a theoretical and empirical basis for interventions and that workers in the field of applied sport psychology not perform interventions for which they do not have the necessary competence. The view that an individual cannot be ethical without being competent (Weiner, 1989) is not only an important guideline, but can be extended to include moral and legal issues as well.

DIRECTIONS FOR FUTURE RESEARCH

Future research in applied sport psychology should be conceptualized and pursued within a theoretical framework. Inquiry in this area should possess internal validity in the sense that instruments employed for assessment purposes, for example, should possess demonstrated construct validity. In addition, future inquiry should possess external validity; that is, samples of participants in studies should be representative of the target population. In the case of laboratory research, it is important that ecological validity be established (i.e., the generalizability of findings from the laboratory to the field setting must be considered if this is the investigator's goal) and this requirement would extend to the type of task(s) employed in the laboratory. Finally, it is important that behavioral artifacts (e.g., Halo effect, Hawthorne effect) be controlled or quantified in future research. This prescription for the future of research may seem rather fundamental, but it is important to emphasize that most of the existing research in this area of inquiry has violated these basic assumptions.

SUMMARY

It is possible to make a strong case in support of the view that maximal physical performance is governed in most cases by factors that have usually been regarded as psychological in nature, but dualistic conceptualizations of this type reflect convenience to a greater extent than fact. Nevertheless, it is understandable that athletes and others have turned to the field of psychology in an effort to maximize physical performance because there are many cases in which "psychological" factors seem to have played an important role in sport performances.

Given the many anecdotes relating to "mind over body," it is remarkable that there is such a limited experimental literature dealing with this subject matter. Furthermore, whether one elects to employ a quantitative or a qualitative analysis of research studies designed to evaluate outcomes of selected psychological interventions, there is an absence of compelling research in support of selected approaches. Indeed, a case is made in this chapter that most of the interventions currently employed in the field of applied sport psychology are based largely on a series of yet-to-be-confirmed hypotheses. This unfortunate state of affairs is due primarily to the emphasis on "intuitive models" in applied sport psychology as opposed to interventions based upon traditional "research models."

The problem with the use of "intuitive models" is that some research has demonstrated the existence of "counter-intuitive" phenomena. One example would be the case of relaxation-induced anxiety; a second would be undesired thermoregulatory responses with relaxation and visualization; and a third would be inhibition of physical performance with relaxation, visualization, autogenic relaxation training, and self-efficacy strategies. It is not uncommon for applied sport psychologists to maintain that a basis (i.e., evidence) actually exists for the interventions they perform. However, a review of this "evidence" usually reveals that it is based upon methodologically unacceptable research, or what has come to be known as "social validity" in the area of applied sport psychology. In other words, an intervention is judged to be valid if providers working in the area employ the intervention. This, of course, is unrelated to the more fundamental question of whether or not the intervention actually works.

There are probably several reasons why applied sport psychologists have opted to rely on intuition rather than research as a basis for interventions. One possible explanation involves the equivocal nature of much of the research that has been attempted in this area. A case in point would be the area of goal-setting and performance. The principal reason for these equivocal results is the exclusive use of problematic nomothetic models. First of all, there are quite a few cases in the literature in which groups of individuals failed to improve with a given intervention such as hypnosis, but some individuals in these groups experienced phenomenal increases in performance. Because it has been shown that some individuals perform best when relaxed, others when anxious, and still others when intermediate on anxiety measures, one would not expect anxiety and performance to be correlated, and this is precisely what the research literature tells us. Also, an intervention designed to increase (i.e., super-psych) or decrease (i.e., relaxation) anxiety would theoretically improve the performance of one subset of individuals, have no effect on another subset of the same group, and probably impair the performance of still a third subset. The net effect would be that the intervention would not have an ergogenic effect, and the null hypothesis would be accepted. Also, even when an intervention is sometimes shown to have a statistically significant but small ergogenic effect, some individuals may achieve enormous gains in performance.

The presence of individual differences coupled with failure to observe group differences and methodological flaws preventing the merger of theory and practice was first described by Dishman (1983b) in a chapter dealing with the ergogenic effects of stress management. Some stress management strategies have been associated with improved performance in about half of the published reports. Dishman interpreted this equivocal state to reflect the problem of individual differences. It is not surprising that applied sport psychologists have relied on nomothetic approaches (e.g., relax or psych everyone) rather than the labor-intensive interventions based on idiographic models. Dishman concluded his chapter with the comment that:

> On the basis of available evidence, stress management as an ergogenic aid must be regarded as an art that can be effective in qualified and skilled hands (p. 309).

This generalization can probably be extended to include most of the interventions currently employed by applied sport psychologists.

Consumers

Several steps should be taken by anyone who is contemplating working with a sport psychologist. First, the credentials of the provider should be a fundamental concern of the consumer. This includes not only the athlete or coach who may be looking for a sport psychologist in an effort, for example, to enhance performance, but also extends to administrators (e.g., athletic directors) and others who might be in a position to subject athletes or coaches to sport psychology services. It is commonly argued by some applied sport psychologists that their sole responsibility is to teach athletes how to improve their performances (i.e., psychological skills training) so these practitioners need not be trained, licensed, or certified in psychodiagnostic or therapeutic domains. The assumption seems to be that all athletes are normal! While there is an absence of sound, systematic epidemiological research involving athletes, it would be quite surprising if at least 5% to 10% of those individuals in the population of athletes being studied did not have problems of clinical significance. In other words, even though an applied sport psychologist may not perform psychotherapy with athletes, he or she should possess the competence necessary to make appropriate referrals. Second, licensure and certification should be viewed as *necessary* rather than *sufficient* evidence of competence. That is, a licensed clinical psychologist may not possess the necessary competencies in exercise and sport science to perform a given intervention. In other words, it is important that applied sport psychologists possess competencies in exercise and sport science as well as in psychology. In those cases in which the provider is actually working with individuals who have clinical problems, the provider should also possess the necessary training and licensure required to function as a competent psychologist.

When a consumer approaches a physician, dentist, or attorney for services, the assumption can be made that the provider is not only trained but also possesses the necessary licensure or certification. Hence, it is not necessary to inquire as to whether or not the individual is actually a physician, dentist, or attorney. It is fair to say that most applied sport psychologists are not licensed or licensable, and even those who are licensed or certified may never have taken a single course in exercise science (including sport psychology) at the doctoral level. An individual can always contact the state licensing board in the state, district, or province in which he or she resides to obtain information regarding the psychologist's licensure status.

Quite independent of competency issues, consumers should also be concerned about whether or not a planned intervention actually has a solid basis. In other words, is there evidence that the intervention in question works? Also, there are some interventions that work reasonably well under certain circumstances, but are also known to have after-effects or side-effects in some situations for some individuals. A consumer should not hesitate to make inquiries about potential problems associated with a particular intervention.

Conclusion

An effort has been made in this chapter to critically analyze the many practices that have become commonplace in the emerging field of applied sport psychology. There is a widely held belief among athletes, coaches, and others involved in sports performance that factors of a psychological nature play a critical role in maximal physical performance. This belief has led to a demand for psychological interventions, and many applied sports psychologists have responded by providing a variety of interventions. Unfortunately, there is a remarkable absence of conventional scientific evidence in support of most of the interventions commonly employed. When there is evidence, it is usually equivocal. Furthermore, there are theoretical rationales and empirical evidence that support the view that some of the interventions might actually impair performance. With very few exceptions, it would seem reasonable to conclude that most of the psychological interventions employed in applied sport psychology are based upon a series of yet-to-be-confirmed hypotheses. There is nothing inherently wrong with employing interventions that are based upon theory rather than research evidence, but it is imperative that providers (e.g., applied sport psychologists) make it clear to consumers (e.g., athletes, coaches) that a given intervention is based upon theory rather than fact, and it is also necessary that undesired negative effects be reviewed with a consumer if this possibility exists. It is not only important that athletes and coaches develop a healthy skepticism regarding many of the psychological interventions that are currently being promoted, but the field of applied sport psychology must also become concerned about the actual efficacy of many applications as well as about the limits and circumstances in which these procedures might be contraindicated. This must be done if the field of applied sport psychology hopes to survive and prosper. The famous naturalist and environmentalist, Aldo Leopold (1938b), commented more than 50 years ago that:

> The public mind is a mirror into which every vocation reflects its image. That image may flatter its subject, or the contrary, depending upon accumulated public impressions of the group and how its members live, think, and work. (p. 249)

The field of applied sport psychology will not only survive, but it will prosper as well if its individual members live, think, and work in a manner consistent with the accepted conventions that have become the foundation and cornerstones of other established vocations.

FOOTNOTE

[1]The 1996 U.S. Men's Olympic Marathon Trial was conducted on Saturday, February 18, 1996, in Charlotte, NC. Even though the 26.2-mi course was regarded as "difficult," it was negotiated in a winning time of 2 h, 12 min and 45 s (2:12.45) by Bob Kempainen. The second and third place finishers were Mark Coogan (2:13.05) and Keith Brantly (2:13.22). These marathon runners represented the U.S. in the 1996 Olympic Summer Games in Atlanta, and these individuals resemble, from a performance standpoint, the elite marathoners described by Morgan and Pollock (1977). It is imperative that runners of this type be included in any efforts to describe the cognitive strategies of "elite" marathon runners. The observation that non-elite runners employ cognitive strategies which do not resemble those of elite runners is not surprising.

ACKNOWLEDGEMENTS

Appreciation is expressed to Rod Dishman, Steve Johnson, David Lamb, Greg Mondin, Sarah Moss, and Dennis Passe for their reviews and helpful comments regarding earlier versions of this chapter. A special thanks is extended to Wendy Dickinson for her expert technical support in the typing of this chapter in draft and final form.

BIBLIOGRAPHY

American Psychological Association (1992). Ethical principles of psychologists and code of conduct. *Amer. Psychol.* 12:1597–1611.
Bannister, R.G. (1981). *The Four-Minute Mile.* New York: Dodd, Mead & Co.
Bannister, R.G. (1956). Muscular effort. *Brit. Med. Bull.* 12:222–225.

Borkovec, T.D. (1985). The role of cognitive cues in anxiety and the anxiety disorders: Worry and relaxation-induced anxiety. In: A.H. Tuma and J. Moser (eds.) *Anxiety and the Anxiety Disorders*. Hillsdale, NJ: Lawrence Erlbaum, pp. 463–478.

Borkovec, T.D., A.M. Mathews, A. Chambers, S. Ebrahimi, R. Lytle, and R. Nelson, (1987). The effects of relaxation training with cognitive or nondirective therapy and the role of relaxation-induced anxiety in the treatment of generalized anxiety. *J. Consult. Clin. Psychol.*, 55:883–888.

Brown, D.R., Y. Wang, A. Ward, C.B. Ebbeling, L. Fortlage, E. Puleo, H. Benson, and J.M. Rippe (1995). Chronic psychological effects of exercise and exercise plus cognitive strategies. *Med. Sci. Sports Exerc.* 27:765–775.

Cavanagh, P.B., M.L. Pollock, and J. Landa (1977). A biomechanical comparison of elite and good distance runners. *Ann. NY Acad. Sci.* 301:328–345.

David-Neel, A. (1967). *Magic and Mystery in Tibet*. London: Souvenir Press.

Dawes, R.M. (1994). *House of Cards: Psychology and Psychotherapy Built on Myth*. New York: The Free Press.

Desharnais, R. (1983). Reaction to the paper by B.S. Rushall: On-site psychological preparations for athletes. In: T. Orlick, J.T. Partington and J.H. Salmela (eds.) *Mental Training for Coaches and Athletes*. Ottawa: Coaching Association of Canada, pp. 150–151.

Dishman, R.K. (1982). Contemporary sport psychology. In: R. Terjung (ed.) *Exercise and Sport Sciences Reviews*. Philadelphia: Franklin Institute Press, pp. 120–159.

Dishman, R.K. (1991). The failure of sport psychology in the exercise and sport sciences. In: R.J. Park and H.M. Eckert (eds.) *The Academy Papers: New Possibilities, New Paradigms*. Champaign, IL: Human Kinetics Publishers, pp. 39–47.

Dishman, R.K. (1983a). Identity crises in North American sport psychology: Academics in professional issues. *J. Sport Psychol.* 5:123–134.

Dishman, R.K. (1989). Psychology of sports competition. In: A.J. Ryan and F. Allman (eds.). *Sports Medicine*. Orlando, FL: Academic Press, pp.129–164.

Dishman, R.K. (1983b). Stress management procedures. In: M.H. Williams (ed.) *Ergogenic Aids in Sports*. Champaign, IL: Human Kinetics Publishers, pp. 275–320.

Dishman, R.K., and F.J. Landy (1988). Psychological factors and prolonged exercise. In: D.R. Lamb and R. Murray (eds.) *Perspectives in Exercise Science and Sports Medicine, Vol. 1: Prolonged Exercise*. Indianapolis: Benchmark Press, pp. 140–167.

Dishman, R.K., W. Ickes, and W.P. Morgan (1980). Self-motivation and adherence to habitual physical activity. *J. Appl. Soc. Psychol.* 10:115–132.

Druckman, D., and R.A. Bjork (1991). Optimizing individual performance. In: D. Druckman and R.A. Bjork (eds.) *In the Mind's Eye—Enhancing Human Performance*. Washington, D.C.: National Academy Press, pp. 193–246.

Druckman, D., and J.A. Swets (eds.) (1988). *Enhancing Human Performance: Issues, Theories, and Techniques*. Washington, D.C.: National Academy Press, pp. 61–101.

Dunn, A.L., and R.K. Dishman (1988). Anxiety and performance on the Tour de France and Tour de France Feminin. *Med. Sci.Sports Exerc.*(Paper presented at the 1988 Annual Convention of the American Psychological Association, Boston, MA.)

Ellickson, K.A. (1986). Precompetitive anxiety states in college athletes. Ph.D. dissertation, University of Wisconsin-Madison.

Eysenck, H.J. (1952). The effects of psychotherapy: An evaluation. *J. Consult. Psychol.* 16:319–324.

Eysenck, H.J., D.K.B. Nias, and D.N. Cox (1982). Sport and personality. *Adv. Behav. Res Ther.* 4:1–56.

Feltz, D.L. (1988). Self-confidence and sports performance. In: K.B. Pandolf (ed.) *Exercise and Sport Sciences Reviews* (Vol. 16). New York: Macmillan Publishing, pp. 423–457.

Feltz, D.L., and D.M. Landers (1983). The effects of mental practice on motor skill learning and performance: A meta-analysis. *J. Sport Psychol.* 5:25–57.

Gallwey, W.T. (1976). *Inner Tennis*. New York: Random House.

Gould, D. (1988). Editorial. *Sport Psychologist*. 2:95–96.

Gould, D. (1993). Goal setting for peak performance. In: J.M. Williams (ed.) *Applied Sport Psychology*. Mountain View, CA: Mayfield Publishing, pp. 158–169.

Gould, D., and E. Udry (1994). Psychological skills for enhancing performance: Arousal regulation strategies. *Med. Sci. Sports Exerc.* 26:478–485.

Greenspan, M.J., and D.L. Feltz (1989). Psychological interventions with athletes in competitive situations: A review. *Sport Psychologist* 3:219–236.

Griffith, C.R. (1925). Psychology and its relation to athletic competition. *Amer. Phys. Educ. Rev.* 30:193–198.

Hall, C.S., and Lindzey, G. (1957). *Theories of Personality*. New York: John Wiley.

Hanin, Y. (1989). Interpersonal and intragroup anxiety in sports. In: D. Hackfort and C.D. Spielberger (eds.) *Anxiety in Sports*. Washington, DC: Hemisphere Publishing, pp. 19–28.

Hanin, Y., and P. Syrjä (1995). Performance affect in junior ice-hockey players: An application of the individual zones of optimal functioning model. *Sport Psychologist*. 9:169–187.

Hanin, Y., and P. Syrjä (1994). Performance affect in soccer players: An application of the IZOF model. *Int. J. Sports Med.* 16:260–265.

Hawkins, R.F. (1992). Self-efficacy: A predictor but not a cause of behavior. *J. Behav. Ther. Exp. Psychiat.* 23:251–256.

Heide, F.J., and T.D. Borkovec (1984). Relaxation-induced anxiety: Mechanisms and theoretical implications. *Behav. Res. Ther.* 22:1–12.

Hilgard, E.R. (1977). *Divided Consciousness: Multiple Controls in Human Thought and Action.* New York: John Wiley & Sons.

Horstman, D.H., W.P. Morgan, A. Cymerman, and J. Stokes (1979). Perception of effort during constant work to self-imposed exhaustion. *Percep. Motor Skills* 48:1,111–1,126.

Ikai, M., and A.H. Steinhaus (1961). Some factors modifying the expression of muscular strength. *J. Appl. Physiol.* 16:157–163.

Kabat-Zinn, J., and B. Beall (1985). A systematic mental training program based on mindfulness meditation to optimize performance in collegiate and olympic rowers. Paper presented at the VIth World Congress of Sport Psychology, Copenhagen, June, 1985.

Kimble, G.A. (1984). Psychology's two cultures. *Amer. Psychologist* 39:833–839.

Kirschenbaum, D., S. McCann, A. Meyers, and J. Williams (1995). The use of sport psychology to improve sport performance. Sport Science Exchange Roundtable, Vol. 6, No. 2. Barrington, IL: Gatorade Sports Science Institute.

Landers, D.M., and S.H. Boutcher (1993). Arousal-performance relationships. In: J.M. Williams (ed.). *Sport Psychology.* Mountain View, CA: Mayfield Publishing, pp. 170–184.

Leopold, A. (1938a). Editorial. *Outdoor America* 3:3.

Leopold, A. (1938b). Engineering and conservation. Lecture presented to the College of Engineering at the University of Wisconsin and dated April 22, 1938. Cited in S.L. Flader and J.B. Callicott (eds.)(1991). *The River of the Mother of God.* Madison, WI: University of Wisconsin Press.

Livermore, B. (1996). Mind games. *Women's Sports Fit.* 18:77–78.

Locke, E.A., and L.G.P. Latham (1985). The application of goal-setting to sports. *J. Sport Psychol.*, 7:205–222.

Locke, E.A. (1991). Problems with goal-setting research in sports—and their solution. *J. Sport Exerc. Psychol.* 8:311–316.

Mahoney, M.J. (1977). Cognitive skills and athletic performance. Paper presented at the 11th Annual Meeting of the Association for the Advancement of Behavior Therapy. Atlanta, GA.

McNair, M., and M. Lorr (1992). *Profile of Mood States.* San Diego: Educational and Industrial Testing Service.

Mittleman, K.D., T.J. Doubt, and M.A. Gravitz (1992). Influence of self-induced hypnosis on thermal responses during immersion in 25° water. *Aviat. Space Environ. Med.* 68:689–695.

Morgan, W.P. (1995). Anxiety and panic in recreational scuba divers. *Sports Med.* 20:398–421.

Morgan, W.P. (1972). Basic considerations. In: W.P. Morgan (ed.) *Ergogenic Aids and Muscular Performance.* New York: Academic Press, pp. 3–31.

Morgan, W.P. (1993). Hypnosis and Sport Psychology. In: J. Rhue, S.J. Lynn, and I. Kirsch (eds.) *Handbook of Clinical Hypnosis.* Washington D.C.: American Psychological Association, pp. 649–670.

Morgan, W.P. (1997). Methodological considerations. In: W.P. Morgan (ed.) *Physical Activity and Mental Health.* Washington, DC: Taylor & Francis, pp. 3–32.

Morgan, W.P. (1984). Mind over matter. In: W.F. Straub and J.M. Williams (eds.) *Cognitive Sport Psychology.* Lansing, NY: Sport Science Associates, pp. 311–316.

Morgan, W.P. (1973). Psychological factors influencing perceived exertion. *Med. Sci. Sports Exerc.* 5:97–103.

Morgan, W.P. (1985a). Psychogenic factors and exercise metabolism: A review. *Med. Sci. Sports Exerc.* 17:309–316.

Morgan, W.P. (1994). Psychological components of effort sense. *Med. Sci. Sports Exerc.* 26:1071–1077.

Morgan, W.P. (1981). Psychophysiology of self-awareness during vigorous physical activity. *Res. Quart. Exerc. & Sport* 52:385–427.

Morgan, W.P. (1985b). Selected psychological factors limiting performance: A mental health model. In: D.H. Clarke and H.M. Eckert (eds.) *Limits of Human Performance (The Academy Papers).* Champaign, IL: Human Kinetics Publishers, pp. 70–80.

Morgan, W.P. (1989). Sport psychology in its own context: A recommendation for the future. In: J.S. Skinner, C.B. Corbin, D.M. Landers, P.E. Martin, and C.L. Wells (eds). *Future Directions in Exercise and Sport Science Research.* Champaign, IL: Human Kinetics Publishers, pp. 97–110.

Morgan, W.P. (1980). The trait psychology controversy. *Res. Quart. Exerc. Sport* 51:50–76.

Morgan, W.P., and D.L. Costill (1972). Psychological characteristics of the marathon runner. *J. Sports Med. Phy. Fitness* 12:42–46.

Morgan, W.P., and D.L. Costill (1996). Selected psychological characteristics and health behaviors of aging marathon runners: A longitudinal study. *Int. J. Sports Med,* 17:305–312.

Morgan, W.P., and K.A. Ellickson. (1989). Health, anxiety and physical exercise. In: C.D. Spielberger and D. Hackbart (eds.) *Anxiety in Sports: An International Perspective.* Washington, D.C.: Hemisphere Publishing, Inc., pp. 165–182.

Morgan, W.P., and M.L. Pollock (1977). Psychologic characterization of the elite distance runner. In: P. Milvy (ed.) *Ann. NY Acad. Sci.* 301:382–403.

Morgan, W.P., and P.B. Raven (1985). Prediction of distress for individuals wearing industrial respirators. *Amer. Ind. Hyg. Assoc. J.* 46:363–368.

Morgan, W.P., D.R. Brown, J.S. Raglin, P.J. O'Connor, and K.A. Ellickson (1987). Psychological monitoring of overtraining and staleness. *Brit. J. Sports Med.* 21:107–114.

Morgan, W.P., D.L. Costill, M.G. Flynn, J.S. Raglin, and P.J. O'Connor (1988a). Mood disturbance following increased training in swimmers. *Med. Sci. Sports Exerc.*, 20:408–414.

Morgan, W.P., D.H. Horstman, A. Cymerman, and J. Stokes (1983). Facilitation of physical performance by means of a cognitive strategy. *Cognitive Ther. Res.* 7:251–264.

Morgan, W.P., P.J. O'Connor, K.A. Ellickson, and P.W. Bradley (1988b). Personality structure, mood states, and performance in elite male distance runners. *Int. J. Sport Psych.* 19:247–263.

Morgan, W.P., P.J. O'Connor, B.P. Sparling, and R.R. Pate (1987). Psychological Characterization of the elite female distance runner. *Int. J. Sports Med.* 8:124–131.

Murphy, S.M. (1988). The on-site provision of sport psychology services at the 1987 U.S. Olympic Festival. *Sport Psychologist.* 2:337–350.

Newsholme, L.E., T. Leech, and G. Duester (1994). *Keep on Running: The Science of Training and Performance.* West Sussex, England: John Wiley & Sons.

O'Connor, P.J. (1992). Psychological aspects of endurance performance. In: R.J. Shephard and P.O. Åstrand (eds.) *Endurance in Sport.* Oxford: Blackwell Scientific, pp. 139–145.

O'Connor, P.J., W.P. Morgan, K.F. Koltyn, J.S. Raglin, J.G Turner, and N.H. Kalin (1991). Air travel across four time zones in college swimmers. *J. Appl. Physiol.* 70:756–763.

Olsen, E. (1984). Dixon's the one. *The Runner*, January: 30–36.

Pen, J.P., C.F, Fisher, G.A. Sforzo, and B.G. McManis (1995). Cognitive strategies and pain tolerance in subjects with muscle soreness. *J. Sports Rehab.* 4:215–222.

Raglin, J.S. (1992). Anxiety and sport performance. In: J.O. Holloszy (ed.) *Exercise and Sport Sciences Reviews (Vol. 20).* Baltimore: Williams and Wilkins, pp. 243–274.

Raglin, J.S. (1996). The mental health model of sport performance: Background and new developments. Tutorial Lecture presented at the Annual Meeting of the American College of Sports Medicine, May 31, 1996, Cincinnati, OH.

Raglin, J.S., and M.J. Morris (1994). Precompetition anxiety in women volleyball players: A test of ZOF theory in a team sport. *Brit. J. Sports Med.* 28:47–51.

Raglin, J.S., and P.E. Turner (1993). Anxiety and performance in track and field athletes: A comparison of the inverted-U hypothesis with zone of optimal function theory. *Personality Individual Differences.* 14:163–171.

Rowley, A.J., D.M. Landers, L.B. Kyllo, and J.L. Etnier (1995). Does the iceberg profile discriminate between successful and less successful athletes? A meta-analysis. *Sport Psychologist* 9:185–196.

Silva, J.M. III, and M.I. Appelbaum (1989). Association-dissociation patterns of United States Olympic trial contestants. *Cognitive Ther. Res.* 13:185–192.

Singer, R.N. (1988). Psychological testing: What value to coaches and athletes? *Int. J. Sport Psychol.* 19:87–106.

Smith, A.L., D.L. Gill, D.J. Crews, R. Hopewell, and D.W. Morgan (1995). Attentional strategy use by experienced distance runners: Physiological and psychological effects. *Res. Quart. Exerc. Sport* 66:142–150.

Sonstroem, R.J., and W.P. Morgan (1989). Exercise and self-esteem: Rationale and model. *Med. Sci. Sports Exerc.* 2:329–337.

Spielberger, C.D., R.L. Gorsuch, and R.E. Lushene (1983). *The state-trait anxiety inventory manual.* Palo Alto (CA): Consulting Psychologists Press.

Straub, W.F., and D.A. Hinman (1992). Profiles and professional perspectives of 10 leading sport psychologists. *Sport Psychologist* 6:297–312.

Suinn, R.M. (1972). Removing emotional obstacles to learning and performance by visuo-motor behavior rehearsal. *Behav. Ther.* 31: 308–310.

Tenenbaum, G., M. Bar-Eli, J.R. Hoffman, R. Jablonovski, S. Sade, and D. Shitrit (1995). The effect of cognitive and somatic psyching-up techniques on isokinetic leg strength performance. *J.Strength Condition. Res.* 9:3–7.

Unestahl, L.E. (1982). Use of Hypnosis in Sports Medicine Workshop. Annual Meeting of the Society for Clinical and Experimental Hypnosis, Indianapolis, IN.

Valenstein, E.S. (1986). *Great and Desparate Cures: The Rise and Decline of Psychosurgery and Other Radical Treatments for Mental Illness.* New York: Basic Books.

Vealey, R.S. (1994). Current status and prominent issues in sport psychology interventions. *Med. Sci. Sports Exerc.* 26:495–502.

Wang, Y., and W.P. Morgan (1992). The effect of imagery perspectives on the psychophysiological responses to imagined exercise. *Behav. Brain Res.* 52:167–174.

Watson, W. (1973). *Super Nature.* New York: Anchor Press/ Doubleday.

Weinberg, R.S. (1994). Goal-Setting and performance in sport and exercise settings: A synthesis and critique. *Med. Sci. Sports Exerc.* 26:469–477.

Weinberg, R., L. Bruya, H. Garland, and A. Jackson (1990). Effect of goal difficulty and positive reinforcement on endurance performance. *J. Sport Exerc. Psych.* 12:144–156.

Weinberg, R., T. Seabourne, and A. Jackson (1987). Arousal and relaxation instructions prior to the use of imagery: Effects on image controllability, vividness and performance. *Int. J. Sport Psychol.* 18:205–214.

Weiner, I.B. (1989). On competence and ethicality in psychodiagnostic assessment. *J. Personal. Assess.* 53:827–831.

Whelan, J.P., M.J. Mahoney, and A.W. Meyers (1991). Performance enhancement in sport: A cognitive behavioral domain. *Behav. Ther.* 22:307–327.

Williamson, R.G. (1996). Improve your concentration. *United States Sports Academy's Sport Supplement* 4:2.

DISCUSSION

LAMB: How would you characterize the research done in this field in the last 10 y or so? Has there been a lot of research? What is the quality of the work that has been done?

MORGAN: I found a lot of research, but the experimentation was largely quasi-experimental in nature, and many of these studies were characterized by numerous methodological problems of a fundamental nature. Rather than bash all of those studies in my chapter, I have simply made some generalizations. For example, it really makes no sense whatsoever to study the effect of some manipulation on elite-level marathon runners, and then generalize to a group of young boys and girls who may never run more than a short distance. Of course, generalizing from results with young boys and girls to elite marathon runners would not make sense either. Why should workers in sport psychology think that using an irrelevant or novel task such as the "ring toss" or accuracy in shooting the basketball while blindfolded with young boys and girls would have any relevance at all for improving the foul-shooting percentage of a professional basketball player? This sort of reasoning is rather bizarre. That is the type of research I came across in my review—research with irrelevant tasks and inappropriate samples rather than samples from the target population. Furthermore, the effects of psychological interventions on the learning of tasks rather than the performance of learned skills has often been the case.

LAMB: One of your messages seems to be that often a group result in sport psychology experimentation doesn't mean very much, and that we have to treat athletes as individuals. Does this mean that qualitative research on individuals is the kind of research that should be done?

MORGAN: Qualitative or ethnographic research is neither good nor bad. Likewise, quantitative research, or the usual kind of research in exercise science, is not good or bad. The question being asked should dictate the methods and model that one elects to employ. I am not trying to dodge your question, and I would like to develop this idea with an example. In the area of hypnosis, for example, with the exception of the early work by Eysenck and a few of Johnson's reports, the quantitative research is largely equivocal from the standpoint of performance enhancement. That is to say, for every study demonstrating that hypnosis improves performance, there is another showing that it does not. On the other hand, when you review those studies that are of a negative nature, where significant effects are not shown, there are always some individuals in those studies who have "psychological breakthroughs" or phenomenal performances. These extraordinary physical performances are simply unexplainable in most cases. In some of the fatigue studies, for example, it's almost as though lactate production was eliminated under hypnosis. A comparison of fatigue curves under control conditions with those under hypnosis suggests that an elimination of the standard fatigue patterns took place, and the individual was able to continue in an apparent steady state under hypnosis. I don't think the two approaches are mutually exclusive. I think you can use both paradigms, and I believe that is why Hanin's work has been so instructive. Hanin demonstrated that anxiety is not correlated with performance, and this finding was based upon his empirical evaluation of hundreds of athletes prior to actual competitions. However, this does not mean that anxiety is not important. Indeed, Hanin's work shows that anxiety is very important, and this finding resulted from the qualitative or ideographic approach rather than the group or nomothetic approach. The challenge is to find out who needs elevated anxiety in the precompetitive setting and who does not.

LAMB: Does this mean that if I am a soccer coach, I need to hire 11 psychologists?

MORGAN: I would suggest that you hire one good one or none at all. Actually, the successful coaches are good practical psychologists in their own right. They will often say that they are not psychologists, but observe the good coaches in action, or read what they are attributed to having said to their teams. Vince Lombardi was such a good motivational speaker that corporations hired him to speak to their top executives. While he is often quoted as having said, "Winning isn't the important thing, it is the only thing," what he actually said was, "Winning isn't the important thing, but the desire to win is." The quote wrongly attributed to Vince Lombardi is a sports writer's mutation of what he actually said. Lombardi's success was undoubtedly due in large measure to the motivational principles he employed, and there are many other examples in the field of coaching. Two that come to mind at once would be Councilman in swimming and Bowerman in track. The point is that successful coaches are successful in large measure because of the psychological principles they employ.

BAR-OR: You have said that some people respond and others do not respond to certain treatments and therefore one cannot generalize about a response pattern. Isn't this then a major challenge for sports psychologists to come up with hypotheses and validate them as to *why* some people would be responders and others will be non-responders? A similar dilemma exists in medical practice. For example, when we treat children who are obese with an exercise-plus-diet intervention, some respond one way, others respond another way. Our challenge is to identify possible mechanisms and patient profiles so that we can predict who will be a good responder and who will not. Shouldn't a similar challenge be given to the sports psychology researchers?

MORGAN: I could not agree more! The first order of business is to recognize that individual differences must be considered. The second step might be to do what Hanin has done, and that is to create a model that actually can enhance performance. I have summarized Hanin's IZOF model in the chapter, and this model actually permits applications. It is one of the few cases in the area of sport psychology that has a sound theoretical rationale along with a compelling empirical data base. However, the approach is labor-intensive, and it requires that each athlete must be treated as an individual. Practitioners who prefer to employ generic models that can be applied to large groups may not find Hanin's IZOF Model to possess sufficient parsimony, but it is probably the most eloquent and successful intervention we have in sport psychology.

KNUTTGEN: You present examples of how psychological techniques have been reported to help athletes like LeMond and Dickson to achieve great success, but do sport psychologists become aware of situations where athletes have tried psychological techniques and have failed miserably?

MORGAN: Sport psychology is no different than physiology, medicine, and most other fields. Practitioners usually do not highlight their failures when giving talks, and journals have a tendency to reject negative results. While there is a disinclination to report negative results, I can give some examples from the field of sport psychology. One is the case of a golfer described by Garver. The golfer was competing at the NCAA Division 1 level, and he would always shoot par or less for 18 holes if he had a par or birdie on the first hole. However, if he had a bogie on the first hole, he would "catastrophize" about this and proceed to have a bad round. So, Garver told the golfer under hypnosis that he should not worry about the first hole. He was advised that "the first hole was not important—a par would be great, a birdie would be even better, but a bogie would be fine as well—don't worry about the first hole." The coach saw the player on the third hole and asked him how he was doing, and he replied that he was doing great. The same query and reply was reported to occur at the sixth and ninth holes. When he completed the round the coach asked him how he did, and he replied that he had a great day. When the coach asked him what he shot that day, he replied that he had an 85! In other words, he felt good about losing. The perception of distress associated with not doing well was eliminated, but the golfer's game was not improved. Garver also reported the case of a gymnast who could perform any routine he tried at a high level in practice, but during competition he always performed below his practice level. This is a very common experience in sports. Garver told him that, "When you mount the horse tomorrow, you are going to feel a surge of strength, and you are going to be the strongest person in the world at that point in time—you will not have any problems tomorrow." Unfortunately, the gymnast took this hypnotic suggestion quite literally, and his "super strength" and force generation carried him beyond the horse and into the bleachers! There are many other examples of this type, but these cases usually do not appear in articles or textbooks.

CLARKSON: Recently I had the opportunity to chair a symposium on the history of training and nutrition in the Olympics at which four Olympians spoke—Al Oerter, Billy Mills, Nicolle Haislett, and Bruce Baumgartner. They were asked why they were successful. They consistently said it was their mental focus and attitude during preparation for the event and during the actual event.

MORGAN: We need to pursue these self-reports and find out what the athletes mean by mental focus. Bannister reports in his book describing events leading up to his breaking of the 4-min mile that he and his running mates were sitting near the track. It was windy and raining, but then the wind died down and the rain stopped. Bannister happened to look up at the flag atop St. George's, and it had stopped blowing in the wind. He reports that he turned to his teammates and said, "It's on!." There was certainly a cognitive component to their record performance. There is no question about the role of psychology in the setting of the world record on that day. So, I think we can learn a great deal from the athlete. But, the tradition in contemporary sport psychology has been to take existing theories in academic psychology, such as those derived from goal-setting theory, and apply this to the athlete. Empirical research by Locke and others involving goal setting in the field of industrial-organizational psychology, using tasks such as card sorting, typing, and so on, has yielded fairly consistent results and principles. However the application of these principles to sport settings is questionable. The goal-setting literature in sport psychology is based largely on fiction, not on fact.

KENNEY: What, if anything, is being done on a national or international level to standardize training and experience for practitioners to delineate those who would fall into the category that you refer to as "ethical and competent" sport psychologists?

MORGAN: In the case of the sport psychologists, it would be my estimate that eight of 10 are not psychologists. But, what is adequate training? Some group can suddenly say it is certifying sport psychologists, but that would not mean that these individuals would necessarily be competent. Also, use of the title psychologist is restricted to licensed psychologists in North America. The ethical and moral issues surrounding the delivery of psychological services by individuals who are not adequately trained could become legal issues in the future.

KANTER: Given your criteria, are there any competent sport psychologists?

MORGAN: Yes, there are a few individuals working in the area of sport psychology who are very effective in what they do. There are very few who have been trained in both psychology and exercise and sport science. I often liken the situation to the field of bioengineering. In this field's early days, individuals who called themselves bioengineers were either biologists or engineers for the most part, but the field evolved to the point where hybridization took place, and scientists pursued advanced training as bioengineers in both biology and engineering. That evolution has not yet occurred in sport psychology. Good training is most critical when dealing with individuals who may have psychological disorders. Some sport psychologists believe that athletes possess "super health" but there is no compelling research in support of this view. Also, most of the athletes we have referred to clinical and counseling psychologists have required short-term or long-term psychotherapy. A smaller number have been referred to out-patient psychiatry by the clinicians we have relied on for referral purposes. Most of these latter cases have involved major depressive episodes, and a few have been regarded as suicidal. Hence, it is imperative that sport psychologists be sensitive to the fact that such possibilities exist, and they must have the minimal competencies necessary to detect problems requiring referrals.

MAUGHAN: You have focused on the elite performer, but I wonder about the effectiveness of psychological intervention in the sub-elite performer. Will these people improve more with psychological intervention because they are further away from the physiological limit?

MORGAN: I have always thought that the answer to your question would be, "Yes," on the grounds that individuals scoring in the basement zone would have a greater potential for improvement because of the greater distance from the ceiling. However, a number of years ago Don Horstman and I were doing research on endurance performance at the Natick Lab, and we showed that an individual with the greatest gain in endurance performance was one who had the highest score to begin with. The participants in the study were young, healthy, male soldiers, and they averaged about 20 min on endurance time to exhaustion at 80% $\dot{V}O_2$max. The individual in question lasted about 40 min at the outset, and yet the psychological intervention resulted in the greatest increase for this individual. In Johnson's early work with hypnosis at the University of Maryland, the top performer in one of his experiments with the barbell press to exhaustion had the greatest gain following hypnotic suggestion. This individual's initial score was 87 repetitions with a 47 lb barbell, which was double the closest performer's score. However, following hypnotic suggestion he was able to increase his performance to over 200 repetitions, and this "psychological breakthrough" persisted into the non-hypnotic state where he peaked at 350 repetitions. In other words, this mesomorphic, weight-trained, professional athlete scored about two standard deviations above the sample mean at baseline and was nevertheless able to experience the greatest gain in performance. It is not easy to explain phenomenal performances of this nature, but here is another example of why we need to look at individual performances as well as group performances; even the best performers can at times have the potential for substantial improvements.

DISHMAN: Perhaps the most significant question in sport psychology when attempting to communicate the evidence that is available to a community outside of the profession of sport psychology, is whether or not there is an available technology that can be implemented. What predictors or principles and methods for applying them are tested with high-level performers and can be communicated to coaches, athletic trainers, administrators, and athletes to utilize for manipulating psychology to reliably enhance performance? There is a huge leap from the recognition that psychology limits performance to changing psychology in a predictable way and explaining how psychology limits performance. Those of us trained in natural science were always taught to take a hierarchical progression from description to prediction to explanation to control. When there is a consumer-based demand for advice, or in some instances a demand created by sport psychologists themselves through self-promotion, then there becomes a market for a profession, and the profession may exist without a valid technology. I think that this largely describes the current state of affairs, which has not changed over the past 15 years. I would say that the energy within the field of sport psychology continues to be disproportionately spent on offering services rather than directed toward improving scientific rationales. It is not that there is no evidence to support the role of psychology, what is lacking is a well-defined technology and a guideline for practice that will insure predictable outcomes that should occur for most people. There are professionals in sport psychology, but if you define a profession by a solid body of knowledge and technology for delivering that body of knowledge, that is where the caveats must be raised. There are very few sport psychologists who are scientist-practitioners, evaluating and improving their professional technology by experimental or controlled case-study research. I don't think Bill or any of us in the field want to convey the message at this meeting that sport psychology does not warrant credibility or does not warrant a place in the sports medicine family. However, there has been a segregation of sport psychology from sport medicine and exercise science. I think most of us would endorse the idea problems in athletes are probably best solved with an integrated effort by a team of sport medicine professionals. Most athletic performances are not limited solely by a shortcoming in a single biological or behavioral system, so they usually require a multi-disciplinary examination. I think we can cast some blame on sport psychology for choosing not to be a part of the exercise and sport science community.

ARROYO: There is no doubt in my mind that we have to work with sport psychologists; they should be part of the team. In Mexico there is a Mexican college of psychologists. Its members have lots of interactions with Europeans, who have an international association for sport psychologists, but there is not much communication between sport psychologists in Mexico and the United States.

MORGAN: Yes, but the difference is that European and Mexican sport psychologists are actually psychologists. This is often not the case in North America.

SCOTT: I think there are some good things resulting from sport psychology. For example, canoeists from Europe were taught how to use the POMS test, and they felt it was probably the most significant improvement in their training programs that they had. They knew when to train harder and when to back off. They were taught a set of skills that allowed them to be their own self-advocates for their own sport motivation and their own sport psychology. I think this is where the cutting edge is. I think athletes can be taught self-monitoring techniques. On another issue, some sports magazines in California have advertisements from sports psychologists stating, for example, that "I treat pro racers X, Y, and Z." People are going to flock to these people because the pros went to them. These practitioners lead the consumers to believe that their interventions were responsible for the athletes' victories. It is not science at all.

MORGAN: That is unethical behavior.

SCOTT: Absolutely, I agree. I would like to see that stopped. I would also like to comment on the association/dissociation issue from my clinical experience as a member of the medical team at the Hawaii Ironman triathlon for the last 8 y. I treated Paula Newby-Fraser this year when she collapsed. She collapsed because she dissociated. You can not do that in a race like the Ironman. She knows exactly what she needs to do, but she ignored her mind, dissociated, and just kept going until she collapsed. Interestingly enough, in this race that lasts 10–20 h, the competitors who are 60–70 years old never come in the medical tent because they do not dissociate during the race.

A final comment about the "monk runners" of Tibet: they do not really run as fast as has been reported because the distance was miscalculated. You can only run 100 mi in 16 h at altitude; 300 mi in 24 h is absolutely impossible.

MANDELBAUM: I must admit that sport psychology has become a hobby of mine the last 5 y. My concern is how to bring the information we have down to the team physician, the coach, the athletic trainer, and the physical therapist. These people have to face practical problems on a daily basis, and they need help. For example, how should they prepare athletes to handle jet lag on long team trips?

MORGAN: I have a concern about your call for practical applications. It seems to me that we should have a research basis for our applications. I think that jet lag is a myth, just as I regard the insomnia-performance link as a myth. The reason I say this is that we have a compelling military literature indicating that traversal of six time zones has no effect on physiological responses during submaximal or maximal treadmill running. Also, we know that athletes who are traveling across multiple time zones improve psychologically. We also know that their perception of effort for fixed bouts of exercise, say swimming 200 m at 90% of maximum velocity is decreased. We know that soldiers running on a treadmill perceive exercise intensity as being easier following traversal of multiple time zones. Why do some sport psychologists perform interventions designed to deal with jet lag or sleep loss in the absence of a research base? These interventions are not based on the type of technology that Dishman suggested we need in his response. We need to first show, for example, that sleep loss leads to performance decrements. Goldman and Soule have shown that sleep loss leads to performance enhancement in soldiers marching on a treadmill while wearing 15 or 30 kg packs. At any rate, before we perform an intervention we should have research evidence regarding its efficacy and possible limitations. A recent issue of *Runner's World* contains a practical prescription for jet lag, and runners are advised that they should plan to arrive at the site of the competition well in advance of their race. They are also told that they should allow one day of recovery for every time zone they traverse. In other words, an athlete traveling across 11 time zones would need to arrive 11 d in advance of the competition. I am unaware of a single study done with athletes that supports such a generalization (see review by O'Connor and

Morgan published in *Sports Medicine* in 1990), and published research argues against the use of practical applications of this nature as a means of coping with jet lag.

MANDELBAUM: Based on my having completed 50 international trips with our national soccer team and having tried every imaginable coping technique, I agree that those techniques don't work, but I totally disagree with your notion that jet lag is a myth.

MORGAN: You and I both have experienced personally the effects of jet lag, but there is at least one other person with us today who informed us at dinner last night that he travels across multiple time zones (10 to 12) on a regular basis and has never had problems with jet lag. Here again we see the common problem of individual differences if we try to make generalizations. One of the problems with the research on jet lag is that the studies were not performed on athletes involved in heavy training. Athletes in heavy training differ from non-athletes when they travel across six or more time zones. Guess what? The athletes are resting and recuperating as they travel. By the time they arrive in the new country their muscle soreness has decreased or even disappeared, their perception of effort is decreased for a standard exercise bout, and they have improvements in mood states such as anxiety and depression. These improvements have been shown to occur for East-West and West-East travel alike. It is possible that jet lag effects are common among sedentary, non-athletes who serve as support personnel and less common among the athletes. However, I am unaware of any research on this subject.

2

Advances in the Evaluation of Sports Training

HARM KUIPERS, M.D., PH.D.

INTRODUCTION
    The Development of Exercise Testing
SPORTS TRAINING
    The Basic Idea of Training
    Training Volume and Performance
EXERCISE TESTING
    Specificity and Validity
    Accuracy and Variability
INDICES OF ENDURANCE CAPACITY
    Maximal Oxygen Uptake ($\dot{V}O_2$max)
    Energy Cost as a Measure of Efficiency
    Power Output or Running Velocity at $\dot{V}O_2$max
    The Plasma Lactate Response to Exercise
        Anaerobic Threshold
        Maximal Lactate Steady State
        Factors That Can Affect Plasma Lactate
        Non Invasive Measurement of the Anaerobic Threshold
    Simulated Time Trials in the Laboratory
MEASUREMENT OF ANAEROBIC ENERGY PRODUCTION
INDICES OF STRENGTH AND SPEED
    Muscular Strength
    Speed
FIELD TESTS OF SPORT PERFORMANCE CAPACITY
    The Use of Heart-Rate Monitors
PRACTICAL IMPLICATIONS
DIRECTIONS FOR FUTURE RESEARCH
SUMMARY
BIBLIOGRAPHY
DISCUSSION

INTRODUCTION

The Development of Exercise Testing

The achievement of peak athletic performance is possible only by training intensively on a daily or near-daily basis; both the coach and the athlete should monitor how the athlete's body responds to the training program and how performance capacity is developing. This requires the availability of valid and reliable tests that will provide information about the training state at various times as training progresses. In this chapter the various laboratory tests that are employed to measure performance capacity will be reviewed.

Experience and intuition guided the training of athletes until the middle of the 20th century when medical doctors and physiologists first became interested in the physiological and medical aspects of sports training. This interest resulted in the first physiological investigations of athletes and the beginning of the rapid development of exercise physiology. Since then, much has been learned about the physiological basis of athletic performance and about training-induced biological adaptations. For example, studies on energy metabolism and gas exchange during exercise revealed that a high maximal oxygen uptake ($\dot{V}O_2$max) is an important prerequisite for success in sports in which a continuous high intensity must be maintained for more than approximately 2 min. Assessment of $\dot{V}O_2$max made it possible to quantify training adaptations and to identify an athlete's potential for endurance sports. However, later research revealed that $\dot{V}O_2$max is not the only determinant for success in endurance sports, and, subsequently, several methods and procedures were developed to quantify performance capacity and to predict the potential for sports performance as reliably and accurately as possible.

Ideally, a simple and sensitive test would yield quantitative information about performance capacity and provide a solid basis for controlling the training process. However, in spite of the many testing methods and testing devices available, the sensitivity and validity of tests for assessing changes in performance capacity need to be improved.

The physiological characteristics that are generally measured in the laboratory to quantify performance capacity are $\dot{V}O_2$max, oxygen costs of given exercise intensities, peak power output, anaerobic threshold, anaerobic power, and strength characteristics. When no laboratory facilities are available, field tests can be used to measure characteristics of endurance, speed, strength, and skill.

SPORTS TRAINING

The Basic Idea of Training

Training for sports is predicated upon the notion that the body will respond to a training-induced disturbance of homeostasis (Viru, 1994). During recovery, homeostasis is restored, biological adaptations occur, and an increased functional capacity for greater exercise intensity and volume results (Viru, 1994). Relatively little is known about the qualitative and quantitative physiological adaptations to training stimuli of various intensities and volumes. Attempts have been made to understand the training process and predict performance with mathematical models (Banister, 1991; Mader, 1991; Morton et al., 1990; Ward-Smith & Mobey, 1995); however, these models are far from accurate and include only a selected number of the many physiological factors that are involved in training and adaptation. Therefore, mathematical models provide only a rough approximation of the complexity of the biological systems involved.

Training Volume and Performance

Some data are available regarding the relationships among training characteristics and their effects on performance capacity. Based on the relatively scarce data, there seems to be an inverse U-shaped relationship between training volume (number of hours spent or total amount of work done during a certain period of time) and the increase in performance (Figure 2-1). As nicely documented by Noakes (1991), a classic example of the inverted U-shaped relationship between training volume and performance is provided by the former long-distance runner, Ron Hill, who was very consistent in his training. When his training distance was plotted against running performance, an optimal performance response appeared to occur when the training distance ranged between 150-170 km/wk (Noakes, 1991). With less than 150 km/wk or more than 170 km/wk, performance declined.

A similar phenomenon may occur in all-round speed skating, which involves four distances, ranging from 500-10,000 m. The duration of these events varies from approximately 40 s-15 min. I was a world-class speed skater from 1972-1975, and my training characteristics and competitive results were recorded daily for several years. Training involved a rather consistent mix of endurance exercise and intermittent exercise at near-competitive intensity. In retrospect, when the total training duration was beyond 15 h/wk, there was a consistent decrement in my competitive performance (Kuipers, unpublished observations). On two occasions, an overtraining syndrome or staleness, as defined by Kuipers

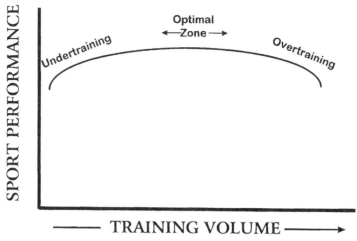

FIGURE 2-1. *Schematic representation of the relationship between training volume and performance capacity.*

and Keizer (1988), was encountered when my training volume exceeded approximately 20 h/wk.

More recent studies provide a similar general picture of the adverse effects of excessive training volume. Costill and co-workers (1991) studied the effect of increasing the training volume on performance capacity in swimmers. Doubling the training volume for 6 wk failed to induce a further increase in swimming power and endurance, but it resulted in a significant decline in sprinting velocity.

Flynn et al.(1994) studied training stress in cross-country runners and collegiate swimmers and found decrements in the performances of both groups of athletes during the period of greatest training volume. However, Vermulst et al.(1991), who studied the relationship between training volume and maximal power output on a rowing ergometer during a rowing season, failed to find such a relationship between training volume and test performance. A possible explanation for these disparate findings is that, with the exception of a training camp, the rowers trained only 60-80 min/d, and it is likely that the training volume was insufficient to induce overtraining. The studies cited above and others (Fry et al., 1991; Lehmann et al.,1992, 1993) support the idea that the relationship between training volume and performance appears to have an inverted U-shape (Figure 2-1). Consequently, there is an optimal zone for the amount of training that leads to a maximal increase in performance. However, this optimal zone is poorly defined, and exceeding it may lead to overtraining. For sports training, knowledge of whether or not an athlete is training in the optimal zone or is overtraining is especially relevant. This is one of the most difficult aspects of training because studies have shown that there is not a specific and reliable indicator for early detection of overtraining (Bruin et al.,1994).

The most sensitive and superior instrument for detecting overtraining is the athlete's body. Signs of increased fatigability and local or generalized stiffening of muscles should be interpreted as incomplete recovery and should lead to adjustment in training volume and/or intensity. This statement is supported by Hooper et al. (1995), who monitored physiological and psychological variables during a 6-mo swimming season in elite swimmers. Although epinephrine concentration and neutrophil number in athletes at rest seemed to be associated with overtraining, the authors concluded that daily logs of training and measures of well-being may assist in programming the appropriate training during periods of intense training.

EXERCISE TESTING

Specificity and Validity

When a laboratory test of performance is developed, the first step is to identify the basic physical and physiologic requirements of the particular sport as accurately as possible. Next, the physical activity performed in the test should resemble as closely as possible the actual sport activity; this is known as test specificity, which is critical to test design (Chin et al., 1995; Dal Monte et al., 1992; Rundell, 1995; Steininger & Wodick, 1987). Several sport-specific ergometers for rowers, swimmers, kayakers, cross-country skiers, and other sport disciplines have been developed (Dal Monte et al., 1992). When the type of ergometer has been chosen, the next step is to identify the variables to be measured and the exercise protocol to be used. The equipment should be calibrated, and the testing should take place under standard conditions. A subject should be well rested before a test and prepared as he or she would be for an important competition.

The validity of a test refers to how accurately a test measures what it intends to measure and can be determined by comparing the test result with a "gold standard" (i.e., the result of competition). Usually the correlation between competitive results and test results is analyzed to assess the degree of relationship between the two. If the results of two tests are very closely related, a correlation coefficient of 0.9-1.0 might be expected; unfortunately, the correlation coefficients between several laboratory tests and performance are only moderate (i.e., 0.5-0.7).

Accuracy and Variability

To decide whether a change over time in the performance of a laboratory test has any physiological significance, the relative accuracy of the test must be known. For example, the accuracy of $\dot{V}O_2$max measurements is between 2% and 6% at best, even with a rigid calibrational discipline (Barbeau et al., 1993). If the error were 6%, a $\dot{V}O_2$max measured as 70 mL·kg^{-1}·min^{-1} could reflect a true $\dot{V}O_2$max as low as 65.8 mL·kg^{-1}·min^{-1} or as high as 74.2 mL·kg^{-1}·min^{-1}. Besides poor calibration, several other measurement problems that reduce accuracy may be encountered. Two such problems are resistance in the breathing valves (leading to air leakage when one uses face masks or mouth pieces) and leakage of tubing that conducts gases to and from the gas analysis equipment. With fully automatic, computerized systems, it is sometimes hard to control and check each step and calculation in the sequence of $\dot{V}O_2$ measurements. In addition to measurement error, day-to-day biologic variability may contribute to the differences in $\dot{V}O_2$max that are often noted on a test-retest basis. Swaine and Zanker (1996) compared peak $\dot{V}O_2$ values between two tests in swimmers who were tested on an isokinetic swim bench. The data showed that peak $\dot{V}O_2$ between the two tests may differ by as much as 12% in some individuals.

The extent to which the variability in $\dot{V}O_2$max may be attributed to biological or methodological variation is presently unclear. Undoubtedly, both biological and methodological variability contribute to the day-to-day variations in test results. For example, Kuipers et al. (1985) conducted a study in which 19 subjects performed an incremental cycle ergometer test once a week during several months to measure variability of maximal power output and some physiological variables such as oxygen uptake and plasma lactate concentration. Depending on the number of weeks the subjects participated in the experiment, subjects completed 15-34 incremental cycle tests. The variability in peak power output ranged from 3-7% among individuals. Changes in peak power output were associated with changes in the physiological responses of heart rate, oxygen uptake, and plasma lactate concentration (Figures 2-2 and 2-3).

Based on these data, we concluded that approximately 80% of the variability in peak power output was of biologic origin. When comparing tests with the same peak power output, we estimated the variability of physiological responses by comparing the physiological responses to given power outputs. With this approach the coefficient of variation (i.e., $100(SD/\bar{x})$) in lactate response at a given power output ranged between 12% and 21%. The coefficient of variation for heart rate response to a given power output during cycling ranged between 1% and 3%

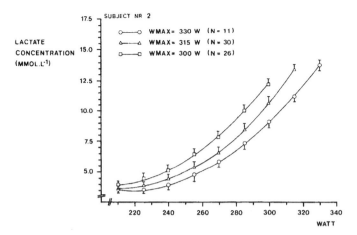

FIGURE 2-2. *Relationship between power outputs (W) and mean plasma lactate concentrations for groups of tests that yielded identical peak power outputs.* The bars represent standard deviations. The number of tests that resulted in the same peak power outputs is indicated in brackets. After Kuipers et al., 1985.

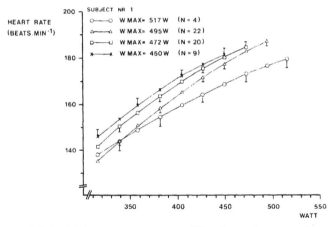

FIGURE 2-3. *Relationship between power outputs (W) and mean heart rates for groups of tests that yielded identical peak power outputs.* The bars represent standard deviations. The number of tests that resulted in the same peak power outputs is indicated in brackets. After Kuipers et al., 1985.

(Kuipers et al., 1985). These data imply that changes in $\dot{V}O_2$max of less than 5% may not be physiologically meaningful. Similarly, for lactate measurements, differences up to 10-15% between tests may well be due to biologic and/or measurement error. Hickey et al. (1992) studied the day to day variation in the cycling performances of well-trained cyclists

EVALUATION OF SPORTS TRAINING **69**

during three time trials on laboratory ergometers for durations of approximately 1 min, 12 min, and 105 min, respectively. Each of the three trials was repeated four times by each individual. The repeatability of these trials, as indicated by coefficients of variation, was approximately 1% for both the 12-min and 105-min trials and 3% for the 1-min trial.

Compared with the relatively large variability of laboratory tests, the difference in performance between winning and losing in actual competitions at the elite level is generally less than 1%. For instance, Snyder and Foster (1994) reported that in the 1988 Olympic speedskating event in Calgary the difference in average velocity between all gold and silver medal performances was 0.3%, whereas the mean difference between all the gold medalists and the 4th place finishers was 1.3%. In the 1991 World Canoeing Championships, a performance decrement of 2.5% would have left the gold medalist ineligible for participation in the event (Fry et al., 1992). In most other sports, similarly small margins determine whether or not a competitor wins a medal. Accordingly, the error inherent in most laboratory measurements makes them unreliable for distinguishing performance changes that can make the difference between winning and losing competitive events.

For estimating intraindividual variability, one can use competitive results during a season. When comparing the results of regional endurance runners throughout a season, Fry et al. (1992) reported coefficients of variation ranging between 1% and 4%, values similar to those previously discussed for repeated tests of peak power output and for repeated time-trial tests.

INDICES OF ENDURANCE CAPACITY

Maximal Oxygen Uptake ($\dot{V}O_2$max)

In endurance events lasting longer than 2 min, most of the energy is delivered aerobically. For several decades, $\dot{V}O_2$max has been the most generally used indicator of endurance capacity. However, $\dot{V}O_2$max is not always the best predictor of competitive results. This is evidenced by the rather low correlations between $\dot{V}O_2$max and actual performance in endurance events (Barbeau et al., 1993; O'Toole, 1989; Ribeiro et al., 1990; Wakayoshi et al., 1992, 1993). Exercise at an intensity that elicits $\dot{V}O_2$max can be maintained for 2-10 min (Billat et al., 1994). Longer-lasting events, such as a triathlon, road-race cycling, and long-distance running, are now conducted at 60-95% of $\dot{V}O_2$max (Wilmore & Costill, 1994). However, a high $\dot{V}O_2$max remains an important prerequisite for success in endurance events, particularly when it is coupled with the capacity to sustain a high percentage of $\dot{V}O_2$max for a prolonged period.

If $\dot{V}O_2$max is measured to evaluate the effectiveness of the training process, it should be measured during a sport-specific activity because this generally yields the highest peak $\dot{V}O_2$ values. This has been shown by Bouckaert et al. (1990), who measured peak $\dot{V}O_2$ on a cycle ergometer as well as on a treadmill in runners and cyclists. The cyclists reached the peak $\dot{V}O_2$ values on a cycle ergometer, whereas the runners attained the highest $\dot{V}O_2$ values on the treadmill. Measuring $\dot{V}O_2$max under competitive sport conditions is difficult, but recently developed, portable, light-weight oxygen measuring systems now permit measurement of $\dot{V}O_2$ during the actual sport activity with an accuracy that is similar to that for laboratory measurements (Crandell et al., 1994; Lucia et al., 1993).

The $\dot{V}O_2$max or peak $\dot{V}O_2$ does respond to training, especially in people who are not well-trained. Therefore, $\dot{V}O_2$max increases mainly during the first weeks or months of the training program. Once an athlete has become highly trained, $\dot{V}O_2$max appears to be a rather stable variable and fails to follow fluctuations in performance capacity (Acevedo & Goldfarb, 1989; Barbeau et al., 1993; Berg et al., 1989). Barbeau and colleagues (1993) suggested that if a decline in $\dot{V}O_2$max occurs in well-trained athletes, it is a reflection of fatigue rather than a reflection of any training adaptation.

In summary, $\dot{V}O_2$max measurement is valuable for determining the basic cardiorespiratory capacity of endurance athletes. The greatest changes in $\dot{V}O_2$max are observed in the first phase of the training process. Therefore, $\dot{V}O_2$max measurements are less suited for evaluation of changes in performance capacity of well-trained endurance athletes.

Energy Cost as a Measure of Efficiency

The oxygen uptake at a given exercise intensity can be used as a measure of efficiency. The lower the oxygen cost at a given intensity, the higher the movement efficiency. Some investigators have shown that, in long-distance runners with a similar $\dot{V}O_2$max, performance is related to the energy cost during running at 12 and 18 km/h (Morgan & Daniels, 1994). For training purposes, it is relevant to know how far oxygen cost can be reduced by training. Brisswalter & Legros (1994) measured ventilatory variables and $\dot{V}O_2$ at training pace in elite long- and middle-distance runners throughout a whole season. They found that $\dot{V}O_2$max significantly increased between test 1 and 3. However, oxygen cost at 12 km/h and at 18 km/h did not change during the whole season. The authors concluded that $\dot{V}O_2$max increases only during the first weeks of the training and that the cost of running at a predetermined submaximal pace failed to show significant changes during an entire season. On the other hand, Barbeau et al.(1993) studied race cyclists during a training season and found that $\dot{V}O_2$max did not change throughout the season, whereas oxygen cost during submaximal exercise declined by approximately 150-250 mL/min. This finding suggests an increase in efficiency of cycling. It is feasible that efficiency increases during training. However, as mentioned before, differences in true oxygen uptake within the $\pm 5\%$ range are difficult to detect.

In summary, oxygen cost at given submaximal exercise intensities may be used as a measure of efficiency. However, this requires accurate measurement of $\dot{V}O_2$. In addition, in activities in which body weight has to be carried (e.g., running) changes in body weight and/or muscle mass throughout a season may affect oxygen cost at a predetermined exercise intensity. A drawback of $\dot{V}O_2$max measurements is that sophisticated, expensive equipment and skilled personnel are required.

Power Output or Running Velocity at $\dot{V}O_2$max

Oxygen is utilized by the body for conversion of metabolic fuel into the mechanical energy required for propulsive speed. Therefore, the power output or exercise intensity at $\dot{V}O_2$max, obtained during an incremental exercise test, is a valuable indicator of endurance capacity. The power output or exercise intensity at $\dot{V}O_2$max can be measured during standard ergometric testing. A calibrated cycle ergometer is very well suited to measure power output (W) at $\dot{V}O_2$max (W_{max}). A major advantage of W_{max} measurement is that no expensive, sophisticated gas-analysis equipment is required.

When an incremental exercise protocol is used, W_{max} is calculated according to the equation:

$$W_{max} = W_{out} + [(t/D)(dW)]$$

in which W_{max} is the power output (W) at $\dot{V}O_2$max, W_{out} is the greatest power (W) sustained for the assigned duration, t is the time (s) the last unfinished load was sustained, D is the assigned duration (s) of each power level, and dW is the last power increment (W). For example, a subject is tested with a protocol in which the power output is increased by 25 W (dW) every 150 s (D). The athlete is able to complete 375 W but can sustain the final power level of 400 W for only 50 s (t). Thus, W_{max} is calculated according to:

$$W_{max} = 375 + [(50/150)(25\ W)],\ \text{yielding}\ 383\ W.$$

Few investigators have studied the relationship between W_{max} and actual sport performance. Jeukendrup et al.(1992) conducted an overtraining study in cyclists, in which the training volume was increased for 2 wk. The subjects were tested each week both in the laboratory with an incremental cycle ergometer test and outdoors with a 8.5 km time

trial. In this study, decline in time-trial performance coi
cline in $W_{max.}$

When Craig et al.(1993) studied the relationship t
mance in endurance track cyclists and several aerobic ana
oratory performance indices, W_{max} was found to be the bes
performance in the individual pursuit over 4000 m. Therefc
formance capacity and changes therein seem to be better ref.   , une
specific power output at $\dot{V}O_2$max (W_{max}) rather than by $\dot{V}O_2$max alone.

Presumably, power output at $\dot{V}O_2$max can also be used in other sports to monitor changes in performance capacity. For example, although $\dot{V}O_2$ was not measured, when Vermulst et al.(1991) studied elite rowers during a rowing season, changes in peak power output during an incremental test on a rowing ergometer suggest that changes in rowing performance were associated with changes in power output at $\dot{V}O_2$max. Running velocity at which $\dot{V}O_2$max is reached can also be used as a marker for endurance capacity. Noakes et al.(1990) demonstrated in ultramarathon runners that the peak treadmill running velocity attained during an incremental $\dot{V}O_2$max test was the best laboratory predictor for running performance in 10-km and 90-km races. This corroborates the findings of Morgan et al.(1989), who studied the relationship between the best 10-km performance and performance indices that were measured in the laboratory. Running speed at $\dot{V}O_2$max showed the highest correlation with the best 10-km performance. Oxygen cost at given speeds, $\dot{V}O_2$max, and running speed at a plasma lactate concentration of 4 mmol/L did not show strong associations with performance. Houmard et al. (1991) and Scott and Houmard (1994) also demonstrated that peak running velocity during an incremental exercise test on the treadmill was a good predictor of running performance in 8-km races in highly trained long-distance runners.

Although there is strong evidence that running velocity at $\dot{V}O_2$max is a valuable predictor for running performance, the velocity at $\dot{V}O_2$max among different studies may vary due to differences in exercise protocols. Hill and Rowell (1996) compared the running speed at $\dot{V}O_2$max as reported in different studies and concluded that the velocity at $\dot{V}O_2$max ($\dot{V}O_2$max) as measured during an incremental $\dot{V}O_2$max test is a valuable and easily measured predictor for endurance performance. However, for comparing $\dot{V}O_2$max data from different studies, the exercise protocol and possible differences in definition of $\dot{V}O_2$max must be taken into account.

In summary, power output and running velocity at $\dot{V}O_2$max are becoming accepted as valuable measures for assessing changes in endurance capacity. The $\dot{V}O_2$max typically changes only during the first few weeks of training; subsequently, only power output or running velocity,

$_2$max, must be measured to calculate the power: $\dot{V}O_2$max index , no expensive, sophisticated gas-analysis equipment is required after the initial phase of training). For detecting changes in endurance capacity in well-trained elite athletes, changes in power output or exercise intensity at $\dot{V}O_2$max seem to be more sensitive indicators than $\dot{V}O_2$max.

The Plasma Lactate Response to Exercise

Anaerobic Threshold. Endurance exercise beyond 10-15 min is not performed at or above $\dot{V}O_2$max intensity but at a submaximal intensity that can be expressed as a certain percentage of $\dot{V}O_2$max (Costill et al., 1973; Morgan & Daniels, 1994), and lactic acid accumulation in the blood is often associated with fatigue in such exercise. The nature of the blood lactate response can be used to assess the exercise intensity that can be sustained for a prolonged time (Anderson & Rhodes, 1989; Guglielmo & Di Prampero, 1995; Loat & Rhodes, 1993; Weltman, 1995). The exercise intensity that is associated with a fixed plasma lactate concentration of 4 mmol/L is often referred to as the "anaerobic threshold" or the "lactate threshold," which has also been defined as 1) the exercise intensity at which the concentration of lactate in plasma is 2 mmol/L, 2) the exercise intensity at which the plasma lactate concentration rises above that at rest, and 3) the exercise intensity associated with an abrupt increase in plasma lactate concentration during an exercise test of progressively increasing intensity (Andersen & Rhodes, 1989). Thus, no unanimity exists about the terminology concerning the lactate response to exercise, and the scientific relevance of these various lactate thresholds is still far from certain. However, studies that have investigated the relationships among anaerobic threshold, $\dot{V}O_2$max, and endurance performance have shown that endurance performance is better correlated with anaerobic threshold than with $\dot{V}O_2$max (Maffulli et al., 1991; Shephard, 1992). In this chapter, the anaerobic threshold is defined as the exercise intensity at which the plasma lactate concentration rises to 4 mmol/L.

Significant advances have been made in the understanding of lactate metabolism. In contrast to the first theory about the origin of the anaerobic threshold, lactate formation during exercise is not merely the reflection of a lack of oxygen. Lactate is a metabolic intermediate rather than the end-product of anaerobic metabolism (Brooks, 1991). Plasma lactate concentration is the result of lactate production, distribution, uptake, and metabolism; therefore, it will be determined by factors such as the plasma volume (Shephard et al., 1989), exercise intensity, the muscle mass producing lactate, and the metabolic activity of various tissues consuming lactate.

Because the muscle mass producing and consuming lactate depends on the type of exercise, the plasma lactate response is exercise specific, as shown by several investigators (Boukaert et al., 1990; Mittelstadt et al., 1995; Weltman, 1995; Withers et al., 1981). Therefore, it is important to note that lactate measurements for training evaluation should always employ an exercise task that is sport specific (i.e., as similar as possible to the sport performance in question for a given athlete) (Beneke et al., 1993; Bunc & Heller, 1991).

Maximal Lactate Steady State. A point that has received little appreciation regarding plasma lactate measurements is that it may take 10-15 min to establish a steady state in plasma lactate concentration at a fixed power output (Aunola & Rusko, 1992). This has led to an additional variable for assessing endurance capacity, the "maximal lactate steady state" (MaxLASS), which is defined as the greatest exercise intensity at which plasma lactate concentration does not increase more than 1 mmol/L during the final 20 min of a 30-min test (Beneke, 1995). A major drawback of MaxLASS measurements is that the procedure is time consuming because repeated 30-min tests with different intensities must be conducted.

By assessing MaxLASS, Jenkins & Quigley (1990) found that cyclists can maintain constant plasma lactate concentrations up to approximately 10 mmol/L. This result is similar to that obtained by Foster et al.(1993), who studied cyclists during a simulated time trial in the laboratory. However, Beneke (1995) showed that rowers tested on a rowing ergometer during a MaxLASS test were on the average only able to sustain much lower plasma lactates (i.e., below 4 mmol/L). In a later study, Beneke and Petelin von Duvillard (1996) compared MaxLASS in rowers, cyclists, and speed skaters during the specific sport activity and showed that MaxLASS values in speed skaters, cyclists, and rowers were on the average 6.5 mmol/L, 5.0 mmol/L, and 3.0 mmol/L, respectively. These differences in MaxLASS among the various sports may be attributable to differences in muscles used that result in different equilibria between lactate production and clearance. No comprehensive data are available about the relationship between MaxLASS and sport performance.

Factors That Can Affect Plasma Lactate. The plasma lactate response during incremental exercise is sensitive to training. Training effects can be detected from shifts in the lactate curve when plotted as a function of exercise intensity (Coen et al., 1991; Weltman, 1995). In general, a lower plasma lactate concentration at a fixed power output or exercise intensity is associated with increased performance capacity (Coen et al., 1991). However, the lactate response during exercise may also be affected by factors such as nutrition and fatigue. Several authors have shown that low carbohydrate intake and low muscle glycogen concentrations result in lower plasma lactate concentrations at fixed exercise intensities (Prusaczyk et al., 1992; Thorland et al., 1994; Weltman, 1995).

Lactate measurements in exercise testing should be done when subjects are well fed and well rested because Foster et al. (1988) showed that athletes undergoing strenuous training are characterized by low plasma lactate levels at given power outputs. Presumably, these low lactate concentrations are a function of low glycogen stores in heavily trained muscles. Thus, in overtrained athletes the plasma lactate response to exercise may be misleading, especially when lactate measurements are made only during submaximal exercise. With overtraining, the lactate curve plotted as a function of exercise intensity shifts paradoxically to the right. To discriminate a positive training effect from overtraining, plasma lactate concentrations should be measured during maximal exercise as well because with overtraining both the maximal plasma lactate concentration and the maximal attained power output or exercise intensity are reduced (Foster et al., 1988; Jeukendrup & Hesselink, 1994).

Protocols for lactate testing that were developed in the laboratory are also often employed under field conditions to assess the physiological challenge of training and competition, but this should be done with caution. For example, it should be taken into account that plasma lactate concentrations may be affected by differences in environmental temperature. Flore et al. (1992) compared the lactate response during an incremental cycle ergometer test at environmental temperatures of 10° and 30°C. The results showed that peak $\dot{V}O_2$ and the peak power outputs were not different between the two conditions, but heart rates and plasma lactate concentrations were significantly lower in the cool environment. The mean power output at a plasma lactate concentration of 4 mmol/L was 35 W greater in the cool environment.

Because heart rate can be measured easily under field conditions, heart rate at the anaerobic threshold previously assessed in the laboratory is often used to advise athletes about the appropriate training intensity. However, the relationship between heart rate and plasma lactate concentration is also sport specific. This is demonstrated by the study of Urhausen et al. (1993), who compared heart rate and lactate responses in rowers on a rowing ergometer and during actual rowing. They found significant differences in the relationship between heart rate and plasma lactate for results obtained during rowing ergometry versus those during free rowing. Similarly, Snyder et al. (1993) demonstrated that heart rates and oxygen uptakes at plasma lactate concentrations of 4 mmol/L are different during in-line skating when compared to running and cycling.

Non-Invasive Measurement of the Anaerobic Threshold. Because lactate measurement requires blood sampling, various attempts have been made to measure a threshold or critical exercise intensity noninvasively. For instance, ventilatory variables can be used to estimate the anaerobic threshold; during an incremental exercise test, pulmonary ventilation and expiratory carbon dioxide (V_{ECO2}) increase linearly until they begin to rise exponentially at a certain exercise intensity. The exercise intensity at which these inflection points in pulmonary ventilation or expiratory carbon dioxide (V_{ECO2}) occur is defined as ventilatory threshold (Anderson & Rhodes, 1989; Peronnet et al., 1987; Schneider & Pollock, 1991). Unfortunately, these measurements require expensive and sophisticated gas-analysis equipment. Similar to the assessment of lactate threshold (MaxLASS), for valid interpretation ventilatory measurements should be made during a sport-specific exercise task.

Breathing frequency has also been used to assess an exercise threshold (Cheng et al.,1992; James et al., 1989), but because ventilatory frequency is difficult to measure under field conditions, no studies have shown how ventilatory frequency behaves during a period of training or how changes in ventilatory frequency coincide with changes in performance capacity. Thus, a drawback of all ventilatory threshold measurements is that ventilatory variables cannot be measured satisfactorily in the field.

Conconi et al.(1982) and Droghetti et al.(1985) have proposed that the anaerobic threshold can be determined during an incremental exercise test by plotting the heart rate as a function of running speed. The speed at which a loss of linearity and a downward deflection in heart rate is found is assumed to coincide with the anaerobic threshold. The "Conconi-test" is basically a field test in which the exercise intensity is increased at fixed distances. For instance, on a 400-m running track, the running speed is increased every 200 m while the heart rate is continuously recorded by a heart-rate monitor.

Several investigators have challenged the validity of the "Conconi test" (Francis et al., 1989; Jones & Doust, 1995; Kuipers et al., 1988). These investigators compared the exercise intensity at which a deflection in heart rate was found using the Conconi protocol with the anaerobic threshold as assessed with invasive determination of plasma lactate concentration. These studies showed that a heart-rate deflection point could not be detected in all subjects, and when a deflection point was observed, it did not occur at the exercise intensity at which a plasma lactate concentration of 4 mmol/L was found. The deflection in heart rate is most likely the result of the protocol used. In the Conconi test, the duration of each consecutive exercise intensity decreases from approximately 1.5 min in the initial phase to approximately 20 s at the higher exercise intensities. As long as the heart rate adjustment to each exercise intensity can be attained, a linear response of heart rate as a function of speed will be found. However, when the duration of the higher exercise intensities becomes too short to allow for heart rate to reach the appropriate level, the heart rate values will decrease and a deflection point may be noticed. No reports were found that noted a relationship between changes in results of the "Conconi test" and changes in sport performance.

In conclusion, there is an insufficient scientific basis for using the anaerobic and lactate thresholds for practical purposes in sports training. The plasma lactate response to exercise is sport-specific, and environmental temperature may affect the plasma lactate concentration at a given exercise intensity and heart rate. This knowledge suggests that if lactate measurements are used for evaluation of training, the standards for their use and evaluation must be stringent, and great caution should be used in interpreting the results of such tests.

Simulated Time Trials in the Laboratory

Because most incremental laboratory tests are quite different from actual sport performances, attempts have been made to simulate competitive conditions as closely as possible in a laboratory setting. With modern ergometers that can be interfaced with a computer to produce a rapid display of power outputs and other test variables, competitions and time trials can be simulated in the laboratory.

Foster et al. (1993) studied cyclists during a simulated 5-km time trial on a racing bicycle attached to a wind simulator. Although the power output could not be measured directly, it was calculated from $\dot{V}O_2$ measurements during the simulated time trial. Peak oxygen uptakes during the time trials were significantly higher than $\dot{V}O_2$max values measured with a conventional $\dot{V}O_2$max test on a cycle ergometer. In addition, peak heart rates, peak plasma lactate levels, and pulmonary ventilations exceeded those obtained during a conventional incremental $\dot{V}O_2$max test.

Jeukendrup et al.(1996) compared three exercise test protocols in well-trained cyclists. Protocol A consisted of cycling to exhaustion on an ergometer at 75% of the peak power output (W_{max}), whereas protocol B consisted of cycling for 45 min at 70% W_{max}, after which the subjects were asked to perform as much work as possible for the next 15 min. Protocol C was a time trial in which an amount of work equivalent to cycling for 1 h at 75% W_{max} was to be completed in the shortest time possible. The coefficient of variation in trial A was approximately 26% but was only approximately 3.5% for protocols B and C.

Coyle et al.(1991) compared a simulated 1-h time trial on a cycle ergometer with an actual 40-km time trial on a flat course and found a correlation of r = 0.88 (P<0.01) between the two performances.

Based on these studies, a simulated time trial seems to be a valuable tool for assessing performance potential in the laboratory in cyclists and for studying training effects. This time-trial approach not only enables one to evaluate performance capacity but also to study athletes under actual competitive conditions, yet in a controlled laboratory setting. Unfortunately, publications about this time-trial approach remain scarce for other endurance sports, such as running, rowing, and cross-country skiing. Further studies are needed to confirm the relationship between lab-based results and actual sport performance results.

MEASUREMENT OF ANAEROBIC ENERGY PRODUCTION

In events lasting up to approximately 2 min, most of the energy is delivered anaerobically. Therefore, several attempts have been made to measure indices of anaerobic energy production during exercise, including anaerobic power and anaerobic capacity. The peak power output during a brief all-out test is referred to as anaerobic power. The total amount of work accomplished during an anaerobic test represents anaerobic capacity. Attempts to estimate anaerobic ATP production during exercise have included measurements of such variables as O_2 debt and maximal blood lactate concentration, but the validity of these estimates has been questioned (Green et al., 1996).

The tests for measuring anaerobic power consist of brief, all-out efforts lasting between a few seconds to approximately 2 min (Bouchard et al., 1991; Green & Dawson, 1993). Studies suggest that the optimal duration for measuring anaerobic power is approximately 30 s (Green & Dawson, 1993, 1996). The most widely used test for determination of anaerobic energy production is the Wingate test, which consists of a 30-s all-out effort on a cycle ergometer against a very high resistance (Bar-Or, 1987). When the equipment is interfaced with a computer, peak power output, mean power output, decline in power output, and total work can be determined. The decline in power output is used as an index of fatigue. Although the Wingate test has been validated extensively as a test for anaerobic performance (Bar-Or, 1987; Winter, 1991), Bar-Or (1987) has stated that "the correlation between the Wingate anaerobic test power indices and anaerobic performance tasks is quite high, but not high enough for using the Wingate anaerobic test as a predictor of success in these specific tasks." Therefore, the Wingate test still has a limited validity for measuring the sport-specific capacities of athletes.

Another approach to measuring anaerobic energy production is measurement of the accumulated O_2 deficit during a brief test of maximal power output lasting approximately 30 s (Medbø et al., 1988). Bangsbo et al. (1993) determined the accumulated O_2 deficit in oarsmen, soccer players, distance runners, and cyclists. They found a large variation in accumulated O_2 deficit, and concluded that this variable is not a valid indicator for sport-specific anaerobic performance capacity and is not related to the maximal activities of glycolytic enzymes in muscle. Further support for this finding was provided by Green and co-workers (1996), who studied accumulated O_2 deficit in cyclists and concluded that it is not related to anaerobic ATP production in muscle.

In summary, valid and reliable laboratory indicators of anaerobic power and capacity specific to performance in anaerobic sport events are unavailable. Therefore, practical field tests are a preferable alternative. Further research is needed to explore the possibilities for measuring anaerobic power in general as well as in specific athletic activities.

INDICES OF STRENGTH AND SPEED

Muscular Strength

Muscular strength is defined as the maximal force or torque a muscle or muscle group can generate at a specified contraction velocity. For many sport activities, muscular strength contributes significantly to performance capacity, so strength training is a common component of modern sports training. Several strength testing methods and devices have been developed to assess maximal isometric strength, the maximal weight that can be lifted for a given number of repetitions (repetitions maximum), and muscular endurance, which is the maximal time during which a given resistance or weight can be displaced (Kraemer & Fry, 1995). Strength measurements can be helpful for evaluation of the effectiveness of resistance training (Abernethy et al., 1995; Kraemer & Fry, 1995; Warren et al., 1992) and for monitoring the progress of rehabilitation after a sport injury.

A lack of specificity is a major problem with strength testing procedures for many sports (Behm & Sale, 1993; Gleeson & Mercer, 1996; Sale, 1991), but for sports such as Olympic weight lifting or power lifting, maximal isometric strength is correlated with sport performance (Warren et al., 1992). Also, for sprinting events, maximal isometric strength is correlated with sprinting qualities (r = 0.79; P<0.03), and the strength that can be delivered during the first 100 ms of a maximal isometric contraction is highly correlated with maximal sprinting velocity (r = 0.80; P<0.0001) (Young et al., 1995).

Changes in strength are not necessarily associated with changes in sport performance. For example, our unpublished measurements in elite sprint speed skaters showed that although a decline in isometric strength coincided with the cessation of weight training, competitive speed skating results were simultaneously improved. Thus, tests to evaluate specific strength characteristics in elite athletes should be developed.

Speed

Maximal speed of a movement can be sustained for only a few seconds and is a critical factor for explosive sports such as shot putting, javelin throwing, and the 100-m dash. As previously described, both maximal isometric strength and strength developed during the first 100 ms of an isometric contraction are significantly related to sprinting success (Young et al., 1995). Because most laboratories are of insufficient size to adequately measure sprinting speed, it is usually measured in field settings (i.e., on an indoor or outdoor running track).

FIELD TESTS OF SPORT PERFORMANCE CAPACITY

Field tests are often used to assess sport performance capacity, particularly when no laboratory facilities are available. The practical problems associated with field tests are numerous. For example, performance can be affected by the weather conditions, making comparison of performances achieved under different conditions problematic. In addition, adequate laboratory facilities for measurement of various biochemical variables in samples of blood, urine, or muscle are usually not present. However, these practical problems should not be a reason to abstain from field tests (Daniels & Foster, 1995). This advice is reflected in the results of Noakes et al.(1990), who demonstrated that, compared with laboratory performance indices such as $\%\dot{V}O_2$max at 16 km/h and lactate threshold, running time in a 10-km race is the best predictor for marathon performance. However, peak treadmill running velocity during a $\dot{V}O_2$max test was the best predictor of triathletes' performance times at ultramarathon distances (Noakes et al., 1990). For sprinting, the most specific test is measuring time to traverse certain distances, for instance, each 10 m of a 100-m sprint. This provides insight into the sprinter's acceleration capabilities and speed profile during the race. Indicators of success for middle-distance running include runs over approximately 200-600 m (Green & Dawson, 1996). However, the validity of such tests for predicting actual sport performance remains to be firmly established.

Field tests can also be employed for cycling. For example, time trials or simulated time trials varying in length between approximately 8 km and 40 km can be used to measure the ability to sustain a high cycling intensity for a prolonged time (Green & Dawson, 1993; Hickey et al., 1992; Jeukendrup et al., 1996; Loftin & Warren, 1994; Neuman, 1992).

Field tests are particularly pertinent for game sports in which performance depends on aerobic power, anaerobic power, speed, skill, agility, and numerous other factors. For sports such as volleyball (Häkkinen, 1993b) and basketball (Häkkinen, 1993a), vertical jumping height, $\dot{V}O_2$max, and isometric strength can be measured during the training season. Häkkinen (1993a, 1993b) found that changes in isometric strength of the knee extensors were correlated with changes in maximal vertical jump performance (r = 0.90; P<0.01). Chin et al. (1995) developed a field test for badminton players in which light bulbs were mounted on posts at different locations around the court, with a shuttlecock suspended from the top of each post. The lights flashed in random order, and the athletes had to react to the flashes and strike the shuttlecocks on the corresponding posts. The number of flashes varied from 16-26/min, and the test consisted of successive 3-min periods. Based on the observation that specific training resulted in better test results, Chin et al.(1995) concluded that this test gives a reasonable estimate of sport-specific physical fitness in elite badminton players. A similar test has been employed in squash players by Steininger & Wodick (1987), yielding similar results.

Bangsbo & Lindquist (1992) conducted various field and laboratory tests in soccer players to study the relationship between test results and performance in soccer matches. The laboratory testing included measurement of $\dot{V}O_2$max on a treadmill and an intermittent exercise test on the treadmill. The intermittent test consisted of high speed running at 18 km/h for 15 s alternated with jogging at 8 km/h for 10 s until exhaustion. The total time until exhaustion was the test score. The field test included an intermittent exercise test consisting of 15 s intensive exercise bouts interspersed with 10 s periods of jogging. During the high intensity exercise bouts the players had to perform various forms of locomotion (i.e., side stepping, and forward and backward running). The test lasted for 16.5 min, and the score was the total distance covered. The results of the interval test on the treadmill were strongly correlated with those for the field test of intermittent exercise. However, the test results were not significantly correlated with the total distance covered during a soccer match. It was concluded that the intermittent field test is a reliable alternative for the intermittent laboratory test and is useful for evaluating the endurance capacity of soccer players. However, the tests failed to predict success in soccer competitions. Balmson (1994) presented an overview of various testing procedures for evaluation of fitness in soccer players and concluded that various tests may provide insight into the components of physical fitness in soccer players but fail to predict success in soccer matches.

Although laboratory and field tests can be valuable tools for evaluation of the general and specific performance capacities in team-sport athletes, test results in these sports should be interpreted with even more caution than for those used in endurance sports. In team sports, performance is not determined by single factors such as peak power output or speed, but by a combination of many factors in addition to the components of individual performance.

The Use of Heart-Rate Monitors

A training tool that has become generally accepted by coaches and athletes during the last decade is the heart-rate monitor. Via a strap around the chest containing electrodes and a transmitter, the heart rate can be displayed continuously and stored into the memory of a computer chip. Leger & Thivierge (1988) and Macfarlane et al. (1989) compared the heart rates recorded by heart-rate monitors with those recorded by electrocardiograph during exercise and found the two measurements to vary by only 0-2 beats/min. For endurance athletes, a heart-rate monitor is an aid for maintaining a proper pace during training and competition (Gilman, 1996; Gilman & Wells, 1993; Hoffman & Street, 1992). As discussed previously, when monitoring heart rates in the field, one must take into account factors such as air temperature and a gradual increase in heart rate ("cardiac drift") as exercise becomes more prolonged (Gilman, 1996). The heart-rate monitor usually presents the option to select certain frequency limits. Exceeding these limits will ring an alarm. Especially in less experienced athletes, a heart-rate monitor can help to maintain a proper pace and to prevent overtraining (Figure 2-4). It can also help monitor progress in training because as the body adjusts to the training, heart rate during a given exercise intensity will decrease.

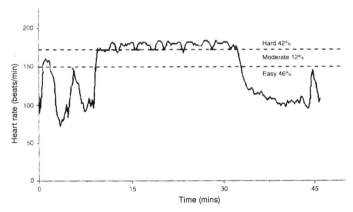

FIGURE 2-4. *Training heart rates of a collegiate cross-country skier during a warm-up and race.* The percentages of the total time that the heart rate was in each of three different intensity zones are indicated on the right. After Gilman, 1996.

PRACTICAL IMPLICATIONS

Testing should be conducted only when it can be made clear why an athlete or team might benefit from such testing and which specific questions should be answered by the tests. General tests of physiological function during exercise (e.g., heart rate, ventilation, and $\dot{V}O_2$max), or tests of body composition, strength, anaerobic power, and flexibility can provide an assessment of some of the basic requirements for sport performance; however, such measurements may be poorly correlated to overall performance capacity in a specific sport. For example, $\dot{V}O_2$max measurements throughout the training season are generally not sufficient to assess changes in performance capacity in specific endurance sports. On the other hand, training-induced changes in the results of certain tests can provide valuable information about changes in performance capacity. For example, changes in power output or running velocity at $\dot{V}O_2$max, measured during an incremental exercise test, are good indicators of corresponding changes in endurance performance.

An incremental exercise test for measuring power output at $\dot{V}O_2$max can be incorporated in a general medical and physiological evaluation at the beginning of a season. The exercise test can yield information about endurance capacity and about electrocardiographic characteristics during exercise. In addition to the general medical examination and maximal exercise test, anthropometry and/or hydrostatic weighing should be used to assess body weight and fat content.

When specific performance capacity is to be assessed in the laboratory, ergometers that mimic the specific sport activity should be used (Bilodeau et al., 1995; Dal Monte et al., 1992), but field tests similar to actual sport performances are often preferred over laboratory tests. Because no standard tests are available for most types of sport performance, the nature of the test is left to the ingenuity, expertise, and experience of the coach, trainer, or team physiologist. When various components of performance capacity are to be evaluated, the test battery may include, for example, measurement of peak power output in an incremental test, anaerobic power, speed, strength, and specific sport skills. A sizeable undertaking awaits researchers who would develop specific and reliable field and laboratory tests for each sport discipline.

In general, it is not necessary to conduct laboratory tests frequently because the practical information for training purposes is usually limited, and the time and costs of laboratory tests can be considerable. Therefore, testing more often than once every 3-4 wk is not recommended, and in many circumstances, even that will be too frequent. If periodization (cyclic variations in volume and intensity) is employed, field and/or laboratory testing can be conducted during the low-volume period of training. As soon as competitions start, testing is less necessary because competition is the best, most-specific, and complete evaluation of the performance capacity.

DIRECTIONS FOR FUTURE RESEARCH

Optimal control of the training process and maximizing performance at the right moment are of vital importance for coaches and athletes. The coach needs information about the progress of the athlete's adaptation to the training so the coach can adjust the training program to the specific needs of the athlete. In addition, the coach must be able to identify the athlete's weaknesses in order to prescribe remedial training programs.

Because little is known about the quantitative relationship between training characteristics and physiological adaptations to the training, research should be focused on explaining this relationship. For example, it is well known that proper training leads to accelerated protein synthesis for maintaining and improving the production of mitochondria, contractile proteins, enzymes for metabolizing fuels, and other cell components. Although measuring variables such as $\dot{V}O_2$max or strength assesses the overall training effect, the basic cellular changes that lead to an increase in oxygen uptake or strength remain obscure. Therefore, measuring protein transcription and synthesis may yield insight into the cellular adaptations to training, enabling the optimization of training. With recent developments in the application of molecular biology to exercise science, great progress in this area is bound to occur. One of the outgrowths of this research may be a greater understanding of the relationships among training frequency, intensity, and duration, and the resulting alterations in cellular protein metabolism.

Unfortunately for the coach, only a few tests give accurate insight into the athlete's specific adaptations to training and have acceptable predictive value for performance. Future research should focus on the development of tests that meet these requirements. In addition, the results of present tests should be compared with actual performance throughout a whole season, in order to study the sensitivity and specificity of these tests. The ability to sustain submaximal power production during endurance events is generally evaluated by measuring the responses of plasma lactate concentration and ventilation to exercise. In spite of a large body of literature, the scientific basis of the application of lactate and ventilatory threshold values to sport performance is not well established. Research should be aimed at extending this foundation for application to various sports.

A great challenge is to develop non-invasive techniques that accurately reflect intramuscular metabolic changes during exercise. One of the techniques that has potential is magnetic resonance spectroscopy, but it is still not possible to use such a technique in a sport-specific way or to study different muscles simultaneously. Nevertheless, the combined use of measurements of anaerobic power plus magnetic resonance spectroscopy may eventually help characterize the anaerobic production of ATP during exercise.

SUMMARY

To facilitate the control of the training process and to be able to plan for peak performance, one needs information about the athlete's adaptation to training. Unfortunately, relatively little is known about the quantitative relationship between training characteristics and physiological adaptations to that training. It appears that the graphical relationship between training volume and performance development has an inverted U-shape. In other words, athletes should try to avoid both undertraining and overtraining.

Endurance capacity is often assessed by measuring maximal aerobic power ($\dot{V}O_2$max), which should be measured in a manner that is as specific to the sport activity as possible. An athlete's $\dot{V}O_2$max increases during the first weeks or months of the training program but fails to parallel changes in performance capacity when a well-trained state is achieved. However, power output or exercise intensity at $\dot{V}O_2$max assessed during an incremental exercise test is a valid indicator of endurance capacity and does parallel changes in performance.

For endurance activities that require a high fraction of $\dot{V}O_2$max, measurements of anaerobic threshold can be employed in a sport-specific manner. Although the scientific basis for applying threshold measurements to sport performance is inadequate, these measurements can yield information about training-induced changes in endurance capacity.

Time trials and simulated time trials are being used more frequently to evaluate sport-specific endurance capacity. The results of such trials parallel changes in specific endurance performance.

In many brief sport activities, anaerobic power is an important characteristic. Assessment of anaerobic power in a sport-specific way in the laboratory is difficult but should be included as a test of training adaptations in athletes who compete in explosive types of sports if the logistics of anaerobic power testing permit.

Strength measurements can yield information about the effects of strength training, but the tests often lack specificity for particular sports and should be interpreted with caution.

Testing of athletes should be conducted only when it gives information that is of practical use. In general, there is no reason to exceed a testing frequency of once per 3-4 wk.

BIBLIOGRAPHY

Abernethy, P., G. Wilson, and P. Logan (1995). Strength and power assessment. *Sports Med.* 19:401–417.

Acevedo, E.O., and A.H. Goldfarb (1989). Increased training intensity effects on plasma lactate, ventilatory threshold, and endurance. *Med. Sci. Sports Exerc.* 21:563–568.

Anderson, G.S., and E.C. Rhodes (1989). A review of blood lactate and ventilatory methods of detecting transition thresholds. *Sports Med.* 8:43–55.

Aunola, S., and H. Rusko (1992). Does anaerobic threshold correlate with maximal lactate steady-state? *J. Sports Sci.* 10:309-323.

Balmson, P. (1994). Evaluation of physical performance. In: B. Ekblom (ed.) *Football.* Oxford: Blackwell Scientific Publ., pp. 102–123.

Bangsbo, J., and F. Lindquist (1991). Comparison of various exercise tests with endurance performance during soccer in professional players. *Int. J. Sports Med.* 13:125–132.

Bangsbo, J., L. Michalsik, and A. Petersen (1993). Accumulated O_2 deficit during intense exercise and muscle characteristics of elite athletes. *Int. J. Sports Med.* 14: 207–213.

Banister, E.W. (1991). Modelling elite athletic performance. In: D. MacDougall, H. Wenger, and H. Green (eds.) *Physiological Testing of the High Performance Athlete.* Champaign, IL: Human Kinetics Publ., pp. 403–424.

Bar-Or, O. (1987). The Wingate anaerobic test, an update on methodology, reliability and validity. *Sports Med.* 4:381–394.

Barbeau, P., O. Serresse, and M.R. Boulay (1993). Using maximal and submaximal aerobic variables to monitor elite cyclists during a season. *Med. Sci. Sports Exerc.* 259:1062–1069.

Behm, D.G., and D.G. Sale (1993). Velocity specificity of resistance training. *Sports Med.* 15:374–388.

Beneke, R., N. Strauss, F. Hartwig, and C. Behn (1993). Die Blutlaktatkonzentration ist bei gegebener Belastungsintensität von der Sportart abhängig. In: Liesen, Weiss, and Baum (eds.) *Regulations- und Repairmechanismen.* Köln: Deutscher Ärtzte Verlag, pp. 170–172.

Beneke, R. (1995). Anaerobic threshold, individual anaerobic threshold, and maximal lactate steady state in rowing. *Med. Sci. Sports Exerc.* 27:863–867.

Beneke, R., and S. Petelin von Duvillard (1996). Determination of maximal lactate steady state response in selected sports events. *Med. Sci. Sports Exerc.* 28:241–246.

Berg, K., R. Olsen, M. McKinney, P. Hofschire, R. Latin, and W. Bell (1989). Effect of reduced training volume on cardiac function, $\dot{V}O_2$max, and running performance. *J. Sports Med. Phys. Fitness* 29:250–252.

Billat, V., J.C. Renoux, J. Pinoteau, B. Petit, and J.P. Koralstein (1994). Reproducibility of running time to exhaustion at $\dot{V}O_2$max in subelite runners. *Med. Sci. Sports Exerc.* 26:254–257.

Bilodeau, B., B. Roy, and M.R. Boulay (1995). Upper-body testing of cross-country skiers. *Med. Sci. Sports Exerc.* 27:1557–1562.

Bouchard, C., A.W. Taylor, and J.A.S. Dulac (1991). Testing anaerobic power capacity. In: D. MacDougall, H. Wenger, and H. Green (eds.) *Physiological Testing of the High Performance Athlete.* Champaign, IL: Human Kinetics Publ., pp. 175–221.

Bouckaert, J., J. Vrijens, and J.L. Pannier (1990). Effect of specific test procedures on plasma lactate concentration and peak oxygen uptake in endurance athletes. *J. Sports Med. Phys. Fit.* 30:13–18.

Brisswalter, J., and P. Legros (1994). Variability in energy cost of running during one training season in high level runners. *J. Sports Med. Phys. Fit.* 34:135–140.

Brooks, G.A. (1991). Current concepts in lactate exchange. *Med. Sci. Sports Exerc.* 23:895–906.

Bruin, G., H. Kuipers, H.A. Keizer, and G.J. VanderVusse (1994). Adaptation and overtraining in horses subjected to increased training loads. *J. Appl. Physiol.* 76: 1908-1913.

Bunc, V., and J. Heller (1991). Ventilatory threshold and work efficiency on a bicycle and paddling ergometer in top canoeists. *J. Sports Med. Phys. Fit.* 31:376–379.

Cheng, B., H. Kuipers, A.C. Snyder, H.A. Keizer, A. Jeukendrup, and M. Hesselink (1992). A new approach for the determination of ventilatory and lactate threshold. *Int. J. Sports Med.* 13:518-522.

Chin, M.K., A.S.K. Wong, R.C.H. So, O.T. Siu, K. Steininger, and D.T.I. Lo (1995). Sport specific fitness testing of elite badminton players. *Br. J. Sports Med.* 29:153–157.

Coen, B., L. Schwarz, A. Urhausen, and W. Kinderman (1991). Control of training in middle- and long-distance running by means of the individual anaerobic threshold. *Int. J. Sports Med.* 12:519-524.

Conconi F., F. Ferrari, P.G. Ziglo, P. Droghetti, and L. Codeca (1982). Determination of the anaerobic threshold by a noninvasive field test in runners. *J. Appl. Physiol.* 52:869-873.

Costill, D.L., H. Thomason, and E. Roberts (1973). Fractional utilization of the aerobic capacity during distance running. *Med. Sci. Sports Exerc.* 5:248-252.

Costill D.L., R. Thomas, R.A. Robergs, D.A. Pascoe, C. Lambert, and W.J. Fink (1991). Adaptations to swimming training: influence of training volume. *Med. Sci. Sports Exerc.* 23:371–377.

Coyle E.F., M.E. Feltner, S.A. Kautz, M.T. Hamilton, S.J. Montain, A.M. Baylor, L.D. Abraham, and G.W. Petrek (1991). Physiological and biomechanical factors associated with elite endurance cycling performance. *Med. Sci. Sports Exerc.* 23:93–107.

Craig, N.P., K.I. Norton, P.C. Bourdon, S.M. Woolford, T. Stanef, B. Squires, T.S. Olds, R.A.J. Conyers, and C.B.V. Walsh (1993). Aerobic and anaerobic indices contributing to track endurance cycling performance. *Eur. J. Appl. Physiol.* 67:150–158.

Crandell, C.G., S.L. Taylor, and P.B. Raven (1994). Evaluation of the Cosmed K2 portable telemetric oxygen uptake analyser. *Med. Sci. Sports Exerc.* 26:108-111.

Dal Monte, A., M. Faina, and C. Menchinelli (1992). Sport specific ergometric equipment. In: R. J. Shephard & P.O. Åstrand (eds.) *Endurance in Sport.* London: Blackwell Scientific Publ., pp. 201–207.

Daniels, P.J., and C. Foster (1995). Practical considerations for fitness field-testing of athletes. In: Maud & Foster (eds). *Physiological Assessment of Human Fitness.* Champaign, IL: Human Kinetics Publ., pp. 245–256.

Droghetti, P., C. Borsetto, I. Casoni, M. Cellini, M. Ferrari, A.R. Paolini, P.G. Ziglio, and F. Conconi (1985). Noninvasive determination of the anaerobic threshold in canoeing, cross-country skiing, cycling, roller and ice-skating, rowing, and walking. *Eur. J. Appl. Physiol.* 53:299-303.

Flore, P., A. Therminarias, M.F. Oddou-Chirpaz, and A. Quirion (1992). Influence of moderate cold exposure on blood lactate during incremental exercise. *Eur. J. Appl. Physiol.* 64:213–217.

Flynn, M.G., F.X. Pizza, J.B. Boone, F.F. Andres, T.A. Michaud, and J.R. Rodriguez-Zayas (1994). Indices of training stress during competitive running and swimming season. *Int. J. Sports Med.* 15:21–26.

Foster, C., A.C. Snyder, N.N. Thompson, and K. Kuettel (1988). Normalization of the blood lactate profile. *Int. J. Sports Med.* 9:198-200.

Foster C., M.A. Green, A.C. Snyder, and N.N. Thompson (1993). Physiological responses during simulated competition. *Med. Sci. Sports Exerc.* 25:877–882.

Francis, K.T., P.R. McClatchey, J.R. Sumsion, and D.E. Hansen (1989). The relationship between anaerobic threshold and heart rate linearity during cycle ergometry. *Eur. J. Appl. Physiol.* 59:273–277.

Fry R.W., A.W. Morton, and D. Keast (1991). Overtraining in athletes: an update. *Sports Med.* 63:228-234.

Fry R.W., A.W. Morton, P. Garcia-Webb, G.P.M. Crawford, and D. Keast (1992). Biological responses to overload training in endurance sports. *Eur. J. Appl. Physiol.* 64:335–344.

Gilman, M.B., and C.L. Wells (1993). The use of heart rates to monitor exercise intensity in relation to metabolic variables. *Int. J. Sports Med.* 14:339-344.

Gilman, M.B.(1996). The use of heart rate to monitor the intensity of endurance training. *Sports Med.* 21:73–79.

Gleeson, N.P., and T.H. Mercer (1996). The utility of isokinetic dynamometry in the assessment of human muscle function. *Sports Med.* 21:18-34.

Green, S., and B. Dawson (1993). Measurement of anaerobic capacities in humans. *Sports Med.* 15:312–327.

Green, S., and B.T. Dawson (1996). The Y-intercept of the maximal work-duration regression and field tests of anaerobic capacity in cyclists. *Int. J. Sports Med.* 17:41–47.

Green, S., B.T. Dawson, C. Goodman, and M.F. Carey (1996). Anaerobic ATP production and accumulated O_2 deficit in cyclists. *Med. Sci Sports Exerc.* 28:315–321.

Gugliemo A., and P.E. Di Prampero (1995). The concept of lactate threshold. *J. Sports Med. Phys. Fit.* 35:6–12.

Häkkinen, K. (1993a). Changes in physical fitness profile in female volleyball players during the competitive season. *J. Sports Med.* 33:223–232.

Häkkinen, K. (1993b). Changes in physical fitness profile in female basketball players during the competitive season including explosive type strength training. *J. Sports Med.* 33:19-26.

Hickey, M.S., D.L. Costill, G.K. McConell, J.J. Widrick, and H. Tanaka (1992). Day to day variation in time trial cycling performance. *Int. J. Sports Med.* 13:467–470.

Hill, D.W., and A.L. Rowell (1996). Running velocity at $\dot{V}O_2$max. *Med. Sci. Sports Exerc.* 28:114–119.

Hoffman, M.D., and G.M. Street (1992). Characterization of the heart rate response during biathlon. *Int. J. Sports Med.* 13:390–394.

Hooper, S.L., L.T. Mackinnon, A.Howard, R.D. Gordon, and A.W. Bachmann (1995). Markers for monitoring overtraining and recovery. *Med. Sci. Sports Exerc.* 27:106–112.

Houmard, J.A., M.W. Craib, K.F. O'Brian, L.L. Smith, R.G. Israel, and W.S. Wheeler (1991). Peak running velocity, submaximal energy expenditure, $\dot{V}O_2$max, and 8-km distance running performance. *J. Sports Med. Phys. Fit.* 31:345–351.

James, N.W., G.M. Adams, and A.F. Wilson (1989). Determination of anaerobic threshold by ventilatory frequency. *Int. J. Sports Med.* 10:192–196.

Jenkins, D.G., and B.M. Quigley (1990). Blood lactate in trained cyclists during cycle ergometry at critical power. *Eur. J. Appl. Physiol.* 61:278-283.

Jeukendrup, A.E., M.K.C. Hesselink, A.C. Snyder, H. Kuipers, and H.A. Keizer (1992). Physiological changes in male competitive cyclists after two weeks of intensified training. *Int. J. Sports Med.* 13:534–541.

Jeukendrup, A.E., and M.K.C. Hesselink (1994). Overtraining, what do lactate curves tell us? *Br. J. Sports Med.* 28:239-240.

Jeukendrup A.E., W.H.M. Saris, F. Brouns, and A.D.M. Kester (1996). A new validated endurance performance test. *Med. Sci. Sport Exerc.* 28:266–270.

Jones, A.M., and J.H. Doust (1995). Lack of reliability in Conconi's heart rate deflection point. *Int. J. Sports Med.* 16:541–544.

Kraemer, W.J., and A.C. Fry (1995). Strength testing: development and evaluation of methodology. In: Maud & Foster (eds). *Physiological Assessment of Human Fitness.* Champaign, IL: Human Kinetics Publ., pp. 115–138.

Kuipers, H., F. Verstappen, H. Keizer, P. Geurten, and G. van Kranenburg (1985). Variability of aerobic performance in the laboratory and its physiological correlates. *Int. J. Sports Med.* 6:197–201.

Kuipers, H., H.A. Keizer, J. de Vries, P. van Rijthoven, and M. Wijts (1988). Comparison of heart rate as a non-invasive determinant of anaerobic threshold with the lactate threshold when cycling. *Eur. J. Appl. Physiol.* 58:303–306.

Kuipers, H., and H.A. Keizer (1988). Overtraining in elite athletes; directions for the future. *Sports Med.* 6:79-92.

Leger, L., and M. Thivierge (1988). Heart-rate monitors; validity, stability and functionality. *Physician Sports Med.* 16:143–151.

Lehmann, M., U. Gastmann, K.G. Petersen, N. Bachl, A. Seidel, A.N. Khalaf, S. Fischer, and J. Keul (1992). Training-overtraining: influence of a defined increase in training volume versus training intensity on performance, catecholamines and some metabolic parameters in experienced middle- and long-distance runners. *Eur. J. Appl. Physiol.* 64:169-177.

Lehmann, M., C. Foster, and J. Keul (1993). Overtraining in endurance athletes: a brief review. *Med. Sci. Sports Exerc.* 25:854–862.

Loat, C.E.R., and E.C. Rhodes (1993). Relationship between the lactate and ventilatory thresholds during prolonged exercise. *Sports Med.* 15:104–115.

Loftin, M., and B. Warren (1994). Comparison of a simulated 16.1 km time trial, VO₂max, and related factors in cyclists with different ventilatory thresholds. *Int. J. Sports Med.* 15:498-503.

Lucia, A., S.J. Fleck, R.W. Gotshall, and J.T. Kearney (1993). Validity and reliability of the Cosmed K2 instrument. *Int. J. Sports Med.* 14:380–386.

Macfarlane, D.J., B.A. Fogarty, and W.G. Hopkins (1989). The accuracy and variablity of commercially available heart-rate monitors. *NZJ Sports Med.* 17:51–53.

Mader, A. (1991). Evaluation of the endurance performance of marathon runners and theoretical analysis of test results. *J. Sports Med. Phys. Fit.* 31:1–19.

Maffulli, N., G. Capasso, and A. Lancia (1991). Anaerobic threshold and performance in middle- and long-distance runners. *J. Sports Med. Phys. Fit.* 31:332–338.

Medbo, J.I., A. Mohn, I. Tabata, R. Bahr, and O. Sejersted (1988). Anaerobic capacity determined by the maximal accumulated oxygen deficit. *J. Appl. Physiol.* 64:50–60.

Mittelstadt, S.W., M.D. Hoffman, P.B. Watts, K.P. O'Hagan, J.E. Sulentic, K.M. Drobish, T.P. Gibbons, V.S. Newbury, and P.S. Clifford (1995). Lactate response to uphill roller skiing: diagonal stride versus double pole techniques. *Med. Sci. Sports Exerc.* 27:1563–1568.

Morgan, D.W., F.D. Baldini, P.E. Martin, and W.M. Kohrt (1989). Ten kilometer performance and predicted velocity at V'O₂max among well-trained male runners. *Med. Sci. Sports Exerc.* 21:78-83.

Morgan, D.W., and J.T. Daniels (1994). Relationship between V'O₂max and the aerobic demand of running in elite distance runners. *Int. J. Sports Med.* 15:426–429.

Morton, R.H., J.R. Fitz-Clarke, and E.W. Bannister (1990). Modelling human performance in running. *J. Appl. Physiol.* 69:1171–1177.

Neuman, G.(1992). Cycling. In: R.J. Shephard & P.O. Åstrand (eds.) *Endurance in Sport.* London: Blackwell, pp. 582–596.

Noakes, T.D., K.H. Myrburgh, and R. Schall (1990). Peak treadmill running velocity during the V'O₂max test predicts running performance. *J. Sports Sci.* 8:35–45

Noakes, T.D.(1991). *Lore of Running.* Champaign, IL: Human Kinetics Publ., pp. 263–361.

O'Toole, M.L. (1989). Training for ultraendurance triathlons. *Med. Sci. Sports Exerc.* 21(5) supplement S209-S213.

Peronnet, F., G. Thibault, E.C. Rhodes, and D.C. Mckenzie (1987). Correlation between ventilatory threshold and endurance capacity in marathon runners. *Med. Sci. Sports Exerc.* 19:610–615.

Prusaczyk, W.K., K.J. Cureton, R.E. Graham, and C.A. Ray (1992). Differential effects of dietary carbohydrate on RPE at the lactate and ventilatory thresholds. *Med. Sci. Sports Exerc.* 24:568-575.

Ribeiro, J.P., E. Cadavid, J. Baena, E. Monsalvete, and A. Barna (1990). Metabolic predictors of middle-distance swimming performance. *Br. J. Sports Med.* 24:196–200.

Rundell, K.W. (1995). Treadmill roller ski test predicts biathlon roller ski race results of elite US biathlon women. *Med. Sci. Sports Exerc.* 27:1677–1685.

Sale, D.G. (1991). Testing strength and power. In: D. MacDougall, H. Wenger, and H. Green (eds.) *Physiological Testing of the High Performance Athlete*. Champaign, IL: Human Kinetics Publ., pp. 21–106.

Schneider, D.A., and J. Pollack (1991). Ventilatory threshold and maximal oxygen uptake during cycling and running in female triathletes. *Int. J. Sports Med.* 12:379-383.

Scott, B.K., and J.A. Houmard (1994). Peak running velocity is highly related to distance running performance. *Int. J. Sports Med.* 15:504–507.

Shephard, R.J., E. Bouhlel, H. Vandewalle, and H. Monod (1989). Anaerobic threshold, muscle volume and hypoxia. *Eur. J. Appl. Physiol.* 58:826–832.

Shephard, R.J. (1992). Muscular endurance and blood lactate. In: R.J. Shephard & P.O. Åstrand (eds.) *Endurance in Sport*. London: Blackwell, pp.215–225.

Snyder, A.C., K.P. O'Hagan, P.S. Clifford, M.D. Hoffman, and C. Foster (1993). Exercise responses to in-line skating: comparison to running and cycling. *Int. J. Sports Med.* 14: 38-42.

Snyder A.C., and C. Foster (1994). Physiology and nutrition for skating. In: D.R. Lamb, H.G. Knuttgen, and R. Murray (eds.) *Perspectives in Exercise Science and Sports Medicine. Vol. 7: Physiology and Nutrition for Competitive Sport*. Carmel, IN:, Cooper Publishing Group, pp. 181–219.

Steininger, K., and R.E. Wodick (1987). Sports-specific fitness testing in squash. *Br. J. Sports Med.* 21:23–26.

Swaine, I.L., and C.L. Zanker (1996). The reproducibility of cardiopulmonary responses to exercise using a swim bench. *Int. J. Sports Med.* 17:140–144.

Thorland, W., D.A. Podolin, and R.S. Mazzeo (1994). Coincidence of lactate and HR-power output threshold under varied nutritional states. *Int. J. Sports Med.* 15:301–304.

Urhausen, A., B. Weiler, and W. Kinderman (1993). Heart rate, blood lactate, and catecholamines during ergometer and water rowing. *Int. J. Sports Med.* 14:20–23.

Vermulst, L.J.M., C. Vervoorn, A.M. Boelens-Quist, H.P.F. Koppeschaar, and W.B.M. Erich (1991). Analysis of seasonal training volume and working capacity in elite female rowers. *Int. J. Sports Med.* 12:567–572.

Viru, A.(1994). Molecular cellular mechanisms of training effects. *J. Sports Med. Phys. Fit.* 34:309-314.

Wakayoshi, K., T. Yoshida, Y. Ikuta, Y. Mutoh, and M. Miyashita (1993). Adaptations to six months of aerobic swim training. *Int. J. Sports Med.* 14:368-372.

Wakayoshi, K., T. Yoshida, M. Udo, T. Kasai, T. Moritani, Y. Mutoh, and M. Miyashita (1992). A simple method for determining critical speed as swimming fatigue threshold in competitive swimming. *Int. J. Sports Med.* 13:367–371.

Ward-Smith, A.J., and A.C. Mobey (1995). Determination of physiological data from a mathematical analysis of the running performance of elite female athletes. *J. Sport Sci.* 13:321–328.

Warren, B.J., M.H. Stone, J.T. Kearney, S.J. Fleck, R.J. Johnson, G.D. Wilson, and W.J. Kraemer (1992). Performance measures, blood lactate and plasma ammonia as indicators of overwork in elite junior weightlifters. *Int. J. Sports Med.* 13:372–376.

Weltman, A. (1995). *The blood lactate response to exercise*. Champaign, IL: Human Kinetics Publ.

Wilmore, J.H., and D.L. Costill (1994). *Physiology of Sport and Exercise*. Champaign, IL: Human Kinetics Publ., pp. 156–158.

Winter, E.M. (1991). Cycle ergometry and maximal intensity exercise. *Sports Med.* 11:351–357.

Withers, R.T., W.M. Sherman, J.M. Miller, and D.L. Costill (1981). Specificity of the anaerobic threshold in endurance trained cyclists and runners. *Eur. J. Appl. Phyiol.* 47:93–104.

Young, W., B. Mclean, and J. Ardagna (1995). Relationship between strength qualities and sprinting performance. *J. Sports Med. Phys. Fit.* 35:13–19.

DISCUSSION

NADEL: I support the conclusion that maximal mechanical power output is a better predictor of endurance capacity and/or performance than is $\dot{V}O_2$max, while recognizing that $\dot{V}O_2$max is an outstanding predictor of performance across the spectrum of $\dot{V}O_2$max from 20 to 80 mL·min^{-1}·kg^{-1}. Maximal mechanical power output is a better predictor because it distinguishes among select populations of athletes who possess different degrees of mechanical efficiency, or what has been called biological economy. When evaluating the linear relationship between $\dot{V}O_2$ and mechanical power output, people who have the same values for $\dot{V}O_2$max can have different slopes describing the relationship between $\dot{V}O_2$ and power output (i.e., those with a steeper slope are less efficient than people with a less steep slope). The textbooks state that the average efficiency across the population is about 24%, indicating that about 24% of the potential energy mobilized can be converted into mechanical work, with the remaining 76% converted to heat, but the range among the population may be rather large—from 20–28% or even greater. Thus, in a group of athletes with identical scores for $\dot{V}O_2$max, those who are less efficient require a higher $\dot{V}O_2$ to produce a given mechanical power output than those with a high efficiency. This might relate to performance, explaining why athletes with identical aerobic capacities do not perform identically.

KUIPERS: You are correct that differences in mechanical efficiency or economy may explain differences in performances by athletes who have similar values for $\dot{V}O_2$max. Let me make one thing clear; a high $\dot{V}O_2$max is an absolute requirement to have high power output, but once an athlete has attained a high level of aerobic fitness through training, $\dot{V}O_2$max is very stable and does not change along with changes in actual performance.

BAR-OR: I, too, am glad you have indicated the importance and the utility of peak mechanical power as an index of performance. We have found it to be useful when testing athletes at the Wingate Institute and more recently with patients in Canada. Obviously, it is much less complex than a test that requires repeated gas collections. A further improvement might be to ask the athlete to perform two different power tests and to report to the coach the results of each test and the relationship between the scores of the two tests. For example, in sports such as rowing, wrestling, and swimming that require good performance both in the upper and lower limbs, the athlete would perform a peak mechanical power test with the arms and, using the same ergometer, a similar test with the legs. This would provide a composite index of power output to the coach whereby the coach could determine if training adaptations were relatively more effective in the arms or legs. Such a mapping of performance could give the coach practical ideas on how to modify the training regimen. Along the same line, for athletes who need both aerobic and anaerobic performance (e.g., rowers and middle-distance runners) one could test peak mechanical power with both aerobic and anaerobic testing and relate the scores to each other, perhaps as a ratio. We have used this approach in research (Blimkie et al., *Europ. J. Appl. Physiol.* 57:677–683, 1988) and in counseling. Some authors used the same approach with athletes of different specialties and found that this ratio could discriminate among people of various specialties.

KUIPERS: I did not find good references related to this issue, but it would be important to establish the validity and practical value of such tests. It is important, for instance, to know if a change in results of one of the test components really means that the athlete should train differently.

KNUTTGEN: It is too bad that there is such a great emphasis in the literature on tests of aerobic conditioning and relatively little attention given to testing anaerobic power, strength, and speed, whereas most Olympic events depend more on coordination and skill, anaerobic power, strength, speed, and factors other than aerobic power. I am thinking of Olympic events such as fencing, gymnastics, baseball, volleyball, all of the field and sprint events in track and field, sailing, diving, synchronized swimming, archery, riflery, and equestrian events, all of which have only modest aerobic demands. Likewise, I am amazed that researchers have so often assessed the strength of various athletes with isometric tests when the performance of the sports of these same athletes involves almost exclusively dynamic muscle actions, both concentric and eccentric.

Also, peak oxygen uptake occurs over a fairly wide range of external power outputs for the particular activity being employed in the testing and not at a single value of power production. How does this phenomenon relate to your use of the term, "maximal power"? Finally, it seems to me that the Wingate test is completely unlike any competitive sport and therefore is unlikely to be a valid test of performance for any sport.

KUIPERS: I completely agree with you that isometric strength is not a useful marker of performance in most sport activities. Even isokinetic test results have poor validity for predicting sport performance. It is also correct that a wide range of power outputs can be obtained at peak $\dot{V}O_2$. Those investigators who advocate the use of peak power output or the maximal exercise intensity or running speed used incremental exercise tests in which peak power output was defined as the final power output achieved by the subject at exhaustion. With a different type of test, the relationship between power output and oxygen uptake may be different. Finally, perhaps Oded Bar-Or will comment on your point about the validity of the Wingate test for predicting performance.

BAR-OR: The validation studies that were included in my 1987 review of the Wingate test were somewhat naive. For example, relating ice hockey performance to performance in the Wingate test is a much too ambitious approach because performance on the ice depends markedly on skill and not exclusively on anaerobic muscle performance or, for that matter, on any other single physiological indicator of fitness. In contrast, for elite cyclists, performance in a modified Wingate test proved highly predictive of their road cycling success.

Not only is it inadvisable to use anaerobic performance as a predictor of athletic success in a task that has a high skill component, it should also not be used a single predictor of success in performing athletic tasks (e.g., running 800 m) that depend greatly on other fitness components (e.g., aerobic performance). That is exactly why I suggest that a testing battery include several physiological functions and that a profile of scores on these items be presented to the coach.

MURRAY: What is the practical value of using heart-rate monitors, particularly considering that heart rate is influenced by such a wide variety of factors? Day-to-day variations and differences in environmental conditions, hydration status, exercise intensity, and fitness levels can all result in widely different heart-rate responses to the same task. Are these devices of any practical relevance?

KUIPERS: I completely agree that the value of heart-rate monitors in sport events is probably overestimated. There is a need to evaluate the use of heart-rate monitors in various sports.

SPRIET: I believe that a test of anaerobic capacity is probably more fruitful than one of anaerobic power for evaluating an athlete's capability to produce energy anaerobically, and the maximal accumulated oxygen deficit is currently the best available estimate of this capability. The best experiments reported that attempt to validate the use of the oxygen deficit for estimating anaerobic capacity and actual anaerobic energy production were the early studies by Jens Bangsbo that were published around 1990. Those were not executed in a whole-body model, which I believe is an inappropriate model for this purpose, but in the isolated quadriceps muscles during leg extension.

MAUGHAN: If we look at the history of track and field, for about 80 y it was common practice for people to perform time trials on a regular basis in preparation for competition and to fix their training loads based on the time trial results. This practice seemed to die out in the late 1950s, not long after the first 4-min mile was run. Why have people stopped this practice when it seems to be the best indicator of performance?

KUIPERS: I think this change can be attributed to the advent of laboratory testing. When I was skating in the late 60s and early 70s, the use of laboratory-based tests became well known, and it was often assumed that these laboratory tests were the ultimate for guiding training; thus, time trials dropped out of favor. We are now back at the beginning, and we realize again that time trials are a valuable way to evaluate performance capacity in the most specific way. I'm very confident that in a couple of years, time trials will again become an important component of the training process.

SHI: Can we use the maximal lactate steady state to predict overtraining?

KUIPERS: We can use it to diagnose overtraining, but not to predict it. When the maximal power output is decreased, the subject is suffering from all the symptoms of overtraining, and when the plasma lactate curve is also shifted to the right it will support the diagnosis of overtraining. But we cannot predict it from plasma lactates. For example, we did an overtraining study in cyclists, and we saw some changes in lactate in subjects who were fatigued but not yet overtrained. The shift in the lactate curve does occur with overtraining, but also with fatigue and carbohydrate depletion.

ARAGON-VARGAS: Competition is what tells you whether things are working or not during training, and it is the best test available. What options or substitutes do we have in evaluating training? Well, we can use short time trials, since we don't want to evaluate a distance runner with a marathon every month. But are the other physiological tests you mentioned useful enough so that after seeing the results the coach can say, "This is the particular part of my training program that I need to adjust for my athlete?"

KUIPERS: I think that plasma lactates can be helpful, but the bottom line is that when an athlete is competing, a test probably will only confirm that he is performing well or not. Some of the physiological tests can be helpful, perhaps in part by providing data that can motivate the athletes to work on certain aspects of performance. The mental aspect is very important in training. Competing and training at a high level for many months and years takes a lot of motivation, a lot of mental strength. Every factor that can increase motivation, including physiological testing, should be used. In the beginning of the season these tests can be helpful to give us a physiological profile of an athlete and an indication of what weaknesses should be addressed. The tests should be repeated later in the season only if a training problem develops with the athlete. We would hope that we could identify what is wrong and advise the coach appropriately. Unfortunately, the importance of tests is often overestimated in sports practice. Coaches too often think that the numbers we produce tell them exactly what should be altered during training and how the athlete is progressing. This is, of course, usually an invalid assumption.

3

Fuels for Sport Performance

Edward F. Coyle, Ph.D.

INTRODUCTION
BODY FAT STORES
BODY CARBOHYDRATE STORES
SUBSTRATE USE DURING EXERCISE OF VARIOUS INTENSITIES
    Low-Intensity Exercise
    Moderate-Intensity Exercise
    High-Intensity Exercise
    Fatty Acid Availability and Exercise Intensity
    Carbohydrate is Essential Because of Muscle's Limited Ability to Oxidize Fat
FAT SUPPLEMENTATION DURING EXERCISE
    Ingestion of Triglycerides
    Intravenous Infusions That Raise Plasma FFA
    Ingestion of Medium Chain Triglycerides
DIETS HIGH IN FAT AND LOW IN CARBOHYDRATE
ENDURANCE TRAINING INCREASES FAT OXIDATION DURING EXERCISE
    Source of the Increase in Fat Oxidation
    Plasma Free Fatty Acid Mobilization and Endurance Training
DIETARY CARBOHYDRATE INFLUENCES FAT OXIDATION DURING EXERCISE
CARBOHYDRATE FEEDING DURING EXERCISE
    Prolonged Moderate-Intensity Exercise
    Type of Carbohydrate Ingested During Exercise
    Timing of Carbohydrate Ingestion During Exercise
    Rate of Carbohydrate Ingestion During Exercise
    Carbohydrate Ingestion During Sport, Recreation, and Intermittent Exercise
METABOLIC RESPONSES TO VARIOUS TYPES OF DIETARY CARBOHYDRATE
MUSCLE GLYCOGEN RESYNTHESIS FOLLOWING EXERCISE
    Rate of Carbohydrate Ingestion
    Carbohydrate Type
    Timing of Carbohydrate Ingestion After Exercise
    Influence of Dietary Fat and Protein on Glycogen Resynthesis
    Practical Considerations and Specific Recommendations
MAXIMIZING MUSCLE GLYCOGEN PRIOR TO COMPETITION
PREEXERCISE NUTRITION
    Carbohydrate Feedings During the Hour Before Exercise

Carbohydrate Ingestion During the 6-h Period Before Exercise
Types of Carbohydrate to Ingest During the 6-h Period Before Exercise
PRACTICAL APPLICATIONS FOR ACTIVE PEOPLE
DIRECTIONS FOR FUTURE RESEARCH
SUMMARY
BIBLIOGRAPHY

INTRODUCTION

This review will describe the extent to which fat and carbohydrate are used for energy during exercise of varying intensity, with a practical emphasis on ingesting fuels to maximize sport performance. Recent findings regarding limitations in the mobilization and oxidation of free fatty acids (FFA) will be presented, findings that further underscore the importance of carbohydrate for energy. The conditions that benefit from exogenous carbohydrate supplementation, the timing of supplementation, and the amount and type of carbohydrate that is most effective will be discussed. The practical recommendations presented will be most applicable to people who exercise intensely or for prolonged periods (i.e., 1 h or more).

Fat and carbohydrate are the fuels predominantly used during steady-state aerobic exercise; protein oxidization does not contribute significantly to energy production (Romijn & Wolfe, 1992). Carbohydrate is also consumed during the anaerobic metabolism required to sustain exercise performed at intensities above maximal oxygen uptake ($\dot{V}O_2$max). The four primary sources of energy for exercise are fat and carbohydrate, supplied from both within the muscle fiber and from the blood (Romijn et al., 1993). Carbohydrate is available within the muscle fiber in the form of muscle glycogen, whereas glucose is supplied from the blood. Fat is available from triglyceride droplets within the muscle fiber (i.e., intramuscular triglyceride) as well as from plasma free fatty acids (FFA) (Martin et al., 1993; Romijn et al., 1993). FFA cannot be oxidized at high enough rates to provide all the energy required by moderate-to-high intensity exercise (i.e., 60–90% $\dot{V}O_2$max). Consequently, carbohydrate oxidation must provide the energy that can not be produced by FFA oxidation (Coggan & Coyle, 1991; Coyle et al., 1986). Not surprisingly, fatigue occurs when muscle glycogen and blood glucose stores become depleted (Coggan & Coyle, 1991). This fundamental understanding provides the rationale for ingesting dietary carbohydrate before, during, and after exercise. Although fat cannot replace carbohydrate as the predominant fuel for intense exercise, an increase in FFA oxidation will slow the reduction in endogenous carbohydrate stores during prolonged exercise at moderate intensities (60–80% $\dot{V}O_2$max) (Costill et al., 1977).

BODY FAT STORES

Triglycerides stored within adipocytes throughout the body represent approximately 50,000–100,000 kcal of energy in men and women who possess 10–30% body fat. That is ample energy to walk or jog 500 to 1000 mi, assuring an energy expenditure of 100 kcal/mi. Triglycerides stored in adipocytes are hydrolyzed (via lipolysis) into glycerol and free fatty acids. FFAs are hydrophilic molecules and must be bound to the protein albumin for transport in the blood to exercising muscles (Bulow & Madsen, 1981; Figure 3-1). The mobilization of fatty acids from adipose issue and their subsequent oxidation by muscle during exercise are limited by several factors that will be discussed in detail later in this chapter.

Approximately 2,000–3,000 kcal of energy in the form of triglycerides are stored within muscle cells and represent an important addition source of FFA. However, relatively little is known about the rates at which intramuscular triglyceride can be oxidized during exercise or how it responds to acute and chronic training (Oscai et al., 1990), primarily because it is difficult to measure intramuscular triglyceride from muscle biopsy samples. Although the rate that intramuscular triglyc-

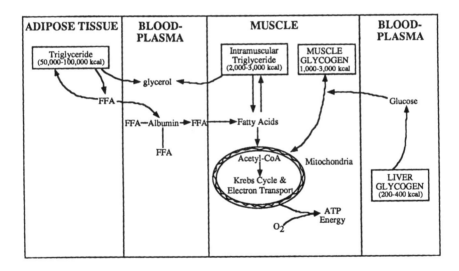

FIGURE 3-1. *Schematic of the storage and mobilization of the body's stored triglyceride (i.e., fat) and glycogen.* Adipose tissue triglyceride can be hydrolyzed to free fatty acids (FFA) and mobilized by binding to plasma albumin and thus transported through blood to skeletal muscle. Intramuscular triglyceride can also be hydrolyzed to fatty acids, which enter the mitochondria for oxidation during exercise. Glycogen in the liver can be hydrolyzed to glucose and delivered to muscle via the blood.

eride can provide energy during exercise is less than one-third the rate of energy production from muscle glycogen (Romijn et al., 1993), intramuscular triglyceride is now acknowledged as a supplementary source of energy. Another source of fat energy available to muscle is plasma triglycerides. In the fasted state, a small amount of triglyceride that is produced by the liver is bound to very-low-density lipoproteins in plasma. Although muscle may be capable of hydrolyzing this triglyceride to some extent during exercise, its contribution to energy production appears very small (Kiens et al., 1993).

Therefore, the two primary sources of FFA for oxidation by muscle during exercise are the adipocyte-derived FFAs found in plasma and the FFAs provided by intramuscular triglycerides. Despite the large amount of potential energy in adipocytes and muscle, the rate at which FFAs can be oxidized is substantially less than that for carbohydrate. However, endurance training markedly increases the contribution of FFA to energy production; this is particularly true of the rate at which intramuscular triglyceride can be oxidized (Martin et al., 1993). An increase in the contribution of FFAs to energy production during exercise at a given intensity results in a slower rate of muscle glycogen degradation. However, training also increases an individual's ability to exercise more intensely (Holloszy & Coyle, 1984), maintaining the reliance on carbohydrate as the primary fuel source during moderate-to-intense exercise.

BODY CARBOHYDRATE STORES

Carbohydrate is stored as glycogen, both within muscle and the liver (Bergstrom, 1966). Depending on diet and activity pattern, approximately 10–30 g of glycogen are stored in each kg of skeletal muscle; thus roughly 1,000–3,000 kcal of glycogen are stored in muscle throughout the body. However, the amount of muscle glycogen available to power exercise will depend upon the amount of muscle mass activated when performing an activity. Additionally, about 80 g (320 kcal) of glycogen are stored in the liver (Figure 3-1). Liver glycogen can be hydrolyzed back to glucose and transported via the blood to the muscles for oxidation. Because a high rate of carbohydrate oxidation is needed to maintain strenuous exercise for prolonged periods, active people can become undernourished in carbohydrate and thus experience muscle fatigue while exercising.

SUBSTRATE USE DURING EXERCISE
OF VARIOUS INTENSITIES

Results of studies employing stable isotope infusion to quantify the contribution of the four major substrates (i.e., blood glucose, muscle glycogen, plasma FFA, muscle triglycerides) to total energy expenditure during exercise over a range of intensities are shown in Figure 3-2 (Romijn et al., 1993). These measures represent values after 30 min of exercise in the fasted state in endurance-trained people. Exercise duration, diet, and fitness level will modify the responses outlined below.

Low-Intensity Exercise

During exercise at 25% $\dot{V}O_2$max, an exercise intensity comparable to walking, muscle derives almost all of its needed energy from plasma FFA, with a small contribution from blood glucose. During this low-intensity exercise, the rate of FFA appearance in plasma (i.e., Ra plasma FFA) is very similar to the rate of FFA oxidation (i.e., 26 μmol·kg^{-1}·min^{-1}) in endurance-trained people. This pattern of energy provision does not change over the course of 2 h of exercise, or perhaps longer, as the majority of the energy requirements at this intensity can be met by mobilization of FFA from the large triglyceride stores in adipocytes throughout the body.

Moderate-Intensity Exercise

As exercise intensity is increased from 25% to 65% and then to 85% $\dot{V}O_2$max, the Ra for plasma FFA declines progressively, and as a result, the concentration of FFA in blood is proportionally reduced (as shown in Figure 3-3). Although the Ra for FFA was reduced as intensity increased from 25% to 65% $\dot{V}O_2$max, it is possible that it might be higher during

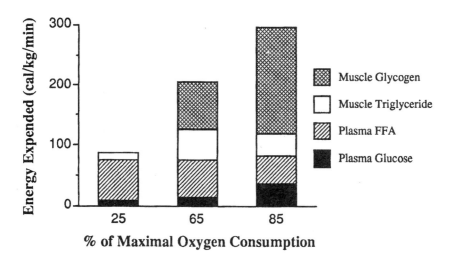

FIGURE 3-2. *Contribution of the four major substrates to energy expenditure after 30 min of exercise at 25%, 65%, and 85% of maximal oxygen uptake when fasted.* Reproduced with permission from Romijn et al. (1993).

exercise at an intermediate intensity (e.g., 45% $\dot{V}O_2$max). This reduced plasma FFA mobilization occurs despite a continued high rate of lipolysis of triglyceride in adipocytes as well as in intramuscular triglyceride droplets, as determined from direct measures of the rate of glycerol appearance (Ra glycerol), an index of lipolysis (Romijn et al., 1993). It seems that the Ra for plasma FFA declines with increasing intensity of exercise due to insufficient blood flow and albumin delivery to carry FFA from adipose tissue and into the systemic circulation (Bulow & Madsen, 1981; Hodgetts et al., 1991). Therefore, it appears that FFAs become trapped in adipose tissue as exercise intensity is increased. This is supported by the observation that cessation of exercise at 65% and 85% results in a large increase in the Ra for plasma FFA as well as in plasma FFA concentration without a concomitant increase in the Ra for glycerol (i.e., lipolysis) (Romijn et al., 1993). Whatever the mechanism, the fact remains that the availability of plasma FFA for oxidation by muscle declines as the intensity of exercise is increased (Figures 3-2 and 3-3).

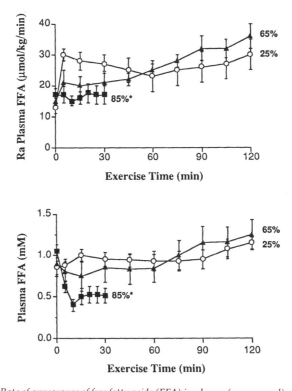

FIGURE 3-3. *Rate of appearance of free fatty acids (FFA) in plasma (upper panel) and plasma FFA concentrations (lower panel) during exercise at 25%, 65%, and 85% $\dot{V}O_2$max.*
* Values during exercise at 85% $\dot{V}O_2$max are significantly lower compared to 25% and 65% $\dot{V}O_2$max (P<0.05). Redrawn with permission from Romijn et al. (1993).

At moderate-exercise intensities (i.e., 65% $\dot{V}O_2$max), comparable to the pace for running or cycling 2–4 h, total fat oxidation increases (compared to exercise at 25% $\dot{V}O_2$max), despite the reduction in the Ra for FFA. This substantially higher rate of total fat oxidation reflects an increased oxidation of intramuscular triglycerides, as shown in Figure 3-2 and emphasized in Figure 3-4 (Romijn et al., 1993). For example, during moderate-intensity exercise, endurance-trained people can oxidize fat at high rates (i.e., >40 μmol/kg/min), with plasma FFA and intramuscular triglyceride contributing equally to fat oxidation (Figure 3-4) (Hurley et al., 1986; Martin et al., 1993). However, even this high rate of fat oxidation cannot provide all of the energy required during moderate-intensity exercise (i.e., 60–75% $\dot{V}O_2$max). About one-half of the total energy must be derived from carbohydrate oxidation (i.e., muscle glycogen and blood glucose) (Figure 3-2). In summary, during moderate-intensity exercise, all four major substrates (i.e., blood glucose, muscle glycogen, plasma FFA, muscle triglycerides) contribute to energy production.

High-Intensity Exercise

High-intensity exercise (i.e., 85% $\dot{V}O_2$max) promotes relatively high rates of muscle glycogen breakdown and thus carbohydrate oxidation (Figure 3-2), with one of the by-products being an accelerated rate of

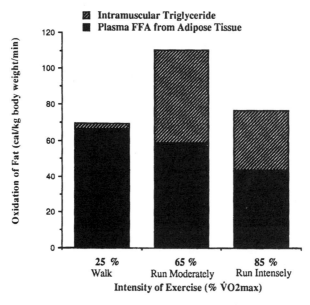

FIGURE 3-4. *Expanded view of the sources of fat for oxidation during exercise at 25% (walking pace), 65% (moderate running or cycling), and 85% (intense running or cycling) $\dot{V}O_2$max when fasted.* Redrawn with permission from Romijn et al. (1993).

production of lactic-acid, which accumulates in muscle and blood. As a result, exercise at 85% $\dot{V}O_2$max can usually be maintained for only about 30-60 min before muscular discomfort and fatigue ensue. At such high exercise intensities, carbohydrate oxidation provides more than two-thirds of the needed energy, with the remainder coming from plasma FFA and intramuscular triglycerides. However, the absolute rate of fat oxidation is significantly decreased when exercise intensity is increased from 65% to 85% $\dot{V}O_2$max (e.g., fat oxidation drops from 43 to 30 μmol/kg/min) (Figures 3-3 and 3-4). Part of this decline appears to be due to the marked suppression of the Ra of plasma FFA during high-intensity exercise and the resulting reduction in FFA concentration in plasma, as shown in Figure 3-3. When the reduction in plasma FFA availability is reversed, fat oxidation is increased and muscle glycogen utilization is decreased (Costill et al., 1977; Dyck et al., 1993, 1996; Romijn et al., 1995). However, in these studies, the restoration of plasma FFA levels was accomplished by intravenous infusion of a triglyceride solution and heparin to allow lipases to hydrolyze plasma triglycerides into FFA. Even despite these extreme measures, fat oxidation does not completely return to the high levels observed during moderate-intensity exercise. This suggests that even when availability of FFA is high, the muscle is limited in its ability to oxidize fat during intense exercise. Theoretically, fat supplementation that elevates plasma FFA above the normally low levels observed during high-intensity exercise could have ergogenic effects by slightly reducing muscle glycogen utilization (Costill et al., 1977; Dycke et al., 1993; Romijn et al., 1995). Realistically, the extent to which this would improve performance at high exercise intensities is unclear because exercise time to fatigue at these intensities appears to result from lactic acid accumulation in the exercising muscles before muscle glycogen becomes sufficiently depleted (Coyle et al., 1988).

Fatty Acid Availability and Exercise Intensity

Is body fat always readily available for oxidation during exercise? The answer to this question depends upon the intensity of the exercise. During low-intensity exercise (i.e., 25% $\dot{V}O_2$max) and when the exerciser is fasted, the answer to the question is yes, as evidenced by the progressive increase in plasma FFA concentration (Figure 3-3). During moderate-intensity exercise (i.e., 65% $\dot{V}O_2$max) in endurance-trained people, adipocyte FFA mobilization is not sufficient to meet the muscle's ability to oxidize fat, and under these conditions intramuscular triglycerides become an important fuel, as do muscle glycogen and blood glucose. For example, during the first 30 min of moderate-intensity exercise (65% $\dot{V}O_2$max), plasma FFA concentration declines, and the Ra of FFA is not high (Figures 3-2, 3-3, and 3-4). Throughout the remainder of moderate-intensity exercise, the Ra of FFA and the plasma FFA concentration increase without proportional increases in fat oxidation, suggesting that plasma FFA availability is adequate. Therefore, with the exception of the early portion of moderate-intensity exercise, the capacity of muscles to oxidize fat appears to be met by a combination of plasma FFA and intramuscular triglycerides, at least in endurance-trained subjects, while carbohydrate oxidation provides the remaining energy. During high-intensity exercise, when muscle glycogenolysis is heavily stimulated, adipocyte FFA mobilization is simultaneously suppressed, and the delivery of FFA to muscle is very low. As a result, muscle glycogenolysis is stimulated slightly more than when plasma FFA concentration is high (Romijn et al., 1995), but this response is in keeping with the muscle's reliance on carbohydrate oxidation.

Carbohydrate is Essential Because of Muscle's Limited Ability to Oxidize Fat

When carbohydrate oxidation declines due to depletion of muscle glycogen and hypoglycemia, FFA oxidation is insufficient to meet the energy requirements of even moderate-intensity exercise (e.g., 60–75% $\dot{V}O_2$max). Under such circumstances, exercise cannot continue unless work rate is reduced to an intensity (e.g., 30–50% $\dot{V}O_2$max) at which muscles can predominantly oxidize fat (Coyle et al., 1983, 1986). This reduction in work rate occurs despite high levels of plasma FFA (Coyle et al., 1983, 1986). That is, fat oxidation appears to be limited by muscle's ability to metabolize FFA. This may explain why further elevation of plasma FFA during low-to-moderate-intensity exercise fails to increase total fat oxidation (Hargreaves et al., 1991; Ravussin et al., 1986).

The reason for muscle's limited ability to oxidize fat, and thus its dependence upon carbohydrate, is not entirely clear. One line of thinking is that the limitation for FFA oxidation is in the transport of FFA into the mitochondria. Traditionally, this step has been thought to be limited by carnitine palmitoyltransferase activity (CPT) required for the transport of FFA across the mitochondrial membrane. Now it is understood that FFA-binding proteins control the transport of FFA through the interstitium and cell membranes as well as through the cytoplasm (Knudsen, 1990; Ockner, 1990), implying that fat oxidation during exercise may be limited by transport at numerous sites within the muscle cell. Additionally, CPT activity is inhibited by malonyl-CoA, the first intermediate in the conversion of glucose to fat (McGarry et al., 1978). Carbohydrate availability in muscle may reduce fat oxidation through malonyl-CoA-induced inhibition of CPT-stimulated FFA transport across the mitochondrial membrane (Elayan & Winder, 1991), although this is an assumption that requires verification.

Given the fact that fat oxidation can provide only about one-half of the energy for exercise at 70% $\dot{V}O_2$max and no more than one-third of the energy for more strenuous exercise lasting 10–30 min (i.e. >85% $\dot{V}O_2$max) (Figure 3-2), the need for adequate muscle glycogen and blood glucose becomes clear and underscores the need for active people to eat sufficient amounts of carbohydrate to maintain glycogen stores.

FAT SUPPLEMENTATION DURING EXERCISE

Ingestion of Triglycerides

It is not possible to ingest free fatty acids because of their acidity and the need for a carrier; thus, the only practical way of significantly raising fat in the blood is via ingestion of triglycerides. Normal dietary triglycerides, containing long carbon chains, enter the blood 2–4 h after ingestion bound to chylomicrons (i.e., lipoprotein carriers). The rate at which trigylcerides are hydrolyzed from plasma chylomicrons by lipoprotein lipase and subsequently taken up by muscle during exercise is relatively low; however, plasma triglycerides do replenish intramuscular triglyceride after exercise (Mackie et al., 1980; Oscai et al., 1990). Therefore, it is unlikely that long-chain-triglyceride ingestion has much potential to provide significant substrate to muscle during exercise (Terjung et al., 1983).

Intravenous Infusions That Raise Plasma FFA

A technique used in research studies to raise plasma FFA is the elevation of plasma triglycerides either by having subjects consume triglycerides or by intravenously infusing a triglyceride emulsion (e.g., Intralipid®). Both procedures should be followed by intravenous infusion of heparin (Vukovich et al., 1993). Heparin causes lipoprotein lipase to be released from tissues into blood where it rapidly hydrolyzes plasma triglyceride and thus raises FFA concentration. Such studies have identified some conditions during exercise when plasma FFA concentration is suboptimal, thereby raising the possibility that there may be a benefit associated with raising plasma FFA. For example, plasma FFA mobilization and concentration are low during intense exercise (as discussed above), as well as during exercise following carbohydrate ingestion (discussed below). Under these conditions, the elevation of FFA via intravenous infusion of triglyceride and heparin has been observed to slightly reduce the rate of muscle glycogen utilization (Costill et al., 1977; Romijn et al., 1995; Vukovich et al., 1993). However, this effect is relatively small, and its benefit to performance has not been determined.

Ingestion of Medium Chain Triglycerides

Unlike long chain triglycerides, medium chain triglycerides (MCT) are rapidly hydrolyzed to free fatty acids and are directly absorbed into the blood via the portal circulation. Therefore, they provide a theoretical means of elevating plasma FFA via ingestion. Another theoretical advantage of MCT is that they appear to be readily transported through muscle cells and into the mitochondria for oxidation. Recent studies have shown that MCT ingestion does result in oxidation of a large percentage of the MCT ingested and that the oxidation increases more rapidly when the MCT is ingested with carbohydrate (Jeukendrup et al., 1995). However, the largest amount of MCT feeding that people seem able to tolerate, due to gastrointestinal discomfort and diarrhea, is less than 30 g. As a result of not being able to eat sufficient amounts, MCT ingestion can only cover 3% to 6% of total energy expenditure during exercise (Jeukendrup et al., 1995). Therefore, it appears that MCT ingestion is not a practical method for significantly raising fat oxidation during exercise. Furthermore, when it is ingested with carbohydrate, the carbohydrate-stimulated insulin secretion partially inhibits endogenous fat mobilization, resulting in large reductions in fat oxidation compared to exercise when fasted.

DIETS HIGH IN FAT AND LOW IN CARBOHYDRATE

Fasting during the two days before an exercise bout, compared to being fed food containing carbohydrate, improves endurance performance in rats, whereas fasting markedly impairs performance in humans (Koubi et al., 1991; Loy et al., 1986). Furthermore, rats appear to perform better on a chronic high-fat diet compared to a very high-carbohydrate diet when the performance task is of relatively low intensity, with fatigue occurring after four or more hours (Lapachet et al., 1996). This may be related to the fact that muscle glycogen concentration in rats is only 5% to 20% of that found in people; therefore, they are much more dependent upon FFA and blood glucose. Consequently, the best diet for improving prolonged performance (i.e., 4-6 h) in rats appears to be a chronic high-fat diet, a diet that presumably raises muscle fatty acid oxidation, followed by a high-carbohydrate diet during the three days before the endurance test (Lapachet et al., 1996).

The possible benefits of a high-fat and low-carbohydrate diet for athletes is not clear. In one study, Phinney et al. (1983) fed endurance-trained men a very high-fat diet containing almost no carbohydrate (i.e., less than 20 g/d) for 4 wk. This diet caused muscle glycogen concentration to be reduced by one-half, and it markedly increased fat oxidation during exercise at moderate intensities (62–64% $\dot{V}O_2$max). However, the diet did not increase the length of time that moderate-intensity exercise could be maintained, despite the fact that fat oxidation was increased. Furthermore, these subjects were not capable of exercising at higher intensities (Dr. Phinney's lecture at ACSM meeting, Minneapolis, 1995). Even with such an extreme diet, it appears that fat oxidation cannot increase sufficiently to fully replace muscle glycogen as a source of energy for intense exercise. Furthermore, high-fat diets over prolonged periods are not healthy from a cardiovascular perspective.

For 2 wk Lambert et al. (1994) fed cyclists a high-fat diet (fat intake = 70% of total energy) that lowered muscle glycogen, compared to a high-carbohydrate diet (74% of total energy). The investigators found that time to fatigue at 90% $\dot{V}O_2$max was 8.3 min after the high-fat diet compared to 12.5 min after the high-carbohydrate diet. However, this sizable difference was not statistically significant. Subsequent to that high-intensity fatigue test, the researchers measured time to fatigue at 60% $\dot{V}O_2$max and found it was 42.5 min on the high-carbohydrate diet and 79.7 min on the high-fat diet, which was significantly longer. However, the validity of these observations is unclear because endurance-trained cyclists should be able to cycle for 240 min or more at 60% $\dot{V}O_2$max (Coyle et al., 1986). These results indicate that the prior high-intensity bout exerted some confounding effect upon subsequent low-intensity performance. Another study claiming an advantage to a 7-d diet with 38% of total energy from fat compared to 15% of total energy from fat is also difficult to interpret because the diets were not randomized, and prolonged performance was also evaluated after a high-intensity exercise bout was performed to fatigue (Muoio et al., 1994).

A recent well-controlled study compared the improvements in exercise performance when untrained men consumed a diet high in carbohydrate (62% of energy) versus a diet high in fat (62% of energy) (Helge et al., 1996). The reported time to exhaustion after 7 wk of training increased from 35 min to 102 min on the high-carbohydrate diet, whereas it increased a lesser amount on the high-fat diet (from 35 to 65 min). Switching from the high-fat to the high-carbohydrate diet for 1 wk further improved performance from 65 to 77 min, but performance still did not approach that experienced by the group training continuously on the high-carbohydrate diet. These results clearly demonstrate that a high-carbohydrate diet is superior to a high-fat diet for inducing improvements in endurance performance during the first 2 mon of training.

ENDURANCE TRAINING INCREASES FAT OXIDATION DURING EXERCISE

Source of the Increase in Fat Oxidation

One of the most functional adaptations to endurance training is an increase in muscle mitochondria (i.e., aerobic metabolism) (Holloszy & Coyle, 1984). During exercise at a given submaximal intensity (i.e., same absolute caloric expenditure), endurance-trained people experience less muscular fatigue, less disturbance of energy balance, and less stimulation of muscle glycogenolysis. The reduction in glycogen use is accompanied by an increase in fat oxidation. There has been much interest in the source of this fat. Two studies have directly addressed this question by measuring the contribution of intramuscular triglyceride and plasma FFA during exercise at 64% pretraining $\dot{V}O_2$max, before and after 12 wk of strenuous running and cycling (Hurley et al., 1986; Martin et al., 1993). The fuel-use characteristics are displayed in Figure 3-5. The reduction in muscle glycogen oxidation (i.e., carbohydrate; CHO) as a result of endurance training was due exclusively to an increase in intra-

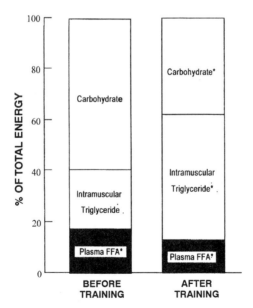

FIGURE 3-5. *Energy substrates during exercise at a given absolute intensity (64% of pre-training $\dot{V}O_2$max).* Measurements were made when subjects were untrained and trained (after training for endurance for 12 wk). After training, carbohydrate oxidation was reduced, as was oxidation of plasma free fatty acids (FFA), whereas estimated intramuscular triglyceride use was significantly increased (*). Redrawn for Martin et al. (1993) with permission.

muscular triglyceride oxidation. The mechanisms accounting for the increased intramuscular triglyceride use are not clear. Increases in intramuscular triglyceride concentration with training may be one potential mechanism, but that did not appear to take place in these studies, although it has been observed previously (Morgan et al., 1969). Surprisingly, plasma FFA disappearance was significantly reduced following training. This suggests that adipose tissue mobilization and oxidation do not demonstrate remarkable adaptation to endurance training during moderate-intensity exercise (Martin et al., 1993). This finding agrees with cross-sectional studies comparing untrained and endurance-trained people during low-intensity exercise (Klein et al., 1994), as discussed below. Therefore, it appears that intramuscular triglyceride is the primary source of fat accounting for the increase in fat oxidation with endurance training, an adaptation that is associated with a reduction in muscle glycogen utilization and improved performance (Hurley et al., 1986; Martin et al., 1993).

Plasma Free Fatty Acid Mobilization and Endurance Training

We have compared the rates of plasma FFA mobilization (i.e., Ra plasma FFA) and whole body lipolysis (i.e., Ra glycerol) in untrained compared to endurance-trained men (Klein et al., 1994). During this experiment, both groups walked on a treadmill for 4 h at a brisk pace that elicited a given absolute rate of oxygen consumption (i.e., 20 mL/kg/min). This elicited about 28% $\dot{V}O_2$max in the trained subjects compared to 43% VO_2max in the untrained subjects. As expected, total body fat oxidation was about one-third higher in the trained compared to untrained subjects. Interestingly, at this low intensity little intramuscular triglyceride use is expected; however, it appeared that the rate of plasma FFA disappearance very closely matched the rate of total fat oxidation in the trained subjects. This suggests that the endurance-trained individuals have the ability to oxidize fat at the same rate at which it was mobilized from adipose tissue. In the untrained subjects, even though the rates of whole body lipolysis and plasma FFA mobilization were identical to that of the trained subjects, the rate of fat oxidation was lower compared to trained subjects. Although the rate of plasma FFA disappearance was similar, trained subjects appeared capable of oxidizing a greater percentage of the FFA leaving the circulation. This indicates that untrained subjects have greater ability to mobilize FFA than they have to oxidize FFA, and, therefore, a sizable portion of the mobilized FFA is reesterified into triglyceride in some tissues. The major adaptation allowing trained subjects to oxidize more fat while walking seems to center around the increase in muscle oxidative capacity rather than on an increased mobilization of plasma FFA from adipose tissue.

The exercise intensity that elicits the highest rates of plasma FFA mobilization and oxidation is presently unknown. It is also not known if the highest rates of FFA mobilization and oxidation can be altered with training. However, this does not appear to be a particularly important question given the fact that the increase in fat oxidation following endurance training is derived from intramuscular triglyceride and not plasma FFA (Hurley et al., 1986; Martin et al., 1993). When exercising at approximately 70% $\dot{V}O_2$max, endurance-trained subjects generate more power compared to untrained subjects and have higher rates of both fat and carbohydrate oxidation. Accordingly, they also have higher rates of whole body lipolysis (i.e., Ra glycerol) (Klein et al., 1996), probably due to augmented intramuscular lipolysis (Hurley et al., 1986; Martin et al., 1993).

DIETARY CARBOHYDRATE INFLUENCES FAT OXIDATION DURING EXERCISE

Fat oxidation during exercise is influenced by exercise duration and by how recently carbohydrate was ingested. The carbohydrate effect on fat oxidation is due in part to the carbohydrate-induced elevation in plasma insulin and the associated inhibition of endogenous triglyceride lipolysis, thus blunting the rise in plasma FFA. This inhibitory effect is evident for at least 4 h after eating 140 g of high-glycemic carbohydrate (Montain et al., 1991). As a result, both total fat oxidation and plasma FFA concentration are reduced significantly during the first 50 min of moderate-intensity exercise. However, this suppression of fat oxidation is reversed as the duration of exercise is increased, so that after 100 min of exercise fat oxidation is comparable to that seen during exercise in the fasted state (Coyle et al., 1985). These results indicate that it is likely that insulin plays a role in regulating the mixture of carbohydrate and fat oxidized during exercise. As discussed below, the reduction in fat oxidation and increase in carbohydrate oxidation are not usually detrimental if most or all of the increase in carbohydrate oxidation is derived from plasma glucose provided by the meal, thus having little influence on muscle glycogen use. Therefore, there is little basis for recommending that people refrain from eating carbohydrates before exercise, especially if a sufficient amount is eaten, as discussed below.

Plasma FFA mobilization is remarkably sensitive to even small increases in plasma insulin (Jensen et al., 1989), and it seems that lipolysis is diminished for a long time after eating carbohydrates (Montain et al. 1991). Diets that are lower in carbohydrate, or that contain carbohydrates that cause less insulin secretion, likely still elicit enough of an insulin response to reduce plasma FFA mobilization. Therefore, it is unlikely that a particular product or diet can increase the mobilization and oxidation of FFA during exercise. To do so would require elimination of the insulin response that accompanies the ingestion of most foods. At the very least, it is incumbent upon the developers of these products to demonstrate that 1) FFA mobilization is increased by consumption of their products or as a result of a specific dietary regimen, and 2) that increased FFA mobilization benefits performance. However, neither possibility is likely because the carbohydrate content of the products or diets will inhibit FFA mobilization. Furthermore, as previously discussed, the oxidation of FFA is determined by the muscle's enzymatic capacity for FFA metabolism and not by the availability of plasma FFA.

CARBOHYDRATE FEEDING DURING EXERCISE

Prolonged Moderate-Intensity Exercise

Humans normally fatigue after 1–3 h of continuous exercise at moderate intensities (i.e., 60–80% $\dot{V}O_2$max), primarily due to carbohydrate depletion. Carbohydrate feedings (e.g., glucose, maltodextrins, or sucrose) during exercise will improve cycling and running performance (Coggan & Coyle, 1991; Tsintzas et al., 1993). However, the delay of fatigue during cycling does not appear to be due to a sparing of muscle glycogen during exercise (Coyle et al., 1986; Fielding et al., 1985; Flynn et al., 1987; Hargreaves & Briggs, 1988; Mitchell et al., 1989; Noakes et al., 1988; Slentz et al., 1990). Instead, it appears that the exercising muscles rely mostly upon blood glucose for energy late in exercise (Coggan & Coyle, 1991; Coyle et al., 1986).

These concepts are summarized in Figure 3-6, displaying the substrate shifts during prolonged exercise at 65–75% $\dot{V}O_2$max in endurance-trained subjects who fasted overnight (Coggan & Coyle, 1991; Coyle et al., 1986; Romijn et al., 1993). Approximately 50% of the energy for exercise at 70% $\dot{V}O_2$max is derived from fat, with equal contributions from plasma FFA and intramuscular triglycerides and with a small increase in plasma FFA contribution over time. The remaining 50% of the energy is derived from carbohydrate (muscle glycogen and blood glucose). During the early portions of exercise, the majority of carbohydrate energy is from muscle glycogen. As exercise progresses, muscle glycogen concentration is reduced and contributes less to the carbohydrate requirements of exercise, with a concomitant increase in blood glucose oxidation.

Figure 3-7 displays the actual plasma glucose and muscle glycogen responses to prolonged cycling, as well as the rates of carbohydrate oxidation. After 3 h of exercise and consumption of only flavored water (i.e., placebo), muscle glycogen concentration is low, and the majority of

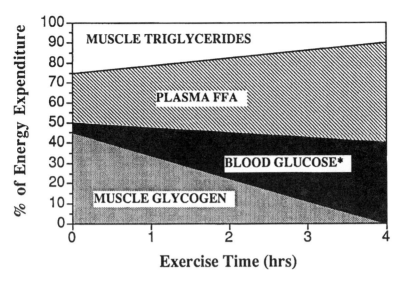

FIGURE 3-6. *Percentage of energy derived from the four major substrates during prolonged exercise at 65–75% VO_2max.* Initially, approximately one-half of the energy requirement is derived from carbohydrate and the other half from fat. As muscle glycogen concentration declines, blood glucose becomes an increasingly important source of carbohydrate energy for muscle. After 2 h of exercise, carbohydrate ingestion is needed to maintain blood glucose concentration and carbohydrate oxidation. Drawn from data in Coyle et al. (1986) and Romijn et al. (1933).

carbohydrate energy is derived from the metabolism of glucose transported from the blood into the exercising muscles. Under these conditions, fatigue occurs after approximately 3 h due to a decrease in blood glucose that causes an inadequate supply of carbohydrate energy for oxidation, as shown in Figure 3-6. However, when carbohydrate is ingested throughout exercise, plasma glucose concentration is maintained and fatigue is delayed by 1 h (i.e., from 3 h to 4 h; Figure 3-7). Remarkably, muscle glycogen use was minimal during the additional hour of exercise despite the fact that carbohydrate oxidation was maintained (Figure 3-7). This suggests that blood glucose was the predominant carbohydrate fuel during the latter stages of exercise.

More-recent studies have employed isotopic tracers to directly measure the rates of glucose entry into blood throughout exercise when fed carbohydrate compared to a placebo (Bosch et al., 1994; McConell et al., 1994). These data indicate that carbohydrate ingestion causes endogenous hepatic glucose production to be greatly suppressed, with the glucose entry into blood being derived predominantly from the ingested carbohydrate (Bosch et al., 1994; McConell et al., 1994). In support of the finding that blood glucose becomes the predominant source of carbohy-

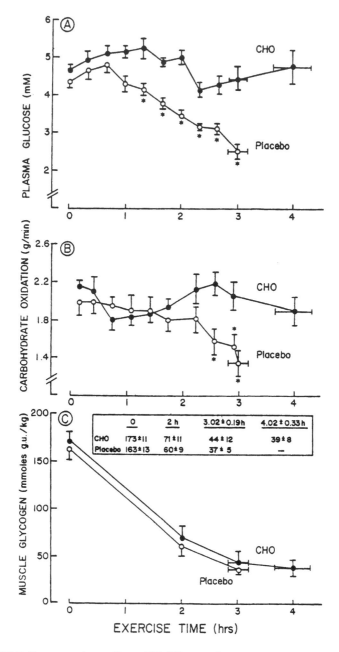

FIGURE 3-7. *Responses when cycling at 74% V̇O₂max. when ingesting a placebo (flavored water) or when ingesting carbohydrate (CHO) every 20 min.* *Placebo significantly different from carbohydrate; P<0.05. From Coyle et al. (1986).

drate after 2–3 h, researchers have found that the ingested carbohydrate is oxidized at approximately 1 g/min late in exercise (Bosch et al., 1994; McConell et al., 1994; Wagenmakers et al., 1993). Interestingly, this rate of exogenous glucose oxidation does not increase appreciably when the rate of carbohydrate ingestion is increased above 60 g/h (i.e., 1 g/min) (Wagenmakers et al., 1993).

It has been observed that carbohydrate feeding during exercise that alternates between moderate and low intensity, and thus promotes hyperglycemia and hyperinsulinemia, does result in a slightly higher muscle glycogen concentration at the end of exercise (Yaspelkis et al., 1993). This is probably due to glycogen resynthesis from glucose taken up by muscles during the periods of low-intensity exercise. Furthermore, carbohydrate ingestion during 60 min of running also appears to result in slightly higher glycogen concentration within Type I fibers in the vastus lateralis muscle, which is somewhat involved in running (Tsintzas et al., 1995). It is reasonable to hypothesize that when athletes ingest carbohydrate during exercise, some of the glucose that disappears from the blood but is not oxidized might be converted to glycogen in certain muscle fibers. However, the mechanism by which carbohydrate feeding delays fatigue or improves power output during the latter stages of exercise appears to be related to the oxidation of the ingested carbohydrate (Bosch et al., 1994, Coggan & Coyle, 1991) rather than to any sparing of muscle glycogen.

Type of Carbohydrate Ingested During Exercise

Glucose, sucrose, and maltodextrins appear to be equally effective in maintaining blood glucose concentration and carbohydrate oxidation and in improving performance (Massicotte et al., 1989; Murray et al., 1989a). Therefore, the selection of carbohydrate for ingestion during exercise should be based upon what is best tolerated during exercise. Interestingly, the combination of glucose and fructose seems to result in enhanced exogenous carbohydrate oxidation (Adopo et al., 1994). Liquid and solid forms of carbohydrate are equally effective (Keizer et al., 1986; Mason et al., 1993; Reed et al., 1989). Liquids are obviously easier to ingest during exercise than solids and also reduce the risk of dehydration. Maltodextrins can be used in sports drinks to reduce the perception of sweetness. However, exercising people can generally meet both their carbohydrate and fluid needs by ingesting 600-1,200 mL/h of a sports drink (Coyle & Montain, 1992).

Timing of Carbohydrate Ingestion During Exercise

The most effective approach is to ingest carbohydrate at regular intervals throughout exercise according to the guidelines given below. If carbohydrate feedings are withheld until the point of exhaustion, fatigue can be delayed (by about 45 min) only if glucose is intravenously infused at a high rate (i.e., over 1 g/min) (Coggan & Coyle, 1987). This impractical approach illustrates that the objective of carbohydrate feeding is to provide the exercising muscle with approximately an additional 1 g/min of exogenous glucose (i.e., 60 g/h). Drinking a concentrated carbohydrate solution at or near the point of fatigue is ineffective because the carbohydrate will not be absorbed rapidly enough to maintain the energy needs of the exercising muscles (Coggan & Coyle, 1987). The latest that a person can delay carbohydrate ingestion and still realize a performance benefit is 30 min before the time of fatigue (Coggan & Coyle, 1989).

Rate of Carbohydrate Ingestion During Exercise

Sufficient carbohydrate should be ingested to supply the blood with exogenous glucose at approximately 1 g/min, late in exercise. Therefore, approximately 60 g of exogenous glucose must be readily available within the body. To ensure this, it seems that larger amounts of carbohydrate must be ingested. Most studies that showed an improved performance with carbohydrate ingestion throughout exercise fed subjects at a rate of 30–60 g/h, beginning early in exercise (Coggan & Coyle, 1988, 1991; Murray et al., 1989b, 1991). In some cases of more prolonged and intense exercise, such as during a long triathlon, it may be beneficial to ingest more than 60 g/h (Walberg-Rankin, 1995). This generally agrees with the expected needs and glucose distribution within the body, although it should be recognized that the fate of the ingested glucose that is not oxidized is unclear.

Carbohydrate Ingestion During Sport, Recreation, and Intermittent Exercise

Carbohydrate feedings are also beneficial during sports involving high-intensity intermittent exercise, such as soccer and ice hockey, where fatigue is due to glycogen depletion (Foster et al., 1986; Muckle, 1973; Simard et al., 1988). The ingestion of carbohydrate throughout the game and during the half-time rest period results in higher muscle glycogen and increased sprinting ability toward the end of the game, compared to when no carbohydrate is ingested and muscle glycogen remains low.

There is little doubt that carbohydrate feeding improves performance during prolonged exercise (e.g., > 2 h) that results in hypoglycemia when only water is ingested. Several studies have reported that carbohydrate ingestion results in improved performance when blood glucose availability and muscle glycogen are not limiting (Below & Coyle, 1993; Mitchell et al., 1989; Murray et al., 1987, 1989a, 1989b, 1991). These findings suggest that carbohydrate ingestion can improve performance in events as brief as 60 min in duration. Additionally, if body carbohydrate stores are reduced prior to the onset of exercise, due to inadequate diet or insufficient recovery from previous exercise, carbohydrate feeding can improve performance during exercise of 60-min duration (Neufer et al., 1987).

METABOLIC RESPONSES TO VARIOUS TYPES OF DIETARY CARBOHYDRATE

Glucose is the only type of carbohydrate (i.e., sugar or starch) that skeletal muscle can readily metabolize for energy or store as glycogen. Carbohydrates can be functionally classified according to the extent to which they increase blood glucose concentration (i.e., glycemic index). The glycemic index is generally determined by the rate at which the ingested carbohydrate is made available to intestinal enzymes for hydrolysis and intestinal absorption (Gatti et al., 1987; O'Dea et al., 1980). This is a function of the gastric emptying time (Mourot et al., 1988) and the physical availability of the sugar or starch to hydrolytic enzymes. The availability of glucose from starch is influenced by cooking that alters the integrity of the starch granule (Wursch et al., 1986) and the degree of gelatinization (O'Dea et al., 1980). Another factor affecting glycemic index is the amylose vs. amylopectin content of food (Behall et al., 1988; Goddard et al., 1984). Adding fiber to glucose also slows the rate of carbohydrate entry into the blood and oxidation during exercise (Jarvis et al., 1992). It is a misconception to think that the glycemic index is simply a function of whether the carbohydrate is complex (i.e., starch) or a simple sugar. Some starchy foods produce glycemic responses that are identical to that of glucose (e.g., mashed potato) (Crapo et al., 1977; Guezennec et al., 1989; Horowitz & Coyle, 1993). On the other hand, the rise in blood glucose after ingestion of fructose or sucrose is less than that observed for a wide range of starchy complex carbohydrates (e.g., potato, bread, cornflakes) (Jenkins et al. 1984, 1988). Foods for physically active people should be classified as having a high, moderate or low glycemic index, as outlined by Jenkins et al. (Jenkins et al., 1984, 1988).

The classification of foods according to their glycemic index does not take into account the insulin response. Insulin has large effects on metabolism and regulates glucose disposal. Although blood glucose and insulin responses are generally related, some foods that do not differ in their glycemic responses could differ in insulin secretion, which has potential to alter metabolism (Westphal et al., 1990). Therefore, the classification of foods according the their glycemic index is recognized to be rather simplistic, but it is certainly better than classifying carbohydrates as simple vs. complex. Future classification of carbohydrate foods should consider their functional influences on metabolism, which is in part related to insulin action on tissues such as muscle and adipocytes.

MUSCLE GLYCOGEN RESYNTHESIS FOLLOWING EXERCISE

Muscle glycogen restoration after heavy training and competition often dictates the time needed to recover between intense bouts of exercise. It is commonly stated that muscle glycogen becomes depleted after about 2–3 h of continuous exercise performed at intensities of approximately 60–80% $\dot{V}O_2$max. It is not usually appreciated that muscle glycogen can also become depleted after only 15–30 min of exercise performed intermittently (e.g., 1–5 min) at very high intensities (90–130% $\dot{V}O_2$max) (Keizer et al., 1986). These patterns of intense exercise are typical of many individual and team sports. Therefore, athletes who attempt to train daily at intensities that deplete muscle glycogen must increase their carbohydrate consumption (Costill et al., 1988) in an attempt to optimize muscle glycogen storage (Kirwan et al., 1988).

Even when adequate amounts of carbohydrate are ingested, muscle glycogen can be resynthesized at a rate of only about 4–5 mmol/kg muscle/h, which corresponds to a rate of about 4–5% per h (i.e., 4–5 mmol/kg muscle/h when attempting to increase muscle glycogen by 80–100 mmol/kg) (Burke et al., 1995). Therefore, approximately 24 h are required to replenish muscle glycogen stores by 80–100 mmol/kg. More time will be necessary if the diet is suboptimal in carbohydrate content. However, very high rates of intravenous glucose infusion or carbohydrate ingestion appear to increase the rate of glycogen resynthesis, especially when glycogen is low (Doyle et al., 1993; Price et al., 1994). The important dietary factors are 1) the rate of carbohydrate ingestion, 2) carbohydrate type, and 3) timing of carbohydrate ingestion after exercise.

Rate of Carbohydrate Ingestion

Blom et al. (1987) and Ivy et al. (1988b) fed subjects different amounts of high-glycemic carbohydrates (i.e., glucose or maltodextrins) every 2 h after exercise and measured the rates of muscle glycogen synthesis during the first 6 h. They reported that glycogen synthesis increased from 2%/h (i.e., 2 mmol/kg/h) when 25 g was ingested every 2 h to 5-6%/h (i.e., 5–6 mmol/kg/h) when 50 g was ingested every 2 h. However, they did not observe muscle glycogen synthesis to increase to more than 5–6%/h (i.e., 5-6 mmol/kg/h) when 100, 112, or 225 g were ingested every 2 h. This plateau in glycogen synthesis does not appear to be due to simply an accumulation of carbohydrate in the gastrointestinal tract because Reed et al. (1989) reported that intravenous glucose infusion at about 100 g every 2 h also failed to increase muscle glycogen synthesis above 7–8 mmol/kg/h. Additionally, the failure of muscle glycogen synthesis to increase with increased carbohydrate ingestion or intravenous glucose infusion (100 g/2 h) occurred despite the fact that increased carbohydrate administration promoted progressively greater increases in blood glucose and plasma insulin concentration (Blom et al., 1987; Ivy et al., 1988b; Reed et al., 1989).

These findings suggest that muscle glycogen synthesis is near optimal (4–7 mmol/kg/h) when at least 50 g of glucose is ingested every 2 h. This forms the basis for the recommendation that the amount and type of food to be eaten after exercise for optimal muscle glycogen resynthesis should be that which promotes glucose entry into the blood and systemic circulation at a rate of at least 50 g every 2 h. This goal can be achieved by considering both the glycemic index of the carbohydrate and the amount of carbohydrate ingested.

Carbohydrate Type

As discussed, the rate of glycogen synthesis after exercise and ingestion of glucose, or food with a high glycemic index, is 5–6%/h (i.e., 5–6 mmol/kg/h) (Blom et al., 1987; Ivy et al., 1988a, 1988b; Reed et al., 1989). When sucrose is ingested, it is hydrolyzed to equal amounts of glucose and fructose. Its ingestion elicits a similar rate of glycogen synthesis as glucose ingestion, despite the fact that the glycemic index of sucrose is 60–70% of that of glucose (Blom et al., 1987), which classifies it as having a moderate to high glycemic index. However, fructose ingestion alone promotes muscle glycogen to be resynthesized at only 3%/h (i.e., 3 mmol/kg/h) because of its low glycemic index (20–30% of that of glucose) (Blom et al., 1987). It appears that fructose ingestion, even in large amounts, cannot produce sufficient entry of glucose into the blood (i.e., 50 g every 2 h), probably because of the relatively slow rate with which the liver converts fructose to glucose. Concerning simple sugars, it appears that glucose and sucrose, which possess high and moderate glycemic indices, are equally effective in the partial restoration of muscle glycogen during the 4–6 h period after exercise, yet fructose is only one-half as effective due to a low glycemic index.

A limited amount of information is available about the rates of glycogen synthesis elicited by eating common foods containing various starches and sugars. However, Burke et al. (1993) reported that muscle glycogen resynthesis is 48% greater in a 24-h period when a variety of high-glycemic foods are eaten compared to when only moderate or low glycemic foods are consumed.

Little data exist as to the extent to which carbohydrate foods with a low glycemic index promote muscle glycogen resynthesis. For example, legumes possess a low glycemic index largely because the carbohydrate granule is not as accessible to digestive enzymes (Wursch et al., 1986), a limitation that can be influenced by food processing and cooking. It is possible, however, that legumes can promote a sufficient rate of glucose entry into blood for optimal muscle glycogen synthesis if a larger amount is eaten to offset the slow rate at which each gram is digested. However, until more direct data become available, it is assumed that foods with a low glycemic index should not comprise the bulk of carbohydrate ingested after exercise because it is likely that muscle glycogen synthesis would be compromised.

Timing of Carbohydrate Ingestion After Exercise

During the first 2 h following exercise, the rate of muscle glycogen resynthesis is 7–8%/h (i.e., 7–8 mmol/kg/h), which is somewhat faster than the frequently reported rate of 5–6%/h, but certainly not rapid (Ivy et al, 1988a). To assure rapid muscle glycogen resynthesis, athletes should ingest carbohydrate as soon after exercise as is practical to allow more total time for resynthesis. The total amount of carbohydrate ingested is more important than the frequency at which it is ingested, as illustrated by Costill et al. (1981). They fed subjects 525 g of carbohydrate over the course of 24 h (which comprised 70% of the caloric intake) and reported that muscle glycogen synthesis was similar when two large meals were eaten as compared to when seven smaller meals were eaten.

Influence of Dietary Fat and Protein on Glycogen Resynthesis

The amount of glycogen synthesis following exercise increases with increasing daily carbohydrate ingestion up to a point, after which eating more carbohydrate promotes little further glycogen storage. It is generally recommended that athletes attempt to ingest at least 8–10 g CHO/kg over 24 h in order to maximize glycogen stores. However, Burke et al. (1995) have recently found that eating more than 7 g/kg of carbohydrate over 24 h did not further increase glycogen resynthesis in their subjects. Furthermore, they found that eating moderate amounts of fat and protein with this 7 g/kg of carbohydrate did not reduce glycogen storage. Therefore, carbohydrate does not have to be ingested at the exclusion of fat and protein, provided that the carbohydrate ingestion amounts to at least 7 g/kg over the day. Overconsumption of carbohydrate, resulting in an intake of energy in excess of daily expenditure, will results in fat storage (Acheson et al., 1988).

Practical Considerations and Specific Recommendations

Hunger is often reduced immediately following exhaustive exercise, and athletes usually prefer to drink fluids rather than to eat solid foods (Keizer et al., 1986). Therefore, beverages that contain glucose, sucrose, maltodextrins, or corn syrup solids in concentrations of 6 g/100 mL (i.e., a 6% solution) or higher should be made available. If preferred, there is no reason an athlete cannot eat solid food. However, because appetite is usually suppressed, foods that provide a concentrated source of carbohydrate with a high glycemic index should be available. When the desire to consume solid food returns, athletes should eat enough to ensure an intake of approximately 500 g of carbohydrate (>7 g/kg body weight) within 24 h. Most of the food chosen should possess a moderate or high glycemic index. Meals with high fat and protein content will reduce total carbohydrate ingestion. Realistically, due to other daily activities including sleep, it is usually not possible to eat frequent meals (every 2 h) that contain at least 50 g of carbohydrate. Therefore, when there is an extended period of time between meals, the last meal should contain enough carbohydrate to suffice for that period (i.e., 25 g/h; 250 g for a 10 h period of fasting). When sufficient carbohydrate is consumed (i.e., >7 g/kg/d), muscle glycogen resynthesis is optimized, a high training intensity can be maintained, and performance improves more compared to the ingestion of lesser amounts of carbohydrate (e.g., 5 g/kg/d) (Simonsen et al., 1991).

MAXIMIZING MUSCLE GLYCOGEN PRIOR TO COMPETITION

A few days prior to a prolonged competition, athletes should regulate their diets and training in an attempt to maximize ("supercompensate" or "load") muscle glycogen stores. High pre-exercise glycogen levels will allow athletes to exercise for longer periods by delaying fatigue. The most practical method of "glycogen loading" involves altering training and diet for 7 d prior to competition (Sherman et al., 1981). On days 7,6,5, and 4 before competition, training should be moderately hard (e.g., 1–2 h/d), and athletes should consume a moderate amount of carbohydrate (i.e., 5g/kg/d). This will result in less-than-optimal carbohydrate stores yet will provide enough carbohydrate to keep glycogen levels from dropping too low. During the 3 d prior to competition, training should be tapered (30–60 min/d of low-to-moderate intensity), and a high-carbohydrate diet should be consumed (i.e., 500+ g/d; >7 g/kg/d). This regimen will increase muscle glycogen stores 20-40% or more above normal. This "modified" glycogen loading regimen is as effective as the "classic" regimen (Bergstrom & Hultman, 1966) and more practical because it does not require athletes to attempt training while consuming a high-fat diet.

PREEXERCISE NUTRITION

The goal of a preexercise carbohydrate meal is to optimize the supply of muscle glycogen and blood glucose late in exercise. Specifically, preexercise carbohydrate meals have the following effects: 1) promote additional muscle glycogen synthesis when stores are not already supercompensated, 2) replenish liver glycogen and store glucose in the body (i.e., gastrointestinal tract and glucose space) for potential oxidation during exercise, and 3) increase carbohydrate oxidation and decrease fat oxidation during exercise.

Although these first two responses to preexercise carbohydrate feeding are beneficial because more carbohydrate is stored within the body, some controversy exists as to whether the increase in carbohydrate oxidation, and concomitant decrease in fat oxidation, is a benefit or a detriment. Ingesting carbohydrate prior to exercise would be disadvantageous if the resulting increases in carbohydrate oxidation promoted rapid glycogen depletion.

Carbohydrate Feedings During the Hour Before Exercise

Although there is little debate surrounding the recommendation that athletes should eat ample amounts of carbohydrate the day before exercise, there is less agreement as to when, how much, and what type of carbohydrate should be eaten in the few hours prior to exercise. Eating high-glycemic carbohydrate during the hour before moderately-intense exercise (i.e., 60–75% $\dot{V}O_2$max) is often associated with a decline in blood glucose concentration at the onset of exercise (Costill et al., 1977; Horowitz & Coyle, 1993). This decline in blood glucose concentration is due to the concomitant hyperinsulinemia accompanying carbohydrate ingestion. This response increases glucose uptake by the contracting muscles at a time when liver glucose output may be reduced, resulting in hypoglycemia (Ahlborg & Bjorkman, 1987; Ahlborg & Felig, 1976; Costill et al., 1977; Nelly et al., 1996). Hyperinsulinemia at the start of exercise provokes large increases in glucose disappearance from blood, a response recently documented using stable-isotope techniques (Nelly et al., 1996). The transient hypoglycemia that results is usually not perceived by subjects, and it is not associated with muscle weakness. Preexercise hyperinsulinemia also has the long-lasting effect of reducing the release of free fatty acids (FFA) from adipocytes and the rate of fat oxidation during exercise (Coyle et al., 1985; Montain et al., 1991). As a result, preexercise carbohydrate feeding causes a shift in blood-borne fuels from fat to glucose.

There has been much debate as to whether the shift in favor of carbohydrate oxidation detrimentally affects muscle glycogen use. Theoretically, muscle glycogenolysis would be increased if the decline in fat oxidation was not offset by a proportional increase in blood glucose uptake and oxidation by muscle. The two studies that have found preexercise feedings to slightly increase muscle glycogen use also reported a relatively large decline in blood glucose concentration, which may have limited increases in muscle glucose uptake (Costill et al., 1977; Hargreaves et al., 1985). Several other studies have not found sugar feedings during the hour before exercise to increase muscle glycogen use, possibly because the hypoglycemia was not as pronounced and/or the suppression of FFA mobilization was not as great (Fielding et al., 1987; Gleeson et al., 1986; Hargreaves et al., 1987; Koivisto et al., 1985; Levine et al., 1983).

More importantly, regarding the studies that have measured endurance performance following carbohydrate ingestion during the hour before exercise, only one study has reported a negative effect (Foster et al., 1979); four studies have observed no significant effect (Devlin et al., 1986; Hargreaves et al., 1987; Keller & Schwarzkopf, 1984; McMurray, 1983); and three studies reported improvements in performance (Gleeson et al., 1986; Okano et al., 1988; Peden et al., 1989). Therefore, there is little support for the idea that carbohydrate ingestion before exercise impairs performance.

Out of concern that ingesting high-glycemic carbohydrate during the hour before exercise will cause hypoglycemia and impair performance, it has been erroneously recommended that complex carbohydrate be consumed during the hour before exercise, with the notion that complex carbohydrate will promote less of an insulin response. As discussed, this is not necessarily the case. For example, the glycemic and insulinemic responses to sucrose (i.e., simple) and mashed-potato (i.e., complex) ingestion 30 min before exercise are identical, and blood glucose declined to equally low values during the initial stages of exercise without either eliciting any symptoms of hypoglycemia (i.e., neuroglucopenia) (Horowitz & Coyle, 1993). Although the blood glucose and insulin responses varied somewhat after eating 50 g of these and other moderate and high glycemic foods, all of the meals caused plasma glucose to decline to equally low concentrations, without affecting sensation of fatigue or ability to complete 1 h of exercise at moderate intensities (i.e., 50–70% $\dot{V}O_2max$) (Horowitz & Coyle, 1993).

Carbohydrate Ingestion During the 6 h Period Before Exercise

In an attempt to avoid a decline in blood glucose at the onset of exercise, it is sometimes recommended that carbohydrate meals be eaten

3–4 h before exercise so as to allow enough time for plasma insulin concentration to return to basal levels. However, the insulin-induced metabolic responses to a preexercise meal last for several hours after plasma insulin has returned to basal levels. Consequently, blood glucose still declines when exercise is begun 4 h after a meal (Coyle et al., 1985; Montain et al., 1991). It appears that at least 6 h of fasting is necessary after consuming a 150-g high-glycemic meal before carbohydrate oxidation rates and plasma glucose concentrations are similar to values typical after an 8–12 h fast (Montain et al., 1991). There is no reason, however, to recommend that athletes fast this long before exercise because the transient decline in blood glucose is not problematic (Brouns et al., 1989). In fact, the decline in blood glucose can be prevented simply by having the subjects exercise slightly more intensely, which likely causes liver glucose output to increase enough to match blood glucose uptake by muscle (Montain et al., 1991). Additionally, the elevation in carbohydrate oxidation during exercise should not be problematic provided that enough carbohydrate was stored in the body as a result of the meal. When muscle glycogen is suboptimal, a substantial amount of the preexercise carbohydrate meal can be converted to muscle glycogen in a 4-h period (Coyle et al., 1985; Neufer et al., 1987). Liver glycogen undoubtedly increases as well.

Accumulating evidence suggests that performance is improved when a relatively large carbohydrate meal is eaten 3–4 h before prolonged exercise compared to when nothing is consumed. Neufer et al. (1987) reported that a 200-g carbohydrate meal of bread, cereal, and fruit eaten 4 h before exercise, as well as 43 g of sucrose eaten 5 min before exercise, resulted in a 22% increase in cycling power compared to placebo. Additionally, Sherman et al. (1989) fed cyclists various amounts of carbohydrate 4 h before exercise and found that a 312-g feeding of carbohydrate (maltodextrin) improved power by 15% during the last 45 min of exercise. Mixed meals containing either 45 g or 156 g of carbohydrate did not significantly improve performance. Apparently, eating approximately 150 g of carbohydrate (i.e., bread and juice) 4 h before exercise does not produce a marked elevation of muscle glycogen, blood glucose, or carbohydrate oxidation after 105 min of exercise (Coyle et al., 1985). This may explain why Sherman et al. (1989) did not observe an improvement in performance with this amount. Finally, Wright et al. (1991) have reported that a 350-g feeding of maltodextrin 3 h before exercise dramatically improves performance.

A relatively large preexercise carbohydrate meal (i.e., >200g) appears to improve performance by maintaining the ability to oxidize glucose at high rates late in exercise. It is not clear, however, if this is simply due to a greater availability of muscle glycogen. It could also be due to increased blood glucose uptake and oxidation, despite the observation that blood glucose concentration is not increased (Neufer et al., 1987; Sherman et al., 1989). Large preexercise carbohydrate feedings in combination with continued feeding during exercise, which does increase blood glucose concentration, produce even more dramatic improvements in performance than when carbohydrate is only eaten before exercise or when carbohydrate feedings are provided only after exercise has begun (Wright et al., 1991).

Types of Carbohydrate to Ingest During the 6 h Before Exercise

Foods ingested during this period should be low in fat, fiber, and bulk to minimize the potential for gastrointestinal distress (including the urge to defecate) during exercise. If muscle glycogen stores are not supercompensated, these foods should have a high or moderate glycemic index to stimulate glycogen synthesis. It is sometimes recommended that low glycemic foods be consumed during this period to minimize the insulin response. This would seem advisable only in situations when muscle glycogen cannot be further increased and carbohydrate will not be ingested during exercise. Carbohydrate foods that are slowly absorbed may theoretically provide glucose from the gastrointestinal tract throughout exercise. However, a more practical solution is to simply ingest carbohydrate during exercise.

PRACTICAL APPLICATIONS FOR ACTIVE PEOPLE

Many of the studies cited in this review used athletes as subjects, most often endurance athletes such as cyclists and runners. Do the responses and dietary needs of competitive athletes differ substantially from people who use daily physical activity simply as a means of staying fit? The major difference is that endurance-trained individuals have a greater capacity to oxidize intramuscular triglyceride and spare muscle glycogen (Hurley et al., 1986; Martin et al., 1993). Although the pattern of substrate use during prolonged exercise at various intensities (Figures 3-2, 3-6) would be generally similar, at a given percentage of $\dot{V}O_2max$, normally active people will oxidize less fat and more muscle glycogen compared to endurance-trained subjects (Coggan et al., 1990; Coyle et al., 1988; Martin et al., 1993). Reliance upon carbohydrate in general and blood glucose in particular is not increased with endurance training (Coggan et al., 1990). Therefore, theoretically, blood glucose supplementation should be as important to normally active people as for endurance-trained athletes. On the other hand, normally active people are less likely to perform strenuous exercise for sufficient duration (longer than 1–2 h) to require supplementation. When they do, however, they too should benefit by carbohydrate supplementation (Coggan & Coyle, 1991).

People who exercise at relatively low intensities and for short duration (e.g., < 1 h), and thus do not substantially deplete muscle glycogen, do not need to design their diet along the guidelines given for maximizing muscle glycogen resynthesis after exercise. Additionally, people who allow themselves 48 h or more for recovery between exercise bouts should be able to restore muscle glycogen in that time by consuming a diet containing 60% of energy from carbohydrate, without special attention to carbohydrate type. People who perform aerobic exercise for general fitness and health are recommended to do so 3–5 d/week (American College of Sports Medicine, 1990) with rest days interspersed between training days. This allows ample time for recovery, particularly of muscle glycogen. When normally active people attempt to perform strenuous aerobic exercise training with only 24 h of recovery time, they should follow the guidelines developed for athletes.

DIRECTIONS FOR FUTURE RESEARCH

This review has presented the results of studies on carbohydrate and fat metabolism during exercise. Future research should focus upon the interactions of carbohydrate and fat metabolism and how these interactions might be modified by diet to optimize the availability and oxidation of both fat and carbohydrate during exercise. For example, it is well known that the insulin response from carbohydrate ingestion has potential to reduce the mobilization and oxidation of endogenous FFA (Horowitz & Coyle, 1993). Therefore, a diet that minimizes the insulin inhibition of fat oxidation while maintaining sufficient carbohydrate availability would theoretically appear to be beneficial. This is not an easy challenge because small increases in plasma insulin are sufficient to reduce fat oxidation (Jensen et al., 1989), without providing sufficient carbohydrate to benefit performance.

SUMMARY

As the intensity of exercise is increased, the rate of plasma FFA mobilization declines and the exercising muscles become dependent upon carbohydrate for energy. This shift is not due simply to the limited availability of FFA, but to a limited capacity for fat oxidation in skeletal muscle. Carbohydrate ingestion before and during exercise exerts a large influence on FFA mobilization and oxidation, making muscle even more dependent upon carbohydrate for energy during exercise. The notion that FFA availability is a limiting factor and that dietary interventions that increase endogenous or exogenous FFA levels are beneficial is currently without scientific basis. Therefore, carbohydrate remains the recommended substrate for ingestion before, during, and following exercise.

Considering that fatigue during prolonged exercise is often due to depletion of muscle and liver glycogen, the goal of carbohydrate intake should be to stimulate carbohydrate oxidation throughout exercise. This can be achieved by ingesting at least 200 g of carbohydrate during the 4-h period before exercise. When possible, carbohydrate should be ingested during exercise at a rate of 30–60 g/h. Following exercise, athletes should ingest about 25 g/h of moderate and high glycemic carbohydrate foods, as part of a diet containing about 500 g/d (i.e., >7 g/kg).

FOOTNOTE

Recommendations in this paper are based upon a person weighing 70 kg (154 lb). The application of these recommendations to individuals of different body mass requires the calculation of carbohydrate intake according to the proportion that body weight differs from 70 kg. For example, a person weighing 100 kg should multiply the recommended intake by 1.4 (i.e., 100/70 kg), whereas a person weighing 50 kg should multiply the recommended intake by 0.7 (i.e., 50/70 kg).

This paper is an update of the following previous reviews by the author: *J. Sports Sci.* 9–29, 1991; *Am. J. Clin. Nutr.* 61: 968S–979S, 1995; *Sports Science Exchange* 8(6), 1995.

BIBLIOGRAPHY

Acheson, K.J., Y.S. Schutz, T.B. Bessard, K. Anantharaman, J.P. Flatt, and E. Jequier (1988). Glycogen storage capacity and de novo lipogenesis during massive carbohydrate overfeeding in man. *Am. J. Clin. Nutr.* 48:240–247.

Adopo, E., F. Péronnet, D. Massicotte, G.R. Brisson, and C. Hillaire-Marcel (1994). Respective oxidation of exogenous glucose and fructose given in the same drink during exercise. *J. Appl. Physiol.* 76:1014–1019.

Ahlborg G, and O. Bjorkman (1987). Carbohydrate utilization by exercising muscle following preexercise glucose ingestion. *Clin. Physiol.* 7:181–195.

Ahlborg G, and P. Felig (1976). Influence of glucose ingestion on the fuel-hormone responses during prolonged exercise. *J. Appl. Physiol.* 41:683–688.

American College of Sports Medicine (1990). The recommended quantity and quality of exercise for developing and maintaining cardiovascular and muscular fitness in healthy adults. *Med. Sci. Sports Exerc.* 22:265–274.

Behall, K.M., D.J. Scholfield, and J. Canary (1988). Effect of starch structure on glucose and insulin responses in adults. *Am. J. Clin. Nutr.* 47:428–432.

Below, P.R., R. Mora-Rodriguez, J. Gonzalez-Alonso, and E.F. Coyle (1995). Fluid and carbohydrate ingestion independently improve performance during 1 h of intense exercise. *Med. Sci. Sports Exerc.* 27: 200–210.

Bergstrom J., and E. Hultman (1966). The effect of exercise on muscle glycogen and electrolytes in normals. *Scand. J. Clin. Invest.* 18:16–20.

Blom, P.C., A.T. Hostmark, O. Vaage, K.R. Vardal, and S. Maehlum (1987). Effect of different post-exercise sugar diets on the rate of muscle glycogen synthesis. *Med. Sci. Sports Exerc.* 19:491–496.

Bosch, A.N., S.C. Dennis, and T.D. Noakes (1994). Influence of carbohydrate ingestion on fuel substrate turnover and oxidation during prolonged exercise. *J. Appl. Physiol.* 76(6):2364–2372.

Brouns, F., W.H.M. Saris, and E. Beckers (1989). Metabolic changes induced by sustained exhaustive cycling and diet manipulation. *Int. J. Sports Med.* 10:S49–S62.

Bulow, J., and J. Madsen (1981). Influence of blood flow on fatty acid mobilization from lipolytically active adipose tissue. *Pflügers Arch.* 390:169–174.

Burke, L.M., G.R. Collier, S.K. Beasley, P.R. Davis, P.A. Fricker, P. Heeley, K. Walder, and M. Hargreaves (1995). Effect of coingestion of fat and protein with carbohydrate feedings on muscle glycogen storage. *J. Appl. Physiol.* 78(6):2187–2192.

Burke, L.M., G.R. Collier, and M. Hargreaves (1993). Muscle glycogen storage after prolonged exercise: effect of the glycemic index of carbohydrate feedings. *J. Appl. Physiol.* 75(2):1019–23.

Coggan, A.R., and E.F. Coyle (1991). Carbohydrate ingestion during prolonged exercise: effects on metabolism and performance. *Exerc. Sport Sci. Rev.* 19:1–40.

Coggan, A.R., and E.F. Coyle (1988). Effect of carbohydrate feedings during high-intensity exercise. *J. Appl. Physiol.* 65:1703–1709.

Coggan, A.R., and E.F. Coyle (1989). Metabolism and peformance following carbohydrate ingestion late in exercise. *Med. Sci. Sports Exerc.* 21:59–65.

Coggan, A.R., and E.F. Coyle (1987). Reversal of fatigue during prolonged exercise by carbohydrate infusion or ingestion. *J. Appl. Physiol.* 63:2388–2395.

Coggan, A.R., W.M. Kohrt, R.J. Spina, D.M. Bier, and J.O. Holloszy (1990). Endurance training decreases plasma glucose turnover and oxidation during moderate-intensity exercise in men. *J. Appl. Physiol.* 68:990–996.

Conus, N.M., S. Fabris, J. Proietto, and M. Hargreaves (1996). Preexercise glucose ingestion and glucose kinetics during exercise. *J. Appl. Physiol.* 81(2):000-000 (in press).

Costill, D.F., E.F. Coyle, G. Dalsky, W. Evans, W. Fink, and D. Hoopes. (1977) Effects of elevated plasma FFA and insulin on muscle glycogen usage during exercise. *J. Appl. Physiol.* 43: 695–699.

Costill, D.L., M.G. Flynn, J.P. Kirwan, J.A. Houmard, J.B. Mitchell, R. Thomas, and S.H. Park (1988). Effects of repeated days of intensified training on muscle glycogen and swimming performance. *Med. Sci. Sports Exerc.* 20:249–254.

Costill, D.L., W.M. Sherman, W.J. Fink, C. Maresh, M. Witten, and J.M. Miller (1981). The role of dietary carbohydrates in muscle glycogen resynthesis after strenuous running. *Am. J. Clin. Nutr.* 34:1831–1836.

Coyle, E.F., and S.J. Montain (1992). Carbohydrate and fluid ingestion during exercise: are there trade-offs? *Med. Sci. Sports Exerc.* 24(6):671–678.

Coyle, E.F., A.R. Coggan, M.K. Hemmert, and J.L. Ivy (1986). Muscle glycogen utilization during prolonged strenuous exercise when fed carbohydrate. *J. Appl. Physiol.* 61:165–172.

Coyle, E.F., A.R. Coggan, M.K. Hemmert, R.C. Lowe, and T.J. Walters (1985). Substrate usage during prolonged exercise following a preexercise meal. *J. Appl. Physiol.* 59(2):429–433.

Coyle, E.F., A.R. Coggan, M.K. Hopper, and T.J. Walters (1988). Determinants of endurance in well-trained cyclists. *J. Appl. Physiol.* 64:2622–2630.

Coyle, E.F., J.M. Hagberg, B.F. Hurley, W.H. Martin, A.A. Ehsani, and J.O. Holloszy (1983). Carbohydrate feedings during prolonged strenuous exercise can delay fatigue. *J. Appl. Physiol.* 55:230–235.

Crapo, P.A., G. Reaven, and J. Olefsky (1977). Postprandial plasma glucose and insulin responses to different complex carbohydrates. *Diabetes.* 26(12):1178–1183.

Devlin, J.T., J. Calles-Escandon, and E.S. Horton (1986). Effects of preexercise snack feeding on endurance cycle exercise. *J. Appl. Physiol.* 60(3):980–985.

Doyle, J.A., W.M. Sherman, and R.L. Strauss (1993). Effects of eccentric and concentric exercise on muscle glycogen replenishment. *J. Appl. Physiol.* 74(4):1848–1855.

Dyck, D.J., S.A. Peters, P.S. Wendling, A. Chesley, E. Hultman, and L.L. Spriet (1996). Regulation of muscle glycogen phosphorylase activity during intense aerobic cycling with elevated FFA. *Am. J. Physiol.* 265(Endocrinol. Metab. 33):E116–E125.

Dyck, D.J., C.T. Putman, G.J. Heigenhauser, E. Hultman, and L.L. Spriet (1993). Regulation of fat-carbohydrate interaction in skeletal muscle during intense aerobic cycling. *Am. J. Physiol.* 265(Endocrinol. Metab. 33):E852–E859.

Elayan, I.M., and W.W. Winder (1991). Effect of glucose infusion on muscle malonyl-CoA during exercise. *J. Appl. Physiol.* 70(4):1495–1499.

Fielding, R.A., D.L. Costill, W.J. Fink, D.S. King, M. Hargreaves, and J.E. Kovaleski (1985). Effect of carbohydrate feeding frequency and dosage on muscle glycogen use during exercise. *Med. Sci. Sports Exerc.* 17:472–476.

Fielding, R.A., D.L. Costill, W.J. Fink, D.S. King, J.E. Kovaleski, and J.P. Kirwan (1987). Effects of preexercise carbohydrate feedings on muscle glycogen use during exercise in well-trained runners. *Eur. J. Appl. Physiol.* 56:225–229.

Flynn, M.G., D.L. Costill, J.A. Hawley, W.J. Fink, P.D. Neufer, R.A. Fielding, and M.D. Sleeper (1987). Influence of selected carbohydrate drinks on cycling performance and glycogen use. *Med. Sci. Sports Exerc.* 19:37–40.

Foster, C., D.L. Costill, and W.J. Fink (1979). Effects of pre-exercise feedings on endurance performance. *Med. Sci. Sports* 11:1–5.

Foster, C., N. Thompson, J. Dean, and D. Kirkendall (1986). Carbohydrate supplementation and performance in soccer players. *Med. Sci. Sports Exerc.* 18, S12.

Gatti, E., G. Testolin, D. Noe, F. Brighenti, G.P. Buzzetti, M. Porrino, and C.R. Sirtori (1987). Plasma glucose and insulin responses to carbohydrate food (rice) with different thermal processsing. *Ann. Nutr. Metab.* 31:296–303.

Gleeson, M., R.J. Maughan, and P.L. Greenhaff (1986). Comparison of the effects of preexercise feedings of glucose, glycerol and placebo on endurance and fuel homeostasis in man. *Eur. J. Appl. Physiol.* 55:645–653.

Goddard, M.S., G. Young, and R. Marcus (1984). The effect of amylose content on insulin and glucose responses to ingested rice. *Am. J. Clin. Nutr.* 39:388–392.

Guezennec, C.Y., P. Satabin, F. Duforez, D. Merino, F. Peronnet, and J. Koziet (1989). Oxidation of corn starch, glucose, and fructose ingested before exercise. *Med. Sci. Sports Exer.* 21(1):45–50.

Hargreaves, M., and C.A. Briggs (1988). Effect of carbohydrate ingestion on exercise metabolism. *J. Appl. Physiol.* 65:1553–5.

Hargreaves, M., D.L. Costill, W.J. Fink, D.S. King, and R.A. Fielding (1987). Effect of preexercise carbohydrate feedings on endurance cycling performance. *Med. Sci. Sports Ex.* 19:33–6.

Hargreaves, M., D.L. Costill, A. Katz, W.J. Fink (1985). Effect of fructose ingestion on muscle glycogen usage during exercise. *Med. Sci. Sports Exerc.* 17:360–3.

Hargreaves, M., B. Kiens, and E.A. Richter (1991). Effect of increased plasma free fatty acid concentrations on muscle metabolism in exercising men. *J. Appl. Physiol.* 70(1):194–201.

Helge, J.W., E.A. Richter, and B. Kiens (1996). Interaction of training and diet on metabolism and endurance during exercise in man. *J. Physiol. (Lond.)* 492: 293–306.

Hodgetts, A., S.W. Coppack, K.N. Frayn, and T.D.R. Hockaday (1991). Factors controlling fat mobilization from human subcutaneous adipose tissue during exercise. *J. Appl. Physiol.* 71:445–51.

Holloszy, J.O., and E.F. Coyle (1984). Adaptations of skeletal muscle to endurance exercise and their metabolic consequences. *J. Appl. Physiol.* 56(4):831–8.

Horowitz, .JF., and E.F. Coyle (1993). Metabolic responses to preexercise meals containing various carbohydrates and fat. *Am. J. Clin. Nutr.* 58:235–41.

Hurley, B.F., P.M. Nemeth, W.H. Martin III, J.M. Hagberg, G.P. Dalsky, and J.O. Holloszy (1986). Muscle triglyceride utilization during exercise: effect of training. *J. Appl. Physiol.* 60:562–7.

Ivy, J.L., A.L. Katz, C.L. Cutler, W.M. Sherman, and E.F. Coyle (1988). Muscle glycogen synthesis after exercise: effect of time of carbohydrate ingestion. *J. Appl. Physiol.* 65:1480–5.

Ivy, J.L., M.C. Lee, J.T. Brozinick Jr., and M.J. Reed (1988). Muscle glycogen storage after different amounts of carbohydrate ingestion. *J. Appl. Physiol.* 65:2018–23.

Jarvis, J.K., D. Pearsall, C.M. Oliner, and D.A. Schoeller (1992). The effect of food matrix on carbohydrate utilization during moderate exercise. *Med. Sci. Sports Exerc.* 24(3):320–6.

Jenkins, D.J.A., T.M.D. Wolever, A.L. Jenkins, R.G. Josse, and G.S. Wong (1984). The glycemic response to carbohydrate foods. *Lancet.* 2:388–91.

Jenkins, D.J.A., T.M.S. Wolever, G. Buckley, et al. (1988). Low-glycemic-index starchy foods in the diabetic diet. *Am. J. Clin. Nutr.* 48:248–54.

Jensen, M.D., M. Caruso, V. Heiling, and J.M Miles (1989). Insulin regulation of lypolysis in nondiabetic and IDDM subjects. *Diabetes.* 38:1595–1601.

Jeukendrup, A.E., W.H.M. Saris, P. Schrauwen, F. Brouns and A.J.M. Wagenmakers (1995). Metabolic availability of medium-chaim triglycerides coingested with carbohydrate during prolonged exercise. *J. Appl. Physiol.* 79:756–762.

Keizer, H.A., H. Kuipers, G. Van Kranenburg, and P. Geurten (1986). Influence of liquid and solid meals on muscle glycogen resynthesis, plasma fuel hormone response, and maximal physical working capacity. *Int. J. Sports Med.* 8:99–104.

Keller, K., and R. Schwarzkopf (1984). Preexercise snacks may decrease exercise performance. *Physician Sportsmed.* 12:89–91.

Kiens, B., B. Essen-Gustavsson, N.J. Christensen, and B. Saltin (1993). Skeletal muscle substrate utilization during submaximal exercise in man: effect of endurance training. *J. Physiol. (London)* 469:459–478.

Kirwan, J.P., D.L. Costill, J.B. Mitchell, J.A. Houmard, M.G. Glynn, W.J. Fink, and J.D. Beltz (1988). Carbohydrate balance in competitive runners during successive days of intense training. *J. Appl. Physiol.* 65(6):2601–6.

Klein, S., E.F. Coyle, and R.R. Wolfe (1994). Fat metabolism during low-intensity exercise in endurance-trained and untrained men. *Am. J. Physiol.* 267(Endocrinol. Metab. 30):E934–E940.

Klein, S., J.M. Weber, E.F. Coyle, and R.R. Wolfe (1996). Effect of endurance training on glycerol kinetics during strenuous exercise. *Metabolism.* 45:357–361.

Knudsen, J. (1990). Acyl-CoA-binding proteins (ACBP) and its relation to fatty acid-binding protein (FABP): An overview. *Mol. Cell. Biochem.* 98(1-2):217–23.

Koivisto, V.A., M. Harkonen, S. Karonen, P.H. Groop, R.A. Elovainio, E. Ferrannini, and R.A. DeFronzo (1985). Glycogen depletion during prolonged exercise: influence of glucose, fructose or placebo. *J. Appl. Physiol.* 58:7341–737.

Koubi, H.E., D. Desplanches, C. Gabrielle, J.M. Cottet-Emard, B. Sempore, and R.J. Favier (1991). Exercise endurance and fuel utilization: a reevaluation of the effects of fasting. *J. Appl. Physiol.* 70(3):1337–43.

Lambert, E.V., D.P. Speechly, S.C. Dennis, and T.D. Noakes (1994). Enhanced endurance in trained cyclists during moderate-intensity exercise following 2 weeks adaptation to a high-fat diet. *Eur J Appl Physiol.* 69(4):287–93.

Lapachet, R.B.A., W.C. Miller, and D.A. Arnal (1996). Body fat and exercise endurance in trained rats adapted to a high-fat and/or high-carbohydrate diet. *J. Appl. Physiol.* 80:1173–1179.

Levine, L., W.J. Evans, B.S. Cadarette, E.C. Fisher, and B.A. Bullen (1983). Fructose and glucose ingestion and muscle glycogen use during submaximal exercise. *J. Appl. Physiol.* 55:1767–71.

Loy, S.F., R.K. Conlee, W.W. Winder, A.G. Nelson, D.A. Arnall, and A.G. Fisher (1986). Effects of 24-h fast on cycling endurance time at two different intensities. *J. Appl. Physiol.* 61(2):654–9.

Mackie, B.G., G.A. Dudley, H. Kaciuba-Uscilko, and R.L. Terjung (1980). Uptake of chylomicron triglycerides by contracting skeletal muscle in rats. *J. Appl. Physiol.* 49: 851–855.

Martin, W.H. III, G.P. Dalsky, B.F. Hurley, D.E. Mathews, D.M. Bier, J.M. Hagberg, M.A. Rogers, D.S. King, and J.O. Holloszy (1993). Effect of endurance training on plasma free fatty acid turnover and oxidation during exercise. *Am. J. Physiol.* 265(Endocrinol. Metab. 28):E708–14.

Mason, W.L., G. McConell, and M. Hargreaves (1993). Carbohydrate ingestion during exercise: liquid vs solid feedings. *Med Sci Sports Exerc.* 25(8):966–9.

Massicotte, D., F. Peronnet, G. Brisson, K. Bakkouch, and C. Hilliare-Marcel (1989). Oxidation of a glucose polymer during exercise: comparison of glucose and fructose. *J. Appl. Physiol.* 66:179–83.

McConell, G., S. Fabris, J. Proietto, and M. Hargreaves (1994). Effect of carbohydrate ingestion on glucose kinetics during exercise. *J. Appl. Physiol.* 77(3):1537–41.

McGarry, J.D., M.J. Stark, and D.W. Foster (1978). Hepatic malonyl-CoA levels of fed, fasted, and diabetic rats as measured using a simple radioisotopic assay. *J. Biol. Chem.* 253:8291–3.

McMurray, R.G., J.R. Wilson, B.S. Kitchell (1983). The effects of fructose and glucose on high intensity endurance performance. *Research Q.* 54:156–62.

Mitchell, J.B., D.L. Costill, J.A. Houmard, W.J. Fink, D.D. Pascoe, and D.R. Pearson (1989). Influence of carbohyrate dosage on exercise performance and glycogen metabolism. *J. Appl. Physiol.* 67:1843–9.

Montain, S.J., M.K. Hopper, A.R. Coggan, and E.F. Coyle (1991). Exercise metabolism at different time intervals after a meal. *J. Appl. Physiol.* 70(2):882–888.

Morgan, T.E., F.A. Short, and L.A. Cobb (1969). Effect of long-term exercise on skeletal muscle lipid composition. *Am. J. Physiol.* 216(1):82–86.

Mourot, J., P. Thouvenot, C. Couet, J.M. Antoine, A. Krobicka, and G. Debry (1988). Relationship between the rate of gastric emptying and glucose and insulin responses to starchy foods in young healthy adults. *Am. J. Clin. Nutr.* 48:1035–40.

Muckle, D.S. (1973). Glucose syrup ingestion and team performance in soccer. *British J. Sports Med.* 7:340–3.

Muoio, D.M., J.J. Leddy , P.J. Horvath, A.B. Awad, D.R. Pendergast (1994). Effect of dietary fat on metabolic adjustments to maximal VO$_2$ and endurance in runners. *Med Sci. Sports Exerc.* 26(1):81–88.

Murray, R., D.E. Eddy, T.W. Murray, J.G. Seifert, G.L. Paul, G.A. Halaby (1987). The effect of fluid and carbohydrate feedings during intermittent cycling exercise. *Med. Sci. Sports Exerc.* 19:597–604.

Murray, R., G.L. Paul, J.G. Seifert, and D.E. Eddy (1991). Responses to varying rates of carbohydrate ingestion during exercise. *Med. Sci. Sports Exerc.* 23(6):713–18.

Murray, R., G.L. Paul, J.G. Seifert, D.E. Eddy, and G.A. Halaby (1989a). The effects of glucose, fructose, and sucrose ingestion during exercise. *Med. Sci. Sports Exerc.* 21:275–82.

Murray, R., J.G. Siefert, D.E. Eddy, G.L. Paul, and G.A. Halaby (1989b) Carbohydrate feeding and exercise: effect of beverage carbohydrate content. *Eur. J. Appl. Physiol.* 59:152–8.

Neufer, P.D., D.L. Costill, W.J. Fink, J.P. Kirwan, R.A. Fielding, M.G. Flynn (1986). Effects of exercise and carbohydrate composition on gastric emptying. *Med. Sci. Sports Exerc.* 18:658–62.

Neufer, P.D., D.L. Costill, M.G. Flynn, J.P. Kirwan, J.B. Mitchell, and J. Houmard (1987). Improvements in exercise performance: effects of carbohydrate feedings and diet. *J. Appl. Physiol.* 62:983–8.

Noakes, T.F., E.V. Lambert, M.I. Lambert, P.S. McArthur, K.H. Myburgh, and A.J.S. Benadé (1988). Carbohydrate ingestion and muscle glycogen depletion during marathon and ultramarathon racing. *Eur. J. Appl. Physiol.* 57:482–9.

Ockner, R.K. (1990). Historical overview of studies on fatty acid-binding proteins. *Mol. Cell. Biochem.* 98(1–2):3–9.

O'Dea, K., P.J. Nestel, L. Antonoff (1980). Physical factors influencing postprandial glucose and insulin responses to starch. *Am. J. Clin. Nutr.* 33:760–5.

Okano, G., H. Takeda, I. Morita, M. Katoh, Z. Mu, and S. Miyake (1988). Effect of preexercise fructose ingestion on endurance performance in fed men. *Med. Sci. Sports Ex.* 20:105–9.

Oscai, L.B., D.A. Essig, and W.K. Palmer (1990). Lipase regulation of muscle triglyceride hydrolysis. *J. Appl. Physiol.* 69: 1571–1577.

Peden, C., W.M. Sherman, L. D'Aquisto, and D.A. Wright (1989). 1 h preexercise carbohydrate meals enhance performance. *Med. Sci. Sports Ex.* 21:S59.

Phinney, S.D., W.J. Bistrian, W.J. Evans, E. Gervino, and G.L. Blackburn (1983). The human metabolic response to chronic ketosis without caloric restriction: preservation of submaximal exercise capability with reduced carbohydrate oxidation. *Metabolism.* 32(8):769–776.

Price, T.B., D.L. Rothman, R. Taylor, M.J. Avison, G.I. Shulman, and R.G. Shulman (1994). Human muscle glycogen resynthesis after exercise: insulin-dependent and -independent phases. *J. Appl. Physiol.* 76(1):104–11.

Ravussin, E., C. Bogardus, K. Scheidegger, B. LaGrange, E.D. Horton, and E.S. Horton (1986). Effect of elevated FFA on carbohydrate and lipid oxidation during prolonged exercise in humans. *J. Appl. Physiol.* 60(3):893–900.

Reed, M.J., J.T. Brozinick Jr, M.C. Lee, and J.L. Ivy (1989). Muscle glycogen storage post exercise: effect of mode of carbohyrate administration. *J. Appl. Physiol.* 66:720–6.

Romijn, J.A., and R.R. Wolfe (1992). Effects of prolonged exercise on endogenous substrate supply and utilization. In: D.R. Lamb and C.V. Gisolfi (eds.) *Perspectives in Exercise Science and Sports Medicine Volume 5: Energy Metabolism in Exercise and Sport.* Dubuque: Brown & Benchmark, pp. 207–34.

Romijn, J.A., E.F. Coyle, L.S. Sidossis, A. Gastaldelli, J.F. Horowitz, E. Endert, and R.R. Wolfe (1993). Regulation of endogenous fat and carbohydrate metabolism in relation to exercise intensity and endurance. *Am. J. Physiol.* 265 (Endocrinol. Metab. 28):E380–E391.

Romijn, J.A., E.F. Coyle, L.S. Sidossis, X.-J. Zhang, and R.R. Wolfe (1995). Relationship between fatty acid delivery and fatty acid oxidation during strenuous exercise. *J. Appl. Physiol.* 79:1939–1945.

Sherman, W.M., G. Brodowicz, D.A. Wright , W.K. Allen, J. Simonsen, and A. Dernbach (1989). Effects of 4 h preexercise carbohydrate feedings on cycling performance. *Med. Sci. Sports Ex.* 21:598–604.

Sherman, W.M., D.L. Costill, W.J. Fink, and J.M. Miller (1981). The effect of exercise and diet manipulation on muscle glycogen and its subsequent utilization during performance. *Int. J. Sports Med.* 2:114–8.

Simard, C., A. Tremblay, and M. Jobin (1988). Effects of carbohydrate intake before and during an ice hockey match on blood and muscle energy substrates. *Res. Quart. Exerc. Sport* 59:144–7.

Simonsen, J.C., W.M. Sherman, D.R. Lamb, A.R. Dernbach, J.A. Doyle, and R. Strauss (1991). Dietary carbohydrate, muscle glycogen, and power during rowing training. *J. Appl. Physiol.* 70: 1500–1505.

Slentz, C.A., J.M. Davis, D.L. Settles, R.R. Pate, S.J. Settles (1990). Glucose feedings and exercise in rats: glycogen use, hormone responses, and performance. *J. Appl. Physiol.* 69(3):989–94.

Terjung, R.L., B.G. Mackie, G.A. Dudley, and H. Kaciuba-Uscilko (1983). Influence of exercise on chylomicron triacylglycerol metabolism: plasma turnover and muscle uptake. *Med. Sci. Sports Exerc.* 15:340–347.

Tsintzas, K., R. Liu, C. Williams, I. Campbell, and G. Gaitanos (1993). The effect of carbohydrate ingestion on performance during a 30-km race. *Inter. J. Sport Nutr.* 3(2):127–39.

Tsintzas, K., C. Williams, L. Boobis, and P. Greenhaff (1995). Carbohydrate ingestion and glycogen utilization in different muscle fiber types. *J. Physiol.* 489:243–250.

Vukovich, M.D., D.L. Costill, M.S. Hickey, S.W. Trappe, K.J. Cole, and W.J. Fink (1993). Effect of fat emulsion infusion and fat feeding on muscle glycogen utilization during cycle exercise. *J. Appl. Physiol.* 75: 1513–1518.

Wagenmakers, A.J., F. Brouns, W.H. Saris, and D. Halliday (1993). Oxidation rates of orally ingested carbohydrates during prolonged exercise in men. *J. Appl. Physiol.* 75(6):2774–80.

Walberg-Rankin, J. (1995). Dietary carbohydrate as an ergogenic aid for prolonged and brief competitions in sport. *Int. J. Sport Nutr.* 5 Suppl:S13–28.

Westphal, S.A., M.C. Gannon, and F. Nuttall (1990). Metabolic response to glucose ingested with various amounts of protein. *Am. J. Clin. Nutr.* 52:267–72.

Wright, D.A., W.M. Sherman, and A.R. Dernbach (1991). Carbohydrate feedings before, during, or in combination improve cycling endurance performance. *J. Appl. Physiol.* 71:1082–8.

Wursch, P., S. Del Vedovo, and B. Koellreutter. Cell structure and starch nature as key determinants of the digestion rate of starch in legume. *Am. J. Clin. Nutr.* 43:25–9.

Yaspelkis, B.B. III, J.G. Patterson, P.A. Anderla, Z. Ding, and J.L. Ivy (1993). Carbohydrate supplementation spares muscle glycogen during variable-intensity exercise. *J. Appl. Physiol.* 75(4):1477–85.

DISCUSSION

HARGREAVES: In addition to promoting muscle glycogen storage, it is worth mentioning that another advantage of high-carbohydrate diets in the recovery period is that they hasten recovery from exhaustion so that high-quality athletic performance can be resumed sooner. Also, would you discuss the role of muscle glycogen and increased glycogen availability during high-intensity exercise?

COYLE: With intermittent high-intensity exercise, glycogen will be the predominant source for resynthesizing ATP. Thus, my recommendations regarding the amounts and types of carbohydrates to ingest after exercise definitely apply to high-intensity sports. One can markedly lower muscle glycogen levels by performing only 15–30 min of total exercise as 1–5 min repeat intervals at 90–115% $\dot{V}O_2$max. Athletes know that adoption of a hard/easy training schedule (i.e., one day of hard training followed by a day of easy training) often improves competitive results. I think much of the reason for this is that time is needed to resynthesize glycogen stores, even from only 15–30 min of intense interval training each day.

WILLIAMS: We have conducted a comprehensive set of experiments on intermittent exercise, which has involved cycle ergometry, treadmill running, and free running. We conduct our studies using an activity pattern based on the combination of activities seen in games such as field hockey, soccer, and rugby, each of which involves approximately 90 min of a combination of sprinting, jogging, and walking. During this intermittent high-intensity exercise, soccer players actually perform better with a carbohydrate-electrolyte drink than with a placebo solution. Biopsy results show less glycogen used in the carbohydrate-electrolyte trial than in the placebo trial. Much has been written on glycogen resynthesis; however, what the coach wants to know is whether or not the dietary advice for recovery works. We have addressed this particular question both with intermittent and prolonged exercise. Using the 90-min training session of intermittent exercise as a model, on one occasion we raised the carbohydrate intake from an average of about 5 g/kg body weight up to 8–9 g/kg over a 24-h recovery period. We found that those athletes who increased their carbohydrate intake were able to reproduce and improve on their 90-min performance 24 h later, whereas those who ate only their normal amount of carbohydrate and extra fat and protein to match the energy intake of the carbohydrate group could not reproduce their 90-min training session the next day.

Similarly, if the recovery period after 90 min of constant pace running is limited to only 4 h, and dehydration is minimized by having the runners consume the appropriate amount of fluid, we found that consuming about 50 g of carbohydrate (versus water only) immediately after exercise significantly enhanced the endurance capacity of the runners. However, when we increased the carbohydrate intake to about 3 g/kg body weight, there was no improvement in glycogen resynthesis nor in performance. Thus, carbohydrate intake in the recovery period does in fact work in a practical situation.

WALBERG-RANKIN: I hear a great deal from laypeople who want the inside scoop concerning the use of the 40-30-30 diet (40% carbohydrate, 30% fat, 30% protein). Please discuss this dietary approach, sometimes called "fat loading."

COYLE: Carbohydrate has certainly been well studied over the past 25 y, including the very practical studies of Mark Hargreaves, Louise Burke, Mike Sherman, and Dave Costill, who have shown that athletes need about 500 g of carbohydrate per day to resynthesize glycogen. Eating above 500 g/d does not promote extra glycogen resynthesis; the fate of the extra carbohydrate above 500 g is not certain. Is there room or even a need for adding something other than carbohydrate after an athlete has eaten 500 g/d? That's the major question. Would extra fat have any benefits, such as an additional resynthesis of intramuscular fat stores? We don't know the source of fat for the resynthesis of those intramuscular triglycerides. How much lipogenesis from carbohydrate can the body achieve? The current thinking is that the ability to make fat from dietary carbohydrate is very limited. Certainly it is limited as far as making VLDL triglycerides from dietary carbohydrate. However, we don't know much about other means for lipogenesis. I don't know of any data that justify the 40-30-30 diet. A diet of 40% carbohydrate would create enough of an insulin response to reduce endogenous FFA mobilization, probably to the same degree as a diet with a greater proportion of carbohydrate, so I doubt that a 40% carbohydrate diet improves the mobilization of endogenous fat. A 30% fat diet is relatively high in fat, and there is no evidence that people need that much fat, and the idea that 30% protein is needed for "good eicosinoids" is unsubstantiated.

WILLIAMS: I have a comment related to our search to find out how we can increase fat metabolism during exercise. If we look at the activity patterns of some of the aboriginal people who still populate the world, they engage in activity that consists mostly of prolonged low-intensity exercise, and fat is the best fuel for that type of activity. We may be genetically programmed for habitual activity that is low intensity and fat consuming. I don't think there was ever a golden age when we could burn fat at 85% of $\dot{V}O_2$max.

SPRIET: One practical way to manipulate fat mobilization at the start of exercise is by using caffeine. The evidence seems still fairly strong that caffeine does mobilize the exogenous fat stores and possibly the endogenous stores, albeit in a very short term period before exercise and at the start of exercise. This might be quite important in terms of deciding the mix of carbohydrate and fat early in exercise, when a lot of muscle glycogen is used.

COYLE: You've published studies showing how caffeine can reduce muscle glycogenolysis early in exercise, but I haven't seen any convincing evidence that caffeine has any effects on raising fat mobilization or fat oxidation in people. We have measured fatty acid mobilization with tracers and have not seen any effect of caffeine during exercise; caffeine raises FFA mobilization at rest, but has no effect on fat mobilization and oxidation after 20 min of exercise.

SPRIET: Terry Graham and colleagues have just done a study with arterial and femoral venous catheterization demonstrating that caffeine ingestion 1 h before exercise produced an early but transient large lipolytic effect in the arterial blood. In the non-caffeine trial exercise began with FFA concentrations about 0.4 µM, and in the caffeine trial FFA levels were about 0.8-0.9 µM; this difference was no longer apparent by the 10 min mark. In the first 10 min of the exercise the muscles apparently utilized the extra store of fat that was accumulated in the plasma during the preexercise hour following the caffeine ingestion. The mass of extra fat used is small, but when it is translated into energy, it becomes very important if an equivalent amount of energy as carbohydrate is spared. However, these results should be corroborated with tracer studies.

COYLE: So you see no effect after 10 min of exercise? Our studies have made measurements with the isotopes after 10 min, and we see no effect of caffeine, so we agree. The question is what is happening during the first 10 min?

SPRIET: The reason we are concentrating on the first 10-15 min is that it looks like that is the time during which there are changes in regulators that might be important in attenuating the activities of key enzymes of the glycolytic pathway when fat metabolism is increased.

WALBERG-RANKIN: I am interested in the applicability of the glycemic index of foods consumed just before or after exercise. There has been only limited research on this topic. For example, Louise Burke and colleagues reported that high-glycemic-index foods fed after exercise were superior for muscle glycogen replacement to foods having a lower glycemic index, but in a subsequent study from their laboratory, the total amount of carbohydrate—not the glycemic index—seemed to be critical to muscle glycogen replacement. John Ivy's lab studied a protein-carbohydrate combination compared to carbohydrate alone on glycogen resynthesis and reported that the addition of protein to carbohydrate, which would tend to reduce the glycemic index relative to carbohydrate alone, enhanced glycogen resynthesis. Should we recommend high-glycemic-index foods after exercise? Theoretically, it would make sense to eat foods having a lower glycemic index to induce a more prolonged elevation of blood glucose throughout exercise with a lower insulin response. This would allow plasma fatty acids to rise during exercise and would also provide continuous blood glucose for oxidation.

COYLE: The glycemic index, I think, is a step in the right direction of quantifying the rates of digestion and glucose availability, but it is not perfect. If one adds protein to a carbohydrate meal, a slightly higher insulin response may occur, and that may be better for resynthesizing glycogen to a small extent. Perhaps the next step should be to factor in the insulinemic index along with the glycemic index, with the result being some sort of glycogen-resynthesis index. So the glycemic index is a first step, but it certainly does not answer all of our questions about the relative importance of various carbohydrates for the athlete's diet.

Using the glycemic index to recommend preexercise feedings is a very complex area. My thinking is that carbohydrate should be ingested before exercise largely in an attempt to maintain a normal concentration of glucose in the blood throughout exercise; it's after 2–3 h of exercise that a high rate of glucose entry into the circulation is needed. However, a better way to maintain glucose is to ingest carbohydrate throughout exercise; an athlete does not have to rely on preexercise feedings to do that. So practically speaking, I don't know why a nutritionist or dietician would develop a diet program based on preexercise carbohydrate ingestion if carbohydrate can be consumed during exercise.

WALBERG-RANKIN: There would be some sports and exercise situations where the athlete would not have access to food and drink.

COYLE: It's hard to make a general recommendation for all situations except that the athlete should consume a relatively large amount of carbohydrate (i.e., more than 100 g). For example, Sherman et al. at Ohio State successfully fed 300 g of carbohydrates to cyclists during the 4 h before exercise. That's a lot of food to be ingesting, but the idea is to eat enough before exercise to allow the athlete to maintain a normal concentration of blood glucose throughout exercise; presumably, this will help the athlete to continue to oxidize glucose.

WALBERG-RANKIN: Most research that has lead to these recommendations to ingest large quantities of carbohydrates was conducted with male subjects. How applicable are the absolute gram quantities for women? For example, for a 60 kg female, 10 g of carbohydrate per kg body weight in a meal would be 2,400 kcal, and this is more energy than many women would eat on an average day.

COYLE: You raise a very important point. We recommend that 500-600 g of carbohydrate (2,000–2,400 kcal)be ingested to recover from only 30 min of hard training that expends only 800 kcal of energy. If one does this day after day, fat storage seems likely. Athletes who have tried to follow my advice have come back to me and said, "I'm fat," and they were right. These "recovery" diets should not be consumed every single day. My opinion is that an athlete should eat large amounts of carbohydrate only on the days before the most intense training. The athletes must decide what two or three days per week in their training that are most important. They should get a good night's sleep before each of those days and eat a high-carbohydrate diet to maximize glycogen. Before the easier days of training, less energy should be consumed to balance the high-energy consumption days and to minimize fat storage.

The athlete can't just keep training the same and eating the same things all the time.

SPRIET: There is the potential that there will eventually be large differences in the recommendations on carbohydrate intake for women compared to men. There are now at least two studies that have shown that the ability to glycogen supercompensate in well-trained women is not comparable to that of men. Therefore, the recommendation that women should be taking in 75% carbohydrate when they consume about 2,000 kcal/d may in fact leave them rather short in terms of dietary protein and fat. It is important to determine whether women rely more on fat at certain submaximal power intensities than do men.

SPRIET: In most preexercise feeding studies, it seems to be assumed that the default metabolic situation is fasting prior to exercise, but in the real world athletes are typically ingesting reasonable amounts of carbohydrate in the hours preceding exercise. I wonder whether this concern changes some of your interpretations of the literature on preexercise feedings. For example, basal rates of lipolysis after fasting are quite high (e.g., leading to a plasma FFA concentration of approximately 1 mM), whereas they would be much lower after eating. Are the changes in lipolysis during carbohydrate feeding the same under both conditions? I don't think so. We need to keep the effect of prolonged fasting in mind when we interpret the results of carbohydrate-feeding studies.

COYLE: Fasting has been part of the typical experimental paradigm. We have been doing more recent studies with preexercise carbohydrate feedings, which obviously reduce the oxidation of fat, both from plasma FFA and from intramuscular triglyceride stores.

SPRIET: Some people might see carbohydrate feedings during exercise in a negative light because they decreases the amount of fat oxidized, but this concern is reduced following a preexercise carbohydrate feeding because a higher percentage of carbohydrate would be oxidized right from the beginning of the exercise, which I would argue would be the more normal situation.

SHI: The oxidation of medium chain triglycerides (MCT) increases when carbohydrate is co-ingested. Could you explain the mechanism of this carbohydrate-induced increase of MCT oxidation?

COYLE: When MCT are added to carbohydrate, MCT appear to increase the rate of gastric emptying of the carbohydrate. The rates of glucose appearance into blood at rest may be higher when you add MCT to carbohydrate. It is a strange phenomenon if true. It also appears that the oxidation of the MCT is increased by adding carbohydrate to the MCT. It makes sense that if MCT are going to be ingested, they should be ingested with carbohydrate. The question now is, do MCT add enough substrate to affect metabolism or reduce reliance on other fuels like glycogen. The MCT appear to be readily oxidized, but most people can't tolerate more than about 25 g of MCT without experiencing severe gastrointestinal problems, including abdominal cramps and diarrhea. Thus people just don't seem to be able to tolerate enough MCT energy, at least in one large feeding, for MCT to add enough energy to significantly reduce the oxidation of glycogen. Can one learn to tolerate more MCT? Will a diet chronically high in MCT be of benefit? These are still open questions in my mind. There may be other sources of triglyceride similar to MCT that can be readily absorbed and provide fatty acids for oxidation by muscle.

SPRIET: If you look around for other fuels to use for exercise, an obvious choice would be acetate. Acetate crosses the muscle membrane quickly and crosses the mitochondrial membrane, so why haven't we evolved to the point where we use it during exercise? It is unfortunate because it is clear that when you consume acetate, you can get it into the plasma, and you can get it into the muscle, but something during exercise limits its use. It may be that the activity of the enzyme that converts it to a acetyl-CoA is not high enough. It brings us back to the point that Clyde Williams brought up that it is clear that we are not designed to use fat at high intensities of exercise. On the other hand, there are other animals in the world that rely totally on fat at 85–95% $\dot{V}O_2$max.

COYLE: Human beings rely heavily upon glycogenolysis during high-intensity exercise. The increases in AMP and Pi levels in muscle stimulate enough glycogenolysis that somehow reduces the oxidation of fat. How that happens is not clear. My bias is that the increase in glycolytic flux may produce malonyl-CoA and a reduced transport of long-chain fatty acids. Whether that happens in human beings is debatable; for example, Odland et al. (1996) showed no increase in malonyl-CoA in people.

GISOLFI: I think the mechanism for the rise in blood glucose after ingesting MCT with carbohydrate is that the MCT increases water absorption, which in turn increases luminal glucose concentration and glucose uptake. Related to this issue, would you comment on the observation that ingesting two different forms of carbohydrate, glucose and fructose, increases carbohydrate oxidation when compared with ingesting the same quantity of glucose or the same quantity of fructose?

COYLE: I suspect you believe that the co-transport or the increased transport of different sugars by numerous transporters in the intestines may be partially responsible for the increase in carbohydrate oxidation. How much the liver is involved in all of this is an open question because the glucose and fructose that are absorbed in the portal circulation must first escape and bypass the liver before appearing in the circulation for oxidation. How that is affected by the different sugars that are being presented to the intestine and liver (fructose vs. glucose) is unclear.

EICHNER: Costill and Sherman and others have shown that ultrastructural muscle damage in runners may slow glycogen restocking. When Costill and Morgan suddenly doubled the training load in swimmers, those with low muscle glycogen didn't perform as well, but that seemed related more to low dietary carbohydrate than to muscle damage. Recently, Anne Snyder and others reported in skaters that, in the face of muscle damage, high-carbohydrate diets don't seem as energizing. How firm is that field; how much muscle damage does it take to impair glycogen restocking; and are there practical tips on how and when to eat to repair or prevent chronically sore muscles?

COYLE: I don't know of any studies that have been done to develop any practical tips to minimize these problems. Certainly Sherman and Costill showed that in the postmarathon period there is an impaired glycogen synthesis and muscle damage. What are the best diets for coping with this? I don't know. My practical approach would be first to try to prevent the soreness and injury by reducing the training volume and/or intensity. Whether this approach works or not is another question.

DISHMAN: It is fair to assume there is more variability in performance than there is in substrate availability, certainly in some circumstances. Is there any literature that examines individual differences and responsiveness of subjects to these dietary manipulations that could explain part of the performance variability? I'm thinking of subjective responses such as mood or perceived exertion.

COYLE: People differ in how responsive or sensitive they are to falling blood glucose concentrations. I think that hypoglycemia below 3 mM has a physiological effect on the brain that carries over to other aspects of physiology and performance. In our studies, we use very motivated cyclists; we push them to the physiological end points of muscle fatigue. That doesn't mean that they aren't experiencing central nervous system sensations related to hypoglycemia. We are just pushing them beyond those symptoms to the point where there are additional causes of fatigue, including a lack of energy supply to the muscles. Some times we have undoubtedly lost sight of the central-nervous-system effects of hypoglycemia with our heavy focus on the muscle.

DISHMAN: Anecdotally, champion athletes have been quoted as saying one of the keys to success is the ability to recover each day after an event that leaves the athlete feeling totally wiped out. We descriptively studied this phenomenon with performers on the Tour de France, and there is clearly a relationship between the performance on the Tour and the subjective responses. I'm not proposing that this observation was independent of diet or glycogen replacement, but it seems that the interaction of diet, substrate availability, and subjective responses is very ripe for experimental research. Certainly, the study of diet and performance that excludes the effects of diet on the central nervous system is an incomplete approach.

COYLE: Diet is probably having more effects than just resynthesizing muscle glycogen, and some of those effects may occur in the brain.

NIEMAN: Have you noticed a difference in the effects of dietary carbohydrate manipulations when you study runners versus cyclists? The reason I bring this up is that we have run 60 marathoners in our lab for 2.5–3.0 h, and it is rare to see a drop in their blood glucose concentrations. With cycling it seems to be more common. Has that been your observation?

COYLE: We haven't made direct comparisons of runners and cyclists. Clyde Williams has studied mostly runners and not cyclists.

WILLIAMS: We have the same experience with blood glucose that David Neiman described (i.e., blood glucose falls more in cyclists than in runners).

COYLE: Tim Noakes and colleagues measured glucose use and blood glucose turnover in runners and cyclists and found that cyclists relied more heavily upon carbohydrate than did runners during exercise at a certain intensity. Surprisingly, they didn't see differences in the blood glucose turnover. That is the only study I know of that has made direct comparisons. But you are right, it seems as though runners, compared to cyclists have a smaller decline in blood glucose.

NIEMAN: Do you think that cyclists need to be more careful than runners in replenishing carbohydrate during exercise?

COYLE: Possibly. However, Clyde Williams' work has shown that carbohydrate feedings delay fatigue and improve performance in runners in generally the same way and to the same extent as in cyclists, so carbohydrate ingestion seems to be important for both runners and cyclists.

4

Optimizing Hydration for Competitive Sport

R.J. Maughan, Ph.D.

INTRODUCTION
THERMOREGULATION AND FLUID BALANCE
    Exercise and Temperature Regulation
    Effects of Manipulation of Body Temperature on Exercise Performance
    Effects of Ambient Temperature on Exercise Performance
    Hydration Status and Exercise Performance
    Effects of Fluid Ingestion on Performance
    Possible Mechanisms of Reduced Exercise Tolerance in the Heat
LIMITATIONS TO FLUID REPLACEMENT
    Gastric Emptying
    Intestinal Absorption
    Tracer Methods
    Effects of Exercise on Gastrointestinal Function
PREEXERCISE HYDRATION
POSTEXERCISE REHYDRATION
FORMULATION OF REHYDRATION FLUIDS
    Balancing Water and Carbohydrate Provision
    Water Overload and Hyponatremia
PRACTICAL IMPLICATIONS FOR THE ATHLETE
BIBLIOGRAPHY
DISCUSSION

INTRODUCTION

Many major sports events—the 1994 Soccer World Cup, the 1996 Olympic Games—are often held in hot humid climates, are conducted in the summer months, and are frequently scheduled for the hottest part of the day. No doubt remains that exercise tolerance is impaired in most types of activity in these conditions, yet the athlete has no choice but to

139

compete. All athletes will be affected, but the athlete who has prepared by a period of acclimatization to these conditions, and who has a clear rehydration strategy, is likely to be least affected. Although these preparations are not a substitute for talent, training, or motivation, they are prerequisites if the individual is to realize his or her potential.

The recognition that adequate hydration is essential for the maintenance of health as well as for exercise performance stretches back to antiquity. Scientific investigation has allowed the physiological basis of this requirement to be understood, at least in part, and studies over the course of this century have clearly established the need for an adequate fluid intake before, during, and after exercise if performance is to be optimized. In spite of this, however, it is depressingly common to find athletes who never drink in training, and even some who deliberately restrict fluid intake during training in the erroneous belief that they can adapt; others, either intentionally or inadvertently, arrive at the start of competition in a hypohydrated state. It seems inexcusable that gifted and motivated athletes who have devoted years of effort to preparation should make these errors, and there has clearly been a failure to communicate the results of scientific research to these athletes and their coaches. Although many unanswered questions remain, it is probably fair to say that communication of the available information remains the biggest barrier to minimizing the decrements in performance that occur as a result of inadequate hydration.

This review will focus on recent developments in the area of fluid balance and exercise performance and will be concerned especially with the development of optimum rehydration strategies for athletes. Where there are unreferenced statements, substantiation will generally be found in one of the earlier extensive reviews published in this field. A full appreciation of fluid balance and exercise performance requires an understanding of the need for replacement of fluid and electrolytes, as well as of carbohydrate, in different exercise situations and of the factors that influence the fate of ingested fluids. In particular, the review will be concerned with the following:

1. The factors that influence fluid loss in exercise, including the effects of environmental conditions and of exercise intensity and duration. These factors determine the need for provision of water, electrolytes, and substrate before, during, and after exercise.
2. The effects of hyperthermia, hypohydration, and fluid replacement on exercise performance.
3. The determinants of fluid replacement during exercise, including especially the processes of gastric emptying and intestinal absorption, but also issues relating to the voluntary consumption of fluids.

4. The practical issues that supervene when attempts are made to apply the available information to the sporting environment.

THERMOREGULATION AND FLUID BALANCE

Exercise and Temperature Regulation

Fluid loss during exercise is primarily a consequence of the need to maintain body temperature—or at least the temperature of the body core—within narrow limits. The resting oxygen consumption of the average man is about 250 mL/min, corresponding to a rate of metabolic heat production of about 70 W. The body exchanges heat with the environment, and heat is gained or lost depending on the temperature gradient between the skin and the environment. Because of the low thermal conductivity and low heat capacity of air, limited loss is possible in still air, but where there is a high air flow over the body surface, sufficient heat loss to balance the rate of metabolic heat production is possible. Heat loss is less of a problem in aquatic sports, but water temperature is critical. Thermoregulation is achieved in most situations by behavioral mechanisms (i.e., the amount of clothing worn is adjusted or the ambient temperature is changed so that the rate of heat production or heat gain is balanced by the rate of heat loss.) During exercise, the rate of heat production can be increased to many times the resting level. At very high power outputs, muscle temperature will rise markedly without major changes in body core temperature, but exercise duration is inevitably short, and it is not clear that core temperature will rise sufficiently to limit performance. The importance of maintaining muscle temperature within narrow limits has been discussed by Nadel (1983).

In sustained rhythmic exercise, muscle blood flow is high, and the rise in muscle temperature is limited by convective heat removal. In an event such as running on the level, the rate of heat production is determined primarily by running speed and body mass, with individual variations in mechanical and metabolic efficiency being of secondary importance. The elite marathon runner can achieve an oxygen consumption of 5 L/min or more, and highly trained athletes can sustain a power output of about 80% of this level (equivalent to 80 kJ/min (20 kcal/min)) for more than 2 h (Maughan & Leiper, 1983). Comparable levels of energy expenditure are achieved in cycling, rowing, and cross country skiing.

When the ambient temperature is higher than skin temperature, heat will also be gained from the environment by physical transfer, adding to the heat load on the body. In spite of this, marathon runners normally maintain body temperature within 2–3°C of the resting level, indicating that heat is being lost from the body almost as fast as it is being produced. The highest temperatures in exercising subjects have generally been observed in runners competing in events at distances of 10–15 km. For example, Sutton (1990) reported more than 30 cases where rectal temperature exceeded 42°C in competitors in a 14-km road race; in such conditions, heat illness and collapse are not uncommon. These observations indicate that a high absolute rate of heat production places the greatest stress on the thermoregulatory system.

At high ambient temperatures the only mechanism by which heat can be lost from the body is evaporation, and even at low ambient temperatures, high sweat rates are observed in some individuals (Maughan, 1985). Evaporation is an extremely effective heat loss mechanism, and evaporation of 1 L of water from the skin surface will remove 2.4 MJ (580 kcal) of heat from the body. For the 2.5 h marathon runner with a body mass of 70 kg to balance the rate of metabolic heat production by evaporative loss alone would, therefore, require sweat to be evaporated from the skin at a rate of about 1.6 L/h. At such high sweat rates, an appreciable fraction of the sweat secreted will drip from the skin without evaporating, so a sweat secretion rate of about 2 L/h is likely to be necessary to achieve a sufficient rate of evaporative heat loss. This is possible, but it would result in the loss of 5 L of body water, corresponding to a loss of more than 7% of body mass for a 70 kg runner. Typical body mass losses in marathon runners range from about 1-6% (0.7–4.2 kg) at low (10°C) ambient temperatures to more than 8% (5.6 kg) in warmer conditions (Maughan, 1985).

Sweat losses are determined by a number of factors. The exercise intensity and duration are crucial, but in most sports situations, the environmental temperature and humidity will play major roles. Although attention is focused most often on the environmental temperature, high humidity may pose more of a threat to the endurance athlete, as this will limit the rate of heat loss that can be achieved by evaporation of sweat. In climates such as that of Atlanta, the site of the 1996 Olympic Games, the combination of high temperature and high humidity is particularly problematical. There are large variations between individuals in the thermoregulatory response to exercise even when the environmental and exercise variables are similar (Havenith et al., 1995), and the sweating characteristics of the individual athlete are important when the need for fluid replacement is considered. Both sweat rate and sweat composition vary widely between individuals. The implications of this for replacement are discussed below.

Fluid losses are distributed in varying proportions among the plasma, extracellular water, and intracellular water. The decrease in plasma volume that accompanies dehydration may be of particular importance in influencing work capacity; blood flow to the muscles must be maintained at a high level to supply oxygen and substrates, but a substantial blood flow to the skin is also necessary to convect heat to the body surface where it can be dissipated (Nadel, 1980). When the ambient temperature is high and blood volume has been decreased by sweat loss during prolonged exercise, meeting the requirement for a high blood flow to both these tissues may be difficult. In this situation, skin blood flow is more likely to be compromised, allowing central venous pressure and muscle blood flow to be maintained but reducing heat loss and causing body temperature to rise sharply (Rowell, 1986).

Effects of Manipulation of Body Temperature on Exercise Performance

An understanding of the conditions under which performance is influenced by body temperature, and of the underlying mechanisms, helps to identify the situations where hydration status becomes a possible limitation to exercise performance. Although it has long been known that warm-up prior to exercise may enhance performance (Asmussen & Boje, 1945), it is equally clear that there is an optimum temperature above which a detrimental effect is observed. The process of warming up also has many effects other than simply those on muscle temperature, and these effects may confound the interpretation of studies. The effects of excessive warming up before competition on core temperature may have important implications for athletes competing in hot climates, as an elevated core temperature prior to exercise may result in an increased demand for sweat loss during exercise and may also predispose the athlete to heat illness.

Several investigations have shown that manipulation of the temperature of human limbs, usually by immersion in water at different temperatures, can influence the capacity for exercise performance. Because of the obvious practical difficulties, there are rather few similar studies with whole body exercise. In isometric contractions at high forces, muscle blood flow is reduced or absent. The ability to sustain submaximal isometric contractions of the forearm muscles is related to the pre-exercise muscle temperature, with the greatest duration being observed when the muscle temperature is about 27°C, compared with the normal resting value of about 34°C. Prior immersion in cold water to lower muscle and core temperature can also reduce performance in cycling exercise; this may be considered an abnormal stress for subjects accustomed to exercise, but does indicate the importance of muscle temperature for optimum performance. Cold air exposure (30 min at 5°C) has recently been shown to improve endurance by 21% in a treadmill run lasting less than 30 min; this was associated with an increased heat storage and lower sweat loss after pre-cooling (Lee & Haymes, 1995), and there are obvious implications of these procedures for the requirement for fluid replacement in exercise. As pointed out by Ethan Nadel (1980), however, these studies are never done with the subjects blinded to treatment, and this may confound the results.

In the exercising dog, cooling of the trunk with ice packs attenuates the rise in both muscle and rectal temperatures and extends exercise time by about 45% compared with the mean exercise time without cooling of 57 min (Kozlowski et al., 1985); this study was carried out at an ambient temperature of 20°C. Similar results have recently been observed in the exercising horse (Marlin, personal communication), but these procedures have not been applied to the human athlete, although they might interact with the need for fluid replacement.

Effects of Ambient Temperature on Exercise Performance

Many studies have investigated the effects of alterations in ambient temperature on the capacity to perform different types of exercise. Except where the exercise times have been very brief, the results of these tests have invariably shown that exercise performance is impaired when the environmental temperature is high. Indeed, a reduction in exercise tolerance in the heat is a matter of common experience.

The effects of high ambient temperatures on exercise capacity can be extremely large. For example, Suzuki (1980) reported that exercise time at a work load of 66% $\dot{V}O_2max$ was reduced from 91 min when the ambient temperature was 0°C to 19 min when the same exercise was performed in the heat (40°C). An unpublished study from our laboratory in which six subjects exercised to exhaustion at 70% $\dot{V}O_2max$ on a cycle ergometer showed that exercise time was reduced from 73 min at an ambient temperature of 2°C to 35 min at a temperature of 33°C. Higher intensities of exercise may also be adversely affected. For instance, Nadel (1983) reported that time to exhaustion at 80% $\dot{V}O_2max$ was reduced from 18.7 min at 20°C to 10.5 min at 30°C, and that at 100% of maximum aerobic power, exercise time was reduced from 4.7 min to 3.3 min. Many other studies have observed that performance of exercise in the heat at temperatures around 30–35°C dry bulb may be substantially reduced compared to a cooler (20–25°C) environment.

More recently, we measured the endurance capacity of subjects cycling at an exercise intensity of about 70% $\dot{V}O_2max$ at ambient temperatures of 4, 11, 21, and 31°C (Figure 4-1; Galloway & Maughan, 1995). It is clear from the results that there is an optimum temperature for performance of this type of exercise, and that this optimum occurs at about 10°C, with shorter exercise times being achieved at lower and at higher temperatures.

Although fatigue in cycle ergometer exercise at these work intensities is generally considered to result from depletion of the muscle glyco-

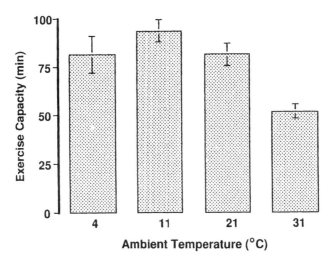

FIGURE 4-1. *Effects of ambient temperature on exercise capacity (mean ± SEM) during cycling at an intensity corresponding to about 70% VO₂max in eight male subjects who were moderately trained but not heat acclimated.* All trials were different from each other (P<0.05), except for those at 4 and 21°C. Based on the data of Galloway and Maughan (1995).

gen stores, this is clearly not the case when the ambient temperature is high because the total amount of carbohydrate oxidized was much less at a high (31°C) ambient temperature because of the brief exercise time, and it seems highly improbable that muscle glycogen stores were exhausted when the subjects stopped exercising.

Maw et al. (1993) have shown that ambient temperature can influence the subjective perception of effort during exercise. Subjects reported a lower level of perceived exertion at an ambient temperature of 8°C or 20°C relative to exercise at the same power output at 40°C. Similar results were obtained by Galloway and Maughan (1995). These subjective responses support the notion of a reduced exercise tolerance in the heat.

Hydration Status and Exercise Performance

It is often reported that exercise performance is impaired when an individual is dehydrated by as little as 2% of body mass and that losses in excess of 5% of body mass can decrease the capacity for work by about 30% (Saltin & Costill, 1988). The original data on which these figures are based have proved elusive, but there are many reports in the literature of reductions in exercise performance resulting from hypohydration induced prior to exercise, and these studies have been comprehensively reviewed (Sawka & Pandolf, 1990).

Several different methods have been used to induce body water loss, including thermal sweating, exercise at high or moderate ambient temperatures, restriction of fluid (and food) intake, and the administration of diuretic agents. The different effects of these various procedures can account for some of the variability in response that has been reported. When exercise is used to provoke sweat loss, hyperthermia and depletion of muscle and liver glycogen stores will also be possible causes of reductions in subsequent exercise performance; therefore, the results of these studies must be interpreted with caution. The early studies in this area have been reviewed in an earlier volume in this series (Maughan, 1991).

Although much of the early evidence on hydration status and exercise performance involved prolonged exercise, there is now good evidence that this may be an important factor even when the exercise intensity is high and the duration is short. Nielsen et al. (1981) showed that prolonged exercise, which resulted in a loss of fluid corresponding to 2.5% of body mass, resulted in a 45% fall in the capacity to perform high-intensity exercise lasting about 7 min. Passive heat exposure in a sauna or similar environment will result in an elevation of body temperature and loss of sweat, but will not affect tissue carbohydrate stores. Sauna exposure has been shown in several early studies to reduce exercise performance when the exercise duration is about 5-10 min, and also to reduce total work output in a task performed for a fixed period. Even when fluid replacement is allowed to reduce the loss in body mass, performance is still impaired. However, as reviewed by Sawka and Pandolf (1990) there are reports that very high-intensity exercise, in which fatigue occurs in less than 1 min, is unaffected by dehydration up to an equivalent of about 5% of body mass.

Diuretic administration (80 mg Lasix, 2.5% reduction in body mass) reduced exercise performance by 18% in the study of Nielsen et al. (1981). When Armstrong et al. (1985) used the same drug (40 mg) to reduce body mass by 1.6–2.1%, mean running speed in simulated races over distances of 1,500, 5,000, and 10,000 m was reduced by 3.1%, 6.7%, and 6.3%, respectively, after dehydration. More recently, Walsh and colleagues (1994) showed that prevention of dehydration by administration of 1 L of dilute saline solution (20 mmol/L) during 1 h of exercise at 70% $\dot{V}O_2$max prolonged exercise time to 9.8 min in a subsequent performance test at 90% $\dot{V}O_2$max, compared with 6.8 min for a control trial in which body mass was reduced by 1.3 kg.

Although there have been many descriptive studies, the mechanism by which hypohydration influences capacity for either prolonged or high-intensity exercise has not been adequately investigated. It is clear that there is a close relationship between the level of hypohydration and the elevation of core temperature, but investigations into the effects of preexercise hypohydration on sweating responses have yielded conflicting results. In 1980, Nadel et al. reported that prior hypohydration reduced cardiac output during exercise by reducing the stroke volume; this increased the threshold temperature for initiation of cutaneous vasodilation and reduced the cutaneous blood flow, resulting in a greater elevation of core temperature than occurred in the euhydrated state.

Montain et al. (1995) confirmed that hypohydration induced prior to exercise in a warm environment increased the threshold temperature for initiation of the sweating response. This occurred in a graded fashion with increasing levels of hypohydration (i.e., for each 1% reduction in body mass, the sweating threshold increased by 0.06°C). The sensitivity of sweating was also attenuated in the hypohydrated state, again in relation to the degree of hypohydration, and this effect was independent of exercise intensity.

Prevention of dehydration by administration of a carbohydrate-electrolyte drink to offset sweat losses during prolonged exercise can attenuate the fall in cardiac output that is normally observed in this situation, allowing better perfusion of the vascular bed of the skin and resulting in improved heat loss and less of a rise in core temperature (Gonzalez-Alonso et al., 1995). In the dehydrated state, vasoconstriction in the skin is necessary to maintain arterial blood pressure in the face of a falling blood volume and a continuing high muscle flow (Nadel et al., 1980). Provision of fluids thus appears to be crucial for the maintenance of stroke volume and for the physiological responses related to a sufficiently large cardiac output during exercise.

There are few reports of the effects of hypohydration on mental performance and cognitive function, but some negative effects have been recorded. Gopinathan et al. (1988) reported a reduction in a variety of tasks involving arithmetic ability, short term memory, and a visual tracking test after dehydration (2–4% of body mass) induced by exercise in the heat and by water restriction; performance was not affected by a 1% reduction in body mass. In spite of the rather clear evidence that exercise in the heat increases subjective assessment of effort, and of the equally clear evidence that hypohydration reduces exercise capacity, it seems surprising that the data of Dengel et al. (1993) indicated that even severe hypohydration (5.6% reduction in body mass) does not increase the subjective perception of effort during exercise in a moderate (22°C) environment.

Effects of Fluid Ingestion on Performance

Fluid replacement during exercise is limited primarily by the volume consumed, and many different factors will limit voluntary intake.

Further potential limitations arise in the stomach; no absorption of water or nutrients (except alcohol, to some extent) occurs in the stomach, but the rate of gastric emptying will determine the rate of delivery to and absorption by the small intestine. A sensation of fullness may also act to limit intake. Another possible restriction to water, electrolyte, and substrate provision may be imposed by the absorptive capacity of the intestine. All of these factors have been investigated to varying degrees in a variety of different experimental models.

The effects of feeding different types and amounts of beverages during exercise have been extensively investigated. Not all of these studies have shown positive effects of fluid ingestion on performance; however, with the exception of a few investigations wherein the composition of the drinks administered was such as to cause gastrointestinal disturbances, there are no studies showing that fluid ingestion will have an adverse effect on performance. These experiments have been the subject of a number of extensive reviews that have concentrated on the effects of administration of carbohydrate, electrolytes, and water on exercise performance; however, the results of the individual studies will not be considered in detail here (Coyle & Coggan, 1984; Lamb & Brodowicz, 1986; Maughan, 1994; Murray, 1987).

Many different fluid replacement regimens have been investigated, and in most studies, drinks administered during exercise trials have contained a variety of types and amounts of carbohydrate as well as electrolytes and other components. The problems in resolving the effects of fluid replacement from those of the supply of exogenous substrate are formidable, and when flavored drinks are ingested the effects of sensory stimulation may also be a factor. This is particularly true as the most effective fluid replacement is known to be achieved with drinks that contain small amounts of glucose and sodium, and the effects of these two components are not easily separated (Leiper & Maughan, 1988). Nonetheless, performance is improved by ingestion of carbohydrate, whether in liquid or solid form (Coyle, 1992), and it seems clear that the most effective way to improve exercise performance is to replace both water and substrate. The precise balance between these two objectives that will be most effective in any given situation will depend on a number of factors, including the exercise intensity and duration, the ambient temperature and humidity, and the physiological and biochemical characteristics and nutritional status of the individual (Maughan, 1994).

There have been rather few systematic investigations of the effects of variations in the composition of ingested fluids or in the amount of fluid ingested on exercise performance. Much of the information in the literature consists of reports of what are effectively tests of candidate solutions for optimizing performance. When two or more solutions are compared, they often differ in several respects, making interpretation of the results difficult. There are more coherent data relating to fluid replacement, and it is clear that increasing the amount of carbohydrate contained in ingested fluids will slow gastric emptying, thus possibly limiting the rate of fluid replacement, while simultaneously increasing the amount of substrate delivered to the small intestine (Vist & Maughan, 1994). The optimum rate of water absorption in the small intestine is achieved with hypotonic (osmolality of about 220–250 mosmol/kg) solutions with relative low glucose concentrations and relatively high sodium concentrations (Leiper & Maughan, 1988; Walker-Smith, 1992). These two sets of observations perhaps set the parameters for optimizing fluid replacement.

As mentioned above, there are many studies showing improvements in performance with the administration of plain water, whereas other studies show that solid carbohydrate feeding can also improve performance. In one investigation, however, several different treatments were compared, and administration of a dilute glucose-electrolyte solution was found to be more effective in improving performance than was either plain water or a concentrated carbohydrate solution (Maughan et al., 1987). Below et al. (1994) also showed that ingestion of carbohydrate and water had separate and additive effects on performance capacity and concluded that ingestion of dilute carbohydrate solutions would optimize performance. Most reviews of the available literature have come to the same conclusion.

It is inevitably the case that most investigations into the effects of fluid ingestion have focused on exercise lasting at least 1 h, and often much longer than this. The delays introduced by gastric emptying and intestinal absorption, especially when the exercise intensity is high, suggest that ingestion of fluid may be of little benefit when the duration of exercise is brief. Fluid administered intravenously, however, appears to be beneficial. Mitchell et al. (1990) found that intravenous infusion of 0.9% sodium chloride or 1.3% sodium bicarbonate in a total volume of 1.5 L during exercise increased exercise time to exhaustion at 80% $\dot{V}O_2$max from 19 min in a trial with no fluid infusion to 32 min on both the trials with fluid infusions. It may still be the case that the gastrointestinal tract will prevent adequate fluid replacement when the exercise duration is brief, but this appears to merit further investigation.

Possible Mechanisms of Reduced Exercise Tolerance in the Heat

With exercise at different temperatures, many studies have shown changes in cardiorespiratory, thermoregulatory, and metabolic functions that were related to the ambient temperature. There are, however, inconsistencies in the reported changes with increases in oxidation rates of both carbohydrate and lipid being reported during exercise in hot or neutral environments compared with a cool environment, and increased oxygen costs of exercise observed in both cold and hot environments. Overall, the reported metabolic responses to heat exposure do not provide strong evidence for substrate depletion as the primary cause of fatigue during exercise in the heat. The results of Galloway and Maughan (1995) showed that subjects exercising at 30°C became exhausted after using only about half of the total amount of carbohydrate that had been oxidized in a test to exhaustion at an ambient temperature of 11°C. This suggests strongly that carbohydrate depletion may not be limiting in exercise at an intensity corresponding to about 70% $\dot{V}O_2$max in the heat. Preliminary results of a muscle biopsy study in which subjects exercised to exhaustion at 3, 20, and 40°C indicate not only that glycogen depletion occurred at a faster rate in the heat, but also that the point of exhaustion was reached before the glycogen stores were depleted (Febbraio et al., 1996). More systematic studies examining the effects of exposure temperature on the metabolic responses to exercise in the heat are required in order to ascertain the major causes of reduced exercise tolerance.

Hypohydration, which may progress to hyperthermia, is the most commonly proposed mechanism for reduced exercise tolerance in the heat. Since the early experiments of Adolph and associates (1947), the effects of hypohydration on exercise performance have been studied extensively. However, it is not clear whether the hypovolemia or the hypertonicity associated with hypohydration is responsible for the subsequent elevations in core temperature, the changes in sweat rate, and the large cardiovascular drift that occur during exercise in the hypohydrated state. Montain and Coyle (1992) highlighted the effects of fluid ingestion on core temperature and sweat rate, showing that core temperature and heart rate typically are reduced and peripheral blood flow is maintained following fluid administration, compared with no fluid ingestion. This, therefore, strongly suggests that fluid balance is a key factor determining exercise tolerance in a hot environment.

During moderate- to intense-exercise in the heat, the combined increased demands for perfusion of the working muscles and of the skin can result in difficulties in meeting both requirements (Rowell, 1986). With hypohydration, heart rate is usually increased and peripheral blood flow reduced in an attempt to maintain arterial blood pressure, but decreasing peripheral blood flow will reduce the ability to lose heat, causing body temperature to rise. The dual circulatory demand of the working muscles and the skin in the heat may also compromise hepatic, splanchnic, and muscle blood flow, which may ultimately limit exercise capacity (Rowell, 1986). This again suggests that fluid balance is a key factor determining exercise capacity. In contrast to this hypothesis, Nielsen (1994) did not observe a reduction in muscle perfusion during exercise and heat stress and suggested that a high core temperature was the more likely cause of fatigue in the heat; a critical limiting temperature was identified as being the most important factor. Also, as early as 1972 Saltin et al. suggested that a high muscle temperature would limit exercise performance in the heat; this has obvious implications for the maintenance of hydration status and the capacity of the circulation to sustain an adequate perfusion of the muscle capillary bed.

It is clear that further investigation of thermoregulation and fluid balance during exercise in hot environments is necessary in order to understand the mechanisms for the reduced exercise tolerance usually observed in the heat. It is also apparent that the thermoregulatory response to exercise varies between individuals. It is unlikely, therefore, that this or any other factor will contribute to the subjective sensation of fatigue to the same degree in all individuals or in all situations. Nonetheless, fluid replacement appears to have a large influence on exercise tolerance during heat exposure, although the mechanisms involved and the interactions with thermoregulation remain obscure.

LIMITATIONS TO FLUID REPLACEMENT

Absorption of ingested water and nutrients occurs primarily, and more or less completely, in the upper part of the small intestine. The function of the stomach is to contain the ingestate and prepare it for delivery to the duodenum. The availability of ingested water or nutrients may therefore be limited by the delay imposed by gastric emptying, or by the absorptive capacity of the intestine. It is easy to demonstrate that either of these processes can, in some situations, limit the rate of exogenous fuel and fluid delivery, but in most exercise situations, fluid replacement is limited by the volume of fluid ingested, and in endurance running events, voluntary intake seldom exceeds about 0.5 L/h (Noakes, 1993). A sensation of "fullness" or of abdominal discomfort is the most commonly cited reason for not ingesting more fluid (Brouns et al., 1987).

Gastric Emptying

The process of gastric emptying and its physiological regulation has been extensively investigated. The first systematic studies in this area were those of Hunt and his colleagues in the 1950s and 1960s; these studies established the basic principles that regulate gastric emptying rates (Table 4-1). The early findings have largely been confirmed by subsequent research, and later refinements are primarily a result of improvements in the methodology used to study gastric emptying in healthy volunteers at rest or during exercise. It is also true, however, that there is no universal agreement on some details of gastric emptying. This conflict is in part due to the characteristics of the different methods used to study gastric emptying and, to some extent, to the frequent use of complex solutions in which many variables were changed simultaneously.

Most of the early studies either aspirated the gastric contents at a single time point or followed the emptying of a gamma-emitting tracer using a scintigraphic detector. The gamma scintigraphy method has been most widely used in clinical settings and can be applied to the study of the gastric emptying of solids, liquids, or mixtures of the two. The major difficulties that are encountered arise only when solid meals are studied and the tracers used may not faithfully follow the test meal; the same is not true for liquid meals when a suitable tracer is used and when appropriate corrections are applied to account for the extrapolation from a two-dimensional image to a process that is occurring in three dimensions. A good agreement between the scintigraphic method and direct measurements by gastric aspiration has been confirmed when dilute or concentrated glucose solutions are studied. There remains the problem of accounting for changes in the gastric volume due to the addition of gastric secretions. In addition, it is also not possible to determine how these secretions change the composition of the gastric contents.

The technique of aspirating the stomach at a single time point has been widely used in exercise studies as well as in resting subjects, and much of the available information has been obtained with this method. The limitations of assessment at a single time point are immediately apparent when it is realized that emptying of liquids, with the possible exception of those with an unusually high energy content, is an exponential rather than a linear process. An example of the limitations to which this can give rise is shown in Figure 4-2, which compares the emptying rates of flavored water and glucose solutions of increasing concentration. The interaction between the two most significant controllers of emptying (volume and energy density) is clearly seen. Water empties faster than

TABLE 4.1. *Factors influencing gastric of liquids.*

Volume of gastric contents	Increasing volume will increase emptying rate, irrespective of composition.
Energy density	Increasing nutrient density will slow gastric emptying; fat, carbohydrate, and protein act independently, and the effects are additive.
Osmolality	Increasing osmolality slows emptying; for carbohydrate solutions, the effect is small, except at high concentrations.
Particulate matter	Presence of solid particles (e.g., fruit pulp) will slow emptying.
Acidity	Emptying is slowed at extremes of pH.

the glucose-containing solutions, so the gastric volume falls more rapidly and the rate of emptying falls over time. At the sampling point of 10 min, it could legitimately be concluded that emptying of all the glucose-containing solutions is delayed relative to water; at the 40 min time point, however, the conclusion would be that only at glucose concentrations in excess of 10% is emptying slowed. The single time point aspiration method effectively allows only one of these answers to be obtained, but when the whole curve is available, the true result is apparent.

The double sampling method, introduced by George (1968) and modified by Beckers et al. (1988), allows measurements to be made at relatively frequent intervals and also allows an estimate to be made of

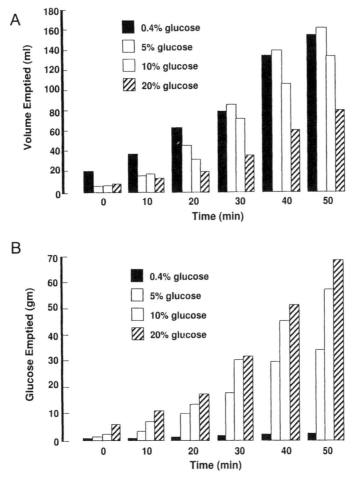

FIGURE 4-2. *Effects of ingestion of 200 mL of flavored water and 5, 10, and 20% glucose solutions on a) volume of fluid emptied from the stomach and b) amount of glucose emptied.*

the volume and composition of gastric secretions added between successive measurements. This should be the method of choice in measurements of the gastric emptying of liquids, and this method is now gradually displacing the others that have been used. This should remove some of the conflict in the literature.

Whatever the composition of the ingested fluid, the volume of the stomach contents has a major influence on the emptying rate. By refilling the stomach at intervals, the volume in the stomach can be kept high. When this has been investigated using dilute carbohydrate-electrolyte solutions, a high rate of gastric emptying was maintained, greatly enhancing both the volume of solution and the amount of carbohydrate delivered to the small intestine for absorption (Mitchell & Voss, 1991; Rehrer et al., 1990). With concentrated carbohydrate solutions, however, the rate of emptying is slow, and care must be taken to ensure that repeated drinking does not lead to accumulation of fluid in the stomach and to subjective sensations of discomfort (Vist et al., 1997).

The composition of ingested fluids also has a major effect on the rate of emptying. Emptying of solutions is slowed by making them markedly hypertonic with respect to the osmolality of body fluids, by increasing their acidity, and by increasing their energy density; all of these factors are relevant to the formulation of drinks to be used during exercise. It seems well established that the emptying rate of carbohydrate solutions is slow relative to that for water or for isotonic saline solutions. The difficulties come in trying to establish at what point the effect of increasing carbohydrate content becomes meaningful, for it is clear that a drastic slowing of gastric emptying will limit rehydration during exercise.

The effect of increasing glucose concentrations on the time course of emptying has been extensively investigated. Dilute glucose solutions (<2.5%) have been reported in several studies to empty from the stomach at the same rate as water, and a number of reports indicate that solutions of 5% carbohydrate will delay the rate of gastric emptying compared with water, suggesting that the critical carbohydrate concentration for an effect is somewhere between these values. Others, however, including a number of recent studies, have found that solutions containing carbohydrates of concentrations up to 7.5% empty from the stomach at rates similar to that for water (Houmard et al., 1991; Mitchell et al., 1988, 1989; Rehrer et al., 1989). There are also published results showing no difference in the rate of gastric emptying between water and a 10% glucose solution (Owen et al., 1986; Zachwieja et al., 1992).

At least part of this apparent discrepancy can probably be traced to the designs of these studies; many used a single time point aspiration method, and most used solutions containing a number of ingredients in addition to carbohydrate, as well as a variety of different carbohydrate sources. If a fixed volume of two different glucose solutions, one dilute and one concentrated, is given, the initial emptying rate for the dilute solution will be more rapid; as the volume falls, so the emptying rate will be reduced, but this effect will be less marked for the more concentrated solution. Recent results obtained using the double sampling gastric aspiration method indicate that glucose concentrations in excess of about 4% will delay gastric emptying (Figure 4-3; Vist & Maughan, 1995). It is also apparent that, although increasing the glucose content of the ingested fluid does slow the rate at which fluid leaves the stomach, it results in a faster delivery of glucose (Hunt et al., 1985, Vist & Maughan, 1995).

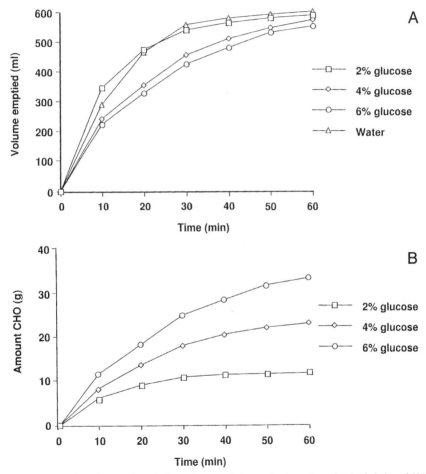

FIGURE 4-3. *Gastric emptying of dilute glucose solutions after ingestion of a single bolus of 600 mL.* a) Total volume emptied from the stomach after ingesting 600 mL of water or 2%, 4%, or 6% glucose solutions. b) The amount of glucose (CHO) delivered to the small intestine after ingesting 600 mL of 2%, 4%, or 6% glucose solutions.

Substitution of maltose, sucrose, or glucose polymers for free glucose may help to promote the emptying of glucose-electrolyte solutions from the stomach by reducing the osmolality of the solution while maintaining the total carbohydrate content, but the studies reported in the literature are by no means in agreement. Sole and Noakes (1989) found that a 15% glucose polymer solution emptied faster than a 15% solution of free glucose, although 5% and 10% solutions of free glucose and polymer appeared to be emptied at the same rates. In another study, Naveri et al. (1989) found that the emptying rates of electrolyte solutions with 3% carbohydrate added in the form of glucose or a polymer were the same. Owen et al. (1986) also found no difference in the rates of emptying of 10% solutions of glucose or glucose polymer, in spite of the higher osmolality of the free glucose solution. Rehrer et al. (1992) also observed similar emptying rates with 18% solutions of glucose polymer (313 mosmol/kg) and free glucose (1,223 mosmol/kg); however, a 4.5% glucose solution emptied faster than an 18% polymer solution with the same osmolality. From this, it might be concluded that osmolality becomes important at high solute concentrations, but the effect is small compared with that of energy density, especially in dilute solutions. Many of the solutions tested in these studies contained a variety of electrolytes and flavorings, which were not always kept the same when different drinks were being compared. In a systematic study, Vist and Maughan (1994) evaluated the effects of osmolality and energy density by comparing solutions of free glucose or glucose polymers. The results showed that a 4% polymer solution (osmolality 42 mosmol/kg) emptied only slightly faster than a 4% glucose solution (osmolality 230 mosmol/kg), whereas an 18.8% polymer solution with the same osmolality as the 4% glucose solution emptied much more slowly, but emptied faster than an 18.8% free glucose solution (osmolality 1,300 mosmol/kg). Even though there are some differences in the results obtained in these studies, in none of the above studies was the emptying rate of polymer solutions slower than that of free glucose solutions with the same energy density, and the polymer solutions were generally emptied faster even when the differences were not statistically significant.

In summary, gastric emptying of liquids is regulated by a number of factors, of which the most important are the volume of the stomach contents, and the energy density and osmolality of drinks consumed. Increasing the carbohydrate content of drinks will delay emptying. Substitution of glucose polymers for free glucose appears to slightly increase the rate of delivery of fluid and substrate to the small intestine. It now seems likely that several other factors that were formerly thought to be important, such as carbonation and the temperature of ingested drinks, do not have a major influence on the rate of emptying. The factors regulating gastric emptying have been the subject of extensive reviews, many of which are cited by Maughan (1991).

Intestinal Absorption

Water absorption occurs largely in the proximal segment of the small intestine and, although water movement is itself a passive process driven by local osmotic gradients, is closely linked to the active transport of solute. The method of choice for measurement of intestinal absorption of water involves placement of a triple-lumen tube in the intestinal region of interest. The test solution, containing a non-absorbable marker, is perfused at a fixed rate within the physiological range for gastric emptying (usually between 5 and 15 mL/min). A sample of the intestinal contents is then aspirated via the second tube from a point 10–20 cm distal to the perfusion port, and the change in composition gives a measure of the effects of mixing of the test solution with the endogenous secretions. Aspiration via the third tube from a site 20–60 cm further along the intestine allows net exchange of solute and water in the test segment to be calculated.

This technique allows reliable measures to be made of the net flux of water and solutes in a well-defined region of the gut. Although the technique is reliable and reproducible in itself, there are some important limitations. Because the test solutions are added directly to the jejunum, the role of the stomach in moderating the delivery rate and in modifying the composition of ingested fluids is ignored. A constant perfusion rate is normally used in perfusion studies, and this may represent an unphysiological situation. A more recent modification to the technique involves repeated ingestion of the test drinks orally in an attempt to maintain a constant rate of gastric emptying, with simultaneous aspiration from three or four sampling sites located in the small intestine. The effects of solute secretion may be important, and there is evidence that, when electrolyte-free solutions are ingested orally, there is a rapid secretion of sodium such that equilibrium is rapidly reached (Gisolfi et al., 1995; Schedl et al., 1994). If this is indeed the case, it confounds the evidence available from the perfusion method that indicates an increased water uptake when sodium-containing fluids are perfused (Leiper & Maughan, 1988). The technique also looks only at a small part of the whole intestinal surface that is available for absorption in the intact individual; thus, concentrated solutions stimulate water secretion in the upper part of the intestine, but absorption will still occur in the distal regions.

Absorption of glucose occurs in the small intestine and is an active, energy-consuming process linked to the transport of sodium. There is no active transport mechanism for water, which will cross the intestinal mucosa in either direction depending on the local osmotic gradients. The rate of glucose uptake is dependent on the luminal concentrations of glucose and sodium, and dilute glucose-electrolyte solutions with an osmolality that is slightly hypotonic with respect to plasma will maximize the rate of water uptake (Wapnir & Lifshitz, 1985). Solutions with a very high glucose concentration will not necessarily promote an increased glucose uptake relative to more dilute solutions but, because of their high osmolality, will cause a net movement of fluid into the intestinal lumen (Gisolfi et al., 1990). This results in an effective loss of body water and will exacerbate any preexisting dehydration. Other sugars, such as sucrose (Spiller et al., 1982) or glucose polymers (Jones et al., 1983; 1987), can be substituted for glucose without impairing glucose or water uptake. In contrast, the absorption of fructose is not an active process in man; it is absorbed less rapidly than glucose and promotes less water uptake (Fordtran, 1975). The use of different sugars that are absorbed by different mechanisms and that might thus promote increased water uptake is supported by recent evidence from an intestinal perfusion study (Shi et al., 1995).

Much of the information in this area is derived from intestinal perfusion studies carried out with the aim of identifying solutions that can effectively replace fluid in individuals, especially children, who suffer from infectious diarrhea (Walker-Smith, 1992). Isotonic glucose-electrolyte oral rehydration solutions (ORS) have been widely promoted for the treatment of dehydration resulting from infectious diarrhea (Elliott et al., 1986). However, rice-based ORS have been reported to be as effective in this treatment as the more common glucose-based ORS (Mohan et al. 1986) and to give a reduced stool volume (Mota-Hernandes et al., 1991). Molla et al. (1989) tried ORS formulations using starch from a number of different sources, including rice, wheat, and potatoes, and found all of them to result in a smaller stool volume and smaller volume of ORS ingested compared with the glucose-based ORS. It is assumed that a decreased stool output in the patient with diarrhea indicates an enhanced water absorption, and there are clearly implications of these results for other situations, such as exercise in the heat, when rapid replacement of fluid losses is essential.

The mechanisms underlying this effect have not been established, but it is known that hypotonic solutions (200–250 mosmol/kg) promote greater rates of water absorption in the small intestine than do isotonic solutions (Elliott et al. 1986; Hunt et al. 1988; Rolston et al. 1987, 1990). Food-based solutions, because of their lower osmolalities compared with isoenergetic glucose-based solutions, may be emptied faster from the stomach and should promote faster water absorption from the small intestine.

Tracer Methods

The rate of gastric emptying and the rate of absorption in segments of the small intestine can be measured separately. Furthermore, by introducing an isotopic tracer for water to ingested solutions and measuring the appearance of this tracer in the circulation, an indication of the combined effect of gastric emptying and intestinal absorption can be obtained. The accumulation in the circulation of a tracer added to the test drink has been used as an index of water absorption from ingested solutions (Davis et al. 1987, Leiper & Maughan 1988). The rate of accumulation in the circulation of deuterium after adding deuterium oxide to the ingested solutions has been shown to follow known gastric emptying and intestinal absorption patterns of the ingested solution (Davis et al. 1987).

Using simultaneous measurements of intestinal absorption with the triple-lumen tube perfusion method and appearance in the circulation of a tracer added to the perfusate, Gisolfi et al. (1990) suggested that results obtained with this method gave little useful information and might actually be misleading. This suggestion was based on the fact that the deuterium tracer method followed only the unidirectional movement of water from the intestinal lumen into the circulation; accumulation of tracer was observed even when a net efflux of water into the intestinal lumen was indicated by the perfusion method. This, however, ignores the fact that the relative rates of water absorption indicated by the tracer method agrees rather well with the results obtained by the more invasive perfusion method. As used by other investigators, the tracer technique has involved addition of the tracer to a bolus of fluid ingested orally. This is quite a different situation from that used by Gisolfi et al. (1990) in which a test solution containing a constant tracer concentration was perfused at constant rate directly into the jejunum, and the available evidence suggests that useful results as to the relative rates of water availability from ingested fluids may be obtained with the bolus tracer method.

Effects of Exercise on Gastrointestinal Function

Several studies have shown that exercise at intensities of less than about 70% $\dot{V}O_2$max has little or no effect on intestinal function, although both gastric emptying and intestinal absorption may be reduced when the exercise intensity exceeds this level. At high exercise intensities, however, when there is likely to be a serious barrier to the availability of ingested food or fluids, the exercise time will probably be too short for there to be any benefit from nutrients ingested during the exercise period. When subjects have been able to sustain high intensity exercise for prolonged periods, attempts to ingest large volumes of fluid have led to gastrointestinal discomfort and impaired exercise tolerance. For example, in the study of Robinson et al. (1995), subjects attempted to ride as far as possible on a bicycle simulator for a period of one hour; the exercise intensity corresponded to about 85% of $\dot{V}O_2$max. When no fluid was consumed, subjects covered 43.1 km, but when 1.5 L of flavored water was consumed during the trial, the distance covered was reduced to 42.3 km (P< 0.05). The reduced performance was ascribed to an uncomfortable feeling of stomach fullness; it seems unlikely that drinking such a volume at rest would produce this effect, suggesting a reduced capacity of the gastrointestinal tract to function at such a high exercise intensity.

The studies investigating gastrointestinal function during exercise have been reviewed and summarized by Brouns et al. (1987) and by Maughan (1991).

Results obtained using an isotopic tracer technique to follow ingested fluids have suggested that there may be a decreased availability of ingested fluids even during low-intensity exercise; a decreased rate of appearance in the blood of a tracer for water added to the ingested drinks was noted at an exercise intensity of 40% VO_2max (Maughan et al., 1990). Clearly, some individuals experience gastrointestinal problems during exercise, and the possible reasons for the susceptibility of these individuals to this potentially debilitating condition have received much attention in recent years. O'Connor et al. (1995) measured the circulating concentrations of a number of gastrointestinal peptide hormones in 26 runners before and after a marathon race. The plasma levels of all the peptides except insulin increased during the race, but there was no relationship between these changes and the incidence of gastrointestinal distress, which affected eight of the runners. The factors associated with gastrointestinal problems during exercise have recently been reviewed (Peters et al., 1995), but there remains no clear indication as to the cause of the problem nor of the best way to avoid its occurrence.

PREEXERCISE HYDRATION

The difficulties of achieving an adequate fluid intake during many competitive sports events and the growing recognition of the negative effects of hypohydration have led to an increasing emphasis on ensuring an optimum hydration status before exercise begins. The kidneys, however, effectively prevent most of the strategies that have been invoked in attempts to increase water storage prior to exercise. Water balance is largely controlled by monitoring of the circulating osmolality, which is intimately linked to the plasma sodium concentration; the osmoreceptor may be in the form of a sodium receptor. Changes in osmolality cause alterations in output of antidiuretic hormone by the pituitary, and antidiuretic hormone in turn controls the reabsorption of water by the distal tubules of the nephrons and by the collecting ducts.

Attempts have been made to induce a state of relative hyperhydration prior to exercise by administration of glycerol solutions. These have the effect of increasing total body water, but result in an increase in plasma osmolality, and so may be considered to result in a relative hypohydration, even though total body water is increased (Gleeson et al., 1986). The elevation of the osmolality of the extracellular space may result in water movements from the intracellular space, and cell dehydration is a well-recognized consequence of the administration of large amounts of glycerol.

Several studies have recently reported that ingestion of glycerol together with water can increase the plasma osmolality and the total body water content, both of which could provide benefits for thermoregulation and exercise performance. Lyons et al. (1990) gave subjects glycerol plus water or water alone 2.5 h prior to a 90-min exercise test at 60% of $\dot{V}O_2$max in a hot (42°C) dry (25% relative humidity) environment. The addition of glycerol decreased urine output over the trial, increased sweat rate, and caused a smaller rise in rectal temperature during the exercise period; there was also a tendency, although not statistically significant, for heart rate to be lower on the glycerol trial. Freund et al. (1995) also reported an enhanced fluid retention and reduced renal flow when glycerol was added to drinks ingested at rest; they proposed that this effect might be mediated by an increased antidiuretic hormone output. Some reports have also indicated improvements in the ability to perform prolonged exercise after glycerol administration (Montner et al., 1996). Although not all individuals showed an improvement in performance, they did find that prior administration of glycerol (1.2 g/kg) plus water resulted in significant improvements in time to exhaustion compared with a water-only trial in two exercise tests lasting about 90 min; the improved exercise performance was associated with a lower heart rate during exercise and a smaller rise in core temperature. The recommendation that endurance athletes competing in the heat should ingest glycerol and water prior to exercise, or that glycerol should be added to drinks, would be premature at this stage, and further developments in this area are awaited with interest.

POSTEXERCISE REHYDRATION

Any athlete beginning exercise in a hypohydrated state will be unable to produce an optimal performance and will also be subject to an increased risk of heat illness. In spite of this, it is not unusual for athletes in weight-category events (e.g., wrestling, boxing, and judo) to undergo severe dehydration in the hours and days prior to competition, and complete restoration of these water losses is not always possible. Because of the increased risk of heat illness, the practice of acute dehydration to make weight should be discouraged. Nonetheless, it will persist, so there is a need to maximize rehydration in the time available. There are other situations, such as tournament competitions, where the interval between rounds may be short and recovery is at a premium. The need for replacement will obviously depend on the extent of the losses incurred during exercise, but will also be influenced by the time and nature of subsequent exercise bouts.

Several studies have investigated the effects of ingestion of water or of commercially available drinks on restoration of fluid balance after exercise-induced dehydration. Costill and Sparks (1973) showed that ingestion of a glucose-electrolyte solution after dehydration resulted in a greater restoration of plasma volume than did plain water; a higher urine output was observed on the water trial. Gonzalez-Alonso et al. (1992) confirmed that a dilute carbohydrate-electrolyte solution (60 g/L carbohydrate, 20 mmol/L Na^+, 3 mmol/L K^+) is more effective in promoting postexercise rehydration than either plain water or a low-electrolyte diet cola; the difference between the drinks was primarily attributed to lesser urine production with the carbohydrate-electrolyte drink. Similar results were obtained by Nielsen et al. (1986). In none of these studies could the mechanism of this action be identified, but they did establish that, because of the high urine flow that ensued, even drinking large volumes of electrolyte-free drinks did not allow subjects to remain in positive fluid balance for more than a very short time.

The first studies to investigate the basis of the reduced urine volume when carbohydrate-electrolyte drinks are consumed versus water showed that the ingestion of large volumes of plain water after exercise-induced dehydration causes a rapid fall in plasma osmolality and in the plasma sodium concentration (Nose et al., 1988a, 1988b), and both of these effects stimulate urine output. A second consequence of ingestion of plain water is to remove the drive to drink by causing plasma osmolality and sodium concentration to fall. When a fixed volume of fluid is given, this is not important, but it will tend to prevent complete rehydration when fluid intake is on a volitional basis. In one of the experiments conducted by the Nose group, subjects exercised at low intensity in the heat for 90–110 min, inducing a mean dehydration of 2.3% of body weight, and then rested for 1 h before beginning to drink. Plasma volume was not restored until after 60 min when plain water was ingested together with placebo (sucrose) capsules. In contrast, when sodium chloride capsules were ingested with water to give a saline solution with an effective concentration of 0.45% (77 mmol/L), plasma volume was restored within 20 min. In the NaCl trial, voluntary fluid intake was higher and urine output was less; 71% of the water loss was retained within 3 h compared with 51% in the plain water trial. The delayed rehydration in the water trial appeared to be a result of renal excretion of sodium, accompanied by water, caused by decreases in both plasma renin activity and plasma aldosterone concentration. When a more severe (4% of body weight) dehydration was induced in resting subjects by heat exposure, consumption over a 3 h period of a volume of fluid equal to that lost did not restore plasma volume or serum osmolality within 4 h. However, ingestion of a glucose-electrolyte solution did restore plasma volume to a greater extent than did plain water; there was a greater urine production in the water trial.

The importance of the addition of sodium to rehydration fluids was systematically evaluated by Maughan and Leiper (1995), who dehydrated subjects by the equivalent of 2% of body mass by intermittent exercise in the heat. Subjects then ingested one of four test drinks over a 60 min period and were followed for a further 6 h; the drink volume was equal to 150% of the body mass lost, and the test drinks contained 0, 25, 50, or 100 mmol/L sodium. Urine output over the subsequent few hours was inversely proportional to the sodium content of the ingested fluid, and only when the sodium content exceeded 50 mmol/L did subjects remain in positive fluid balance throughout the recovery period (Figure 4-4).

These observations were confirmed in a further study that systematically varied the volume of fluid ingested as well as the sodium content of rehydration drinks administered after induced hypohydration (Shirreffs et al., 1996). Even drinking large volumes (twice the sweat loss) did not allow subjects to remain in positive fluid balance for more than 2 h when the sodium content of the drinks was low (20 mmol/L). Increasing the sodium content to 60 mmol/L, however, allowed subjects to remain well hydrated when volumes equal to 1.5 times or twice the sweat loss were ingested.

When the electrolyte content of drinks is the same, it appears that other factors such as the addition of carbohydrate (100 g/L) or carbonation has no effect on the restoration of plasma volume over a 4-h period after sweat loss corresponding to approximately 4% of body weight (Lambert et al., 1992). The need to replace electrolytes after dehydration is linked to the loss of electrolytes in sweat. Sodium and chloride are the main electrolytes lost in sweat, whereas potassium losses are rather small. The composition of human sweat is highly variable, and its electrolyte concentration and total volume will determine the extent of electrolyte loss. At least part of the variability in the reported composition of sweat can be accounted for by methodological problems associated with

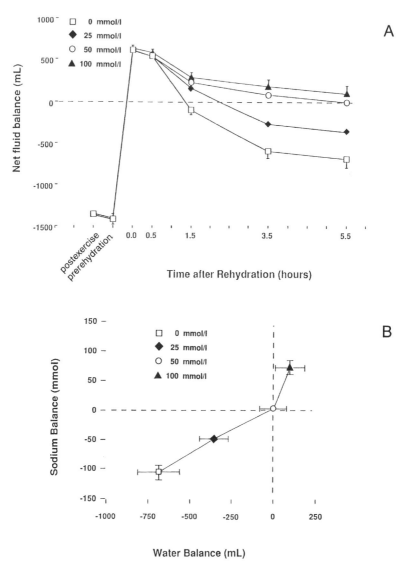

FIGURE 4-4. *Restoration of water balance after exercise-induced sweat loss is strongly influenced by the sodium content of ingested fluids.* Subjects were dehydrated by 2% of body mass and then drank a volume of fluid equal to 1.5 times the sweat loss; drinks contained sodium in concentrations of 0, 25, 50, or 100 mmol/L. Fluid balance was followed for a further 5.5 h after the end of the drinking period. a) Net fluid balance (mean ± SEM, calculated from sweat loss, fluid ingested, and urine output over the whole course of the study. Subjects remained in net fluid balance only when the sodium content of ingested drinks was high. b) There was a close relationship between the means (± SEM) for net fluid balance and net sodium balance (estimated on the assumption that the sweat sodium concentration was 50 mmol/L) at the end of the study period. Data from Maughan and Leiper (1995).

the collection procedure, but there is also a large biological v₊ Training and acclimation result in an enhanced sweating respons the elevated sweating rate is accompanied by a fall in the sodium chloride concentrations of sweat (Kobayashi et al., 1980). Some studies show an increased sodium and chloride concentration with increasing sweat rate within an individual (Costill, 1977), but others show no relationship between sweat rate and concentration (Verde et al., 1982). Typical ranges for sweat sodium and potassium concentrations are 20–80 mmol/L and 4–8 mmol/L, respectively (Maughan, 1991).

It is clear that rehydration after exercise can only be achieved if the sodium lost in sweat is replaced as well as the water, and it might be suggested that rehydration drinks should have a sodium concentration similar to that of sweat. The sodium content of sweat varies widely, and no single formulation will meet this requirement for all individuals in all situations. However, the upper end of the normal range for sodium concentration (80 mmol/L) is similar to the sodium concentrations of many commercially produced oral rehydration solutions (ORS) intended for use in the treatment of diarrhea-induced dehydration, and some of these are not unpalatable. The ORS recommended by the World Health Organization for rehydration in cases of severe diarrhea has a sodium content of 90 mmol/L, reflecting the high sodium losses that may occur in this condition. By contrast, the sodium content of most sports drinks is in the range of 10–25 mmol/L and is even lower in some cases; most commonly consumed soft drinks contain virtually no sodium, and these drinks are therefore unsuitable when the need for rehydration is crucial. The problem with high sodium concentrations is the possible negative effect on taste, resulting in a reduced consumption.

The requirement for sodium replacement stems from its role as the major ion in the extracellular fluid. Expansion of the plasma volume is well recognized as an early response to endurance training, even as soon as following a single bout of hard exercise. Armstrong et al. (1987) found that restriction of the dietary sodium intake attenuated the normal response. A close relationship has also been observed between dietary sodium intake and the expansion of plasma volume that occurred in response to 3 d of endurance cycling (approximately 2 h/d) (Luetkemeier, 1995). These reports emphasize the importance of adequate sodium replacement as well as rehydration after exercise and suggest that normal dietary sodium intake may not be adequate for some individuals when daily sweat losses are high and there is an ongoing expansion of the extracellular volume such as occurs in the early stages of endurance training or heat acclimation.

It had been speculated that inclusion of potassium, the major cation in the intracellular space, would enhance the replacement of intracellu-

xercise and thus promote rehydration (Nadel et al.,
mental investigation suggested that inclusion of potas-
ve as sodium in retaining water ingested after exercise-
ation (Maughan et al., 1994). Addition of either ion will
rease the fraction of the ingested fluid that is retained,
olume of fluid ingested is equal to that lost during the
, there is no additive effect of including both ions as
would be expected if they acted independently on different body fluid
compartments.

FORMULATION OF REHYDRATION FLUIDS

There is still no general agreement on the optimal formulation of rehydration drinks for use in competitive sport. There has been a move
away from the acceptance of plain water as the best drink, but debate
continues on issues relating to the optimal type and concentration of
carbohydrate, the optimal sodium concentration, and the usefulness of
other additives.

Balancing Water and Carbohydrate Provision

The effects of water and of carbohydrate provision are briefly summarized here before considering what might be the most effective combination of these ergogenic components. It seems clear that the provision of exogenous carbohydrate during exercise can increase exercise
capacity, and this effect may be due to a sparing of the endogenous muscle glycogen stores (Hargreaves et al., 1984), although this is by no
means a consistent finding (Coyle et al., 1986; Fielding et al., 1985; Hargreaves & Briggs, 1988). Fatigue during prolonged exercise, at least in cycling exercise, appears to be closely related to the depletion of the glycogen reserves in the exercising muscles, so there is good reason for
supposing that the provision of additional carbohydrate should delay
the onset of fatigue. Ingestion of large amounts of carbohydrate allows
exercise to continue even when the muscle glycogen content has fallen
almost to zero in well-trained cyclists (Coyle et al., 1986), and it is commonly recommended that an intake of at least 30–60 g of carbohydrate
per hour is necessary to achieve the greatest benefit (Coyle, 1992).

Several studies have shown that drinking plain water in a variety of
different situations can improve exercise performance, whereas others
have not reported a significant difference between water and no-drink
trials. The effects of water ingestion have been less thoroughly investigated than those of carbohydrate-electrolyte solutions; early studies in
this area were reviewed by Maughan (1991). Barr et al. (1991) studied
the responses of individuals to prolonged (6 h) low-intensity cycling ex-

ercise in the heat (30°C) who were given water, a sodium chloride solution (25 mmol/L), or no drink during exercise. For the no-drink trial, exercise was terminated after a mean time of 4.5 h, but the 6-h exercise task
was completed by seven of the eight subjects in the other two trials,
clearly suggesting an improved exercise tolerance with water replacement versus no fluid. In another study of prolonged walking (5–6 h),
Strydom et al. (1966) observed sweat losses of about 4.5 L; one group of
subjects, whose fluid intake was restricted, had higher rectal temperatures than the other group who were allowed water ad libitum, but no
measures of performance were made. In shorter duration exercise lasting 70–90 min, it has been reported that endurance time at a workload
of 70% $\dot{V}O_2$max was improved by consumption of an isotonic glucose-
electrolyte solution, but was not significantly improved by drinking solutions containing large amounts of carbohydrate or by the ingestion of
water (Maughan et al., 1987); there was a small (6 min; P = 0.10) increase
in the mean time to exhaustion in the trial in which water was given.
This last finding of a possible benefit from drinking plain water during
prolonged cycling is supported by more recent results of the same authors, which showed a significant improvement in exercise time (from
80.7 to 93.1 min) when water was consumed at a rate of 100 mL every 10
min during exercise compared to a no-drink trial (Maughan et al., 1996).
It is worth noting that in this latter study, ingestion of dilute glucose-
electrolyte solutions was again more effective than plain water in improving performance. In the study of Robinson et al. (1995) already referred to, administration of flavored water in a volume of 1.5 L during a
60-min cycle ergometer exercise test decreased the total distance covered compared with a trial in which no fluid was given. The reduced
performance was ascribed to sensations of gastric discomfort, and the
reluctance to drink such large volumes was clearly apparent as the intake volume was less than that prescribed. It seems clear that the subjects would not voluntarily have chosen to drink such large volumes,
and the effects of ingestion of a smaller, more acceptable, volume of
water were not investigated in this study.

Below et al. (1994) established in a well-controlled study that there
are independent and additive effects of ingesting carbohydrate and
water on performance of a high-intensity performance ride following 50
min of cycling at about 80% $\dot{V}O_2$max. They found that when only a small
volume (200 mL) of water was given during the initial 50-min cycling
period, the mean time required to complete the assigned performance
task was 11.34 min, whereas ingestion of the same volume with the addition of 79 g of carbohydrate and ingestion of a large (1,330 mL) volume of plain water both resulted in significant improvements in performance time, to 10.55 min and 10.51 min, respectively. Ingestion of the

same large fluid volume, but this time as a 6% carbohydrate solution (which contained the same amount of carbohydrate as the small volume of the concentrated solution), was more effective than either of the treatments individually, and the mean exercise time on this trial was 9.93 min. Although the improved performances when a large fluid volume was ingested were associated with a reduced heart rate and core temperature during the prolonged exercise, the improvements associated with carbohydrate ingestion were not.

In contrast to the apparent effectiveness of plain water in improving performance, Burgess et al. (1991) reported that administration of a glucose-electrolyte solution with a low (1.8%) carbohydrate content that provided only 13 g of carbohydrate per hour did not improve performance versus a no-fluid treatment. However, more recent results suggest that dilute glucose-electrolyte solutions may improve exercise capacity in prolonged cycling (Maughan et al., 1996).

This discrepancy with regard to the effects of the administration of dilute carbohydrate-electrolyte solutions is surprising in view of the well-known effects of these solutions in maximizing the rate of rehydration that can be achieved (Leiper & Maughan, 1988), and of the negative effects of dehydration on exercise performance (Walsh et al., 1994). It also conflicts with previous reports showing that provision of even small amounts of carbohydrate in the form of glucose-electrolyte solutions may enhance exercise performance (Maughan et al., 1987, 1996).

Sweat losses during prolonged exercise can reduce circulating blood volume, which may result in a decreased blood flow to the skin (Fortney et al., 1984) and a reduced sweating rate (Sawka et al., 1985), leading to an elevated core temperature (Gisolfi & Copping, 1974). Many studies have shown that fluid ingestion during a range of different exercise intensities and durations can attenuate the rise in body temperature that occurs, whether glucose-electrolyte drinks or plain water are taken. However, there is no good evidence that an elevated core temperature is in itself the cause of fatigue in prolonged exercise, and rather few studies seem to have examined the effects of the ingestion of plain water on endurance capacity.

The composition of drinks to be consumed will thus be influenced by the relative importance of the need to supply fuel and water; this in turn depends on the intensity and duration of the exercise task, on the ambient temperature and humidity, and on the physiological and biochemical characteristics of the individual athlete. Carbohydrate depletion can cause fatigue and reduce the exercise intensity that can be sustained, but is not normally a life-threatening condition. Disturbances in fluid balance and temperature regulation have potentially more serious consequences, and it may be, therefore, that the emphasis for the major-

ity of participants in endurance events should be on proper maintenance of fluid and electrolyte balance.

Water Overload and Hyponatremia

Voluntary fluid intakes are seldom sufficient to balance fluid losses
when sweat rates are high, and it is recognized that this may lead to dehydration and heat illness in prolonged exercise when the ambient temperature is high. Wyndham and Strydom (1969) noted that marathon
runners typically drink only about 100 mL/h, and more recent evidence
confirms that the intakes of other serious runners are not much higher
than this (Noakes, 1988). Accordingly, the advice often given to endurance athletes is that they should make a conscious effort to ensure a
high fluid intake by drinking even when not thirsty and by following a
strict fluid replacement regimen that prescribes fixed volumes at set intervals. It is also recommended that drinks should contain low levels of
glucose and electrolytes so as not to delay gastric emptying (American
College of Sports Medicine, 1984). It is now recognized that the addition
of electrolytes has relatively little effect on the rate of gastric emptying,
and the revised ACSM guidelines for fluid replacement (American College of Sports Medicine, 1996) support the addition of low levels of
sodium. In accordance with these recommendations, most carbohydrate-electrolyte drinks intended for consumption during prolonged exercise have been formulated to have a low electrolyte content, with
sodium and chloride concentrations typically in the range of 10–20
mmol/L. While this might represent a reasonable strategy for providing
substrates and water (although it can be argued that a higher sodium
concentration might confer some benefits and that a higher carbohydrate content would increase substrate provision), these recommendations may not be appropriate in all circumstances.

Cases of collapse among runners at the end of long distance races
are relatively rare, but some of the major city marathons held in recent
years have attracted as many as 30,000 runners, and in some of these
races there have been significant casualties. In most of these individuals,
who typically collapse within a few minutes of completing the race, hyperthermia associated with dehydration and hypernatremia is observed, and the condition is resolved rapidly after oral or intravenous
administration of fluids. However, it is clear that a few individuals at
the end of very prolonged events suffer from hyponatremia in conjunction with either hyperhydration (Frizell et al., 1986; Noakes et al., 1985,
1990; Saltin & Costill, 1988) or dehydration (Hiller, 1989).

All the cases reported in the literature have been associated with ultramarathon or prolonged triathlon events; most of these have occurred in
events lasting in excess of 8 h, and there are few reports of cases where the

exercise duration was less than 4 h. These athletes may actually have encountered difficulties by adhering too closely to inappropriate recommendations for fluid intake. Noakes et al. (1985) reported four cases of exercise-induced hyponatremia; race times were between 7 and 10 h, and post-race serum sodium concentrations were between 115 and 125 mmol/L, so these individuals were clearly hyponatremic. Estimated fluid intakes were 6–12 L and consisted of water or drinks containing low levels of electrolytes; estimated total sodium chloride intakes during the race were 20–40 mmol. These individuals were therefore adhering to the American College of Sports Medicine guidelines, which recommend an intake, at the upper end of the range, of about 1 L/h. Frizell et al. (1986) reported even more astonishing fluid intakes of 20–24 L of fluids (an intake of almost 2.5 L/h) with a mean sodium content of only 5–10 mmol/L in two runners who collapsed after an ultramarathon run and who were found to be hyponatremic (serum sodium concentration 118–123 mmol/L). It seems clear that the fluid requirements of the slower runner are much more variable than those of the elite competitor; because of the lower exercise intensity and longer duration, excessive drinking is possible.

Hyponatremia as a consequence of ingesting large volumes of fluids with a low sodium content has also been recognized in resting individuals. A reduction in serum sodium and osmolality normally stimulates output of copious amounts of dilute urine, but in the case of the individuals referred to above, who clearly replaced water in excess of losses but did not ingest adequate electrolytes, this does not happen. They therefore suffered from a dilutional hyponatremia. However, competitors in the Hawaii Ironman Triathlon who were found to be hyponatremic were also dehydrated (Hiller, 1989). Finally, Fellmann et al. (1988) reported a small but statistically significant fall in serum sodium concentration, from 141 to 137 mmol/L, in runners who completed a 24-h run, but food and fluid intakes were neither controlled nor measured.

These reports are interesting and indicate that some supplementation with sodium chloride may be required in extremely prolonged events when large sweat losses can be expected and when it is possible to consume large volumes of fluid. This should not, however, divert attention away from the fact that electrolyte replacement during exercise is not a priority for most participants in most sporting events, although it is certainly helpful after the event to restore body water and electrolyte content.

PRACTICAL IMPLICATIONS FOR THE ATHLETE

Although the basic principles that govern fluid replacement strategies for athletes are well established, there are some real difficulties in putting these into practice. Athletes and their advisers want a prescription for the composition, amount, and timing of fluid intake that will cover all situations. Even within a single event, however, the requirement will vary so much between individuals, depending on the physiological and biochemical characteristics of the individual as well as on the training load and on other factors such as taste preference, that such recommendations can only be made on an individual basis. When the possible effects of different climatic conditions and different training and competition schedules are added, the problems in making a simple recommendation are multiplied.

These difficulties are immediately apparent when any of the published guidelines for fluid intake during exercise is examined. Guidelines are generally formulated to include the needs of most individuals in most situations, with the results that the outer limits become so wide as to be, at best, meaningless, and at worst, positively harmful. The guidelines of the American College of Sports Medicine, published in its 1984 Position Statement on the prevention of heat illness in distance running, were more specific than an earlier (1975) version of these guidelines. The recommendation for marathon runners was for an intake of 100–200 mL every 2–3 km, giving a total intake of 1,400–4,200 mL at the extremes. Again, taking these extreme values, it is unlikely that the elite runners, who take only a little over 2 h to complete the distance, could tolerate a rate of intake of about 2 L/h, and equally unlikely that an intake of 300 mL/h would be adequate for the slowest competitors except perhaps when the ambient temperature was low. These same guidelines also recommended that the best fluid to drink during prolonged exercise is cool water. In view of the accumulated evidence presented above, this recommendation seems even less acceptable than it was in 1984. This has been recognized, and the updated version of the Guidelines (American College of Sports Medicine, 1996) are in accord with the current mainstream thinking: For events lasting more than 60 min, the use of drinks containing "proper amounts of carbohydrates and/or electrolytes" is favored. The evolution of this series of ACSM Position Stands demonstrates the progress made in our understanding of this complex area.

Because of the difficulty in making specific recommendations that will meet the needs of all individuals in all situations, the only possible approach is to formulate some general guidelines and to indicate how these should be modified in different circumstances. Assuming that athletes are willing and able to take fluids during training, the recommendations for fluid use in training will not be very different for training and competition, except in events of very short duration. The sprinter or pursuit cyclist, whose event lasts a few seconds or minutes, has no opportunity or need for fluid intake during competition, but should drink during training sessions that may stretch over two hours or more. The body does not adapt to repeated bouts of dehydration; training in the dehydrated state will impair the quality of training, and confers no advantage. The choice of the fluid to be used is again a decision for the individual. Water ingestion is better than fluid restriction, but dilute carbohydrate-electrolyte drinks will provide greater benefits than water alone. The optimum carbohydrate concentration in most situations will be in the range of about 2–8%, and several different carbohydrates, either alone or in combination, are effective. Glucose, sucrose, maltose, and glucose oligomers are all likely to promote improved performance; addition of small amounts of fructose to drinks containing other carbohydrates seems to be acceptable, but high concentrations of fructose alone are best avoided. Some sodium should probably be present, with the optimum concentration somewhere between 10 and 60 mmol/L, but there is also a strong argument that, in events of short duration, this may not be necessary. There is little evidence to suggest that small variations in the concentrations of these components of ingested fluids will significantly alter their efficacy. No evidence at present supports the addition of other components (e.g., potassium, magnesium, other minerals, or vitamins) to drinks intended to promote or maintain hydration status. Palatability is, however, an important issue, and flavoring of drinks to promote consumption is crucial.

In almost every exercise situation, but especially when there is a heat stress imposed by the environmental conditions, individuals who begin exercise in a hypohydrated state will demonstrate a reduced exercise capacity. Full hydration prior to exercise is therefore essential, although it is not at present clear how beneficial attempts to over-hydrate might be. Evidence continues to accumulate that acute restoration of fluid losses after dehydration induced by exercise and by restriction of food and fluid ingestion may not restore exercise capacity (Burge et al., 1993). When large sweat losses are incurred, it seems clear that more effective restoration is achieved by ingestion of solutions containing electrolytes, especially sodium, and evidence indicates that carbohydrate ingested at this time is also beneficial.

Restoration of fluid and electrolyte losses is a crucial part of the recovery process. Athletes should be encouraged to record body mass changes during training as an estimate of sweat losses. Full replacement requires an intake of water in excess of the sweat loss and restitution of electrolyte losses. When no solid food is consumed, these electrolytes must be present in the drinks consumed.

BIBLIOGRAPHY

Adolph, E.D., and Associates (1947). *Physiology of Man in the Desert*. New York: Wiley.
American College of Sports Medicine (1984). Position stand on prevention of thermal injuries during distance running. *Med. Sci. Sports Exerc.* 16:ix–xiv.

American College of Sports Medicine (1996). Exercise and fluid replacement. *Med. Sci. Sports Exerc.* 28:i–vii.

Armstrong, L.E., D.L. Costill, and W.J. Fink (1987). Changes in body water and electrolytes during heat acclimation: effects of dietary sodium. *Aviat. Space Environ. Med.* 58:143–148.

Armstrong, L.E., D.L. Costill, and W.J. Fink (1985). Influence of diuretic-induced dehydration on competitive running performance. *Med. Sci. Sports Exerc.* 17:456–461.

Asmussen, E., and O. Boje (1945). Body temperature and capacity for work. *Acta Physiol. Scand.* 10:1–22.

Barr, S.I., D.L. Costill, and W.J. Fink (1991). Fluid replacement during exercise: effects of water, saline or no fluid. *Med. Sci. Sports Exerc.* 23:811–817.

Beckers, E.J., N.J. Rehrer., F. Brouns, F. ten Hoor, and W.H.M. Saris (1988). Determination of total gastric volume, gastric secretion and residual meal using the double sampling technique of George. *Gut* 29:1725–1729.

Below, P., R. Mora-Rodriguez, J. Gonzalez-Alonso, and E.F. Coyle (1994). Fluid and carbohydrate ingestion independently improve performance during 1 h of intense cycling. *Med. Sci. Sports Exerc.* 27:200–210.

Brouns, F., W.H.M. Saris, and N.J. Rehrer (1987). Abdominal complaints and gastrointestinal function during long-lasting exercise. *Int. J. Sports Med.* 8:175–189.

Burge, C.M., M.F. Carey, and W.R. Payne (1993). Rowing performance, fluid balance, and metabolic function following dehydration and rehydration. *Med. Sci. Sports Exerc.* 25:1358–1364.

Burgess, W.A., J.M. Davis, W.P. Bartoli, and J.A. Woods (1991). Failure of low dose carbohydrate feeding to attenuate glucoregulatory hormone responses and improve endurance performance. *Int. J. Sport Nutr.* 1:338–352.

Costill, D.L. (1977). Sweating: its composition and effects on body fluids. *Ann. N.Y. Acad. Sci.* 301:160–174.

Costill, D.L., and K.E. Sparks (1973). Rapid fluid replacement following thermal dehydration. *J. Appl. Physiol.* 34:299–303.

Coyle, E.F. (1992). Timing and method of increased carbohydrate to cope with heavy training, competition and recovery. In: C. Williams and J.T. Devlin (eds.) *Foods, Nutrition and Sports Performance.* London: Spon, pp. 35–62.

Coyle, E.F., and A.R. Coggan (1984). Effectiveness of carbohydrate feeding in delaying fatigue during prolonged exercise. *Sports Med.* 1:446–458.

Coyle, E.F., A.R. Coggan, M.K. Hemmert, and J.L. Ivy (1986). Muscle glycogen utilisation during prolonged strenuous exercise when fed carbohydrate. *J. Appl. Physiol.* 61:165–172.

Davis, J.M., D.R. Lamb, W.A. Burgess, and W.P. Bartoli (1987). Accumulation of deuterium oxide (D2O) in body fluids following ingestion of D2O-labelled beverages. *J. Appl. Physiol.* 63:2060–2066.

Dengel, D.R., P.G. Weyand, D.M. Black, and K.J. Cureton (1993). Effects of varying levels of hypohydration on ratings of perceived exertion. *Int. J. Sport Nutr.* 3:376–386.

Elliott, E.J., J.A. Walker-Smith, and M.J.G. Farthing (1986). Relationship between glucose and sodium in oral rehydration solutions (ORS); studies in a model of secretory diarrhoea. *Pediatr. Res.* 20:690.

Febbraio, M.A., J.A. Parkin, J. Baldwin, S. Zhao, and M.F. Carey (1996). Metabolic indices of fatigue in prolonged exercise at different ambient temperatures. *J. Sports Sci.* (Abstract) In Press.

Fellmann, N., M. Sagnol, M. Bedu, G. Falgairette, E. Van Praagh, G. Gaillard, P. Jouanel, and J. Coudert (1998). Enzymatic and hormonal responses following a 24 h endurance run and a 10 h triathlon race. *Eur. J. Appl. Physiol.* 57:545–553.

Fielding, R.A., D.L. Costill, W.J. Fink, D.S. King, M. Hargreaves, and J.E. Kovaleski (1985). Effect of carbohydrate feeding frequencies on muscle glycogen use during exercise. *Med. Sci. Sports Exerc.* 17:472–476.

Fortney, S.M., C.B. Wenger, J.R. Bove, and E.R. Nadel (1984). Effect of hyperosmolality on control of blood flow and sweating. *J. Appl. Physiol.* 57:1688–1695.

Freund, B.J., S.J. Montain, A.J. Young, M.N. Sawka, J.P. DeLuca, K.B. Pandolf, and C.R. Valeri (1995). Glycerol hyperhydration: hormonal, renal and vascular fluid responses. *J. Appl. Physiol.* 79:2069–2077.

Frizell, R.T., G.H. Lang, D.C. Lowance, and S.R. Lathan (1986). Hyponatraemia and ultramarathon running. *J. Am. Med. Assoc.* 255:772–774.

Galloway, S.D.R., and R.J. Maughan (1995). Effects of ambient temperature on the capacity to perform prolonged exercise in man (abstract). *J. Physiol.* 489:35–36P.

George, G. (1968). New clinical method for measuring the rate of gastric emptying: the double sampling test meal. *Gut* 9:237–242.

Gisolfi, C.V., and J.R. Copping (1974). Thermal effects of prolonged treadmill exercise in the heat. *Med. Sci. Sports Exerc.* 6:108–113.

Gisolfi, C.V., R.D. Summers, H.P. Schedl, and T.L. Bleiler (1995). Effect of sodium concentration in a carbohydrate-electrolyte solution on intestinal absorption. *Med. Sci. Sports Exerc.* 27: 1414–1420.

Gisolfi, C.V., R.W. Summers, H.P. Schedl, T.L. Blieler, and R.A. Oppliger (1990). Human intestinal water absorption: direct vs indirect measurements. *Am. J. Physiol.* 258:G216–222

Gleeson, M., R.J. Maughan, and P.L. Greenhaff (1986). Comparison of the effects of preexericse feeding of glucose, glycerol and placebo on endurance and fuel homeostasis in man. *Eur. J. Appl. Physiol.* 55:645–653.

Gonzalez-Alonso, J., C.L. Heaps, and E.F. Coyle (1992). Rehydration after exercise with common beverages and water. *Int. J. Sports Med.* 13:399–406.

Gonzalez-Alonzo, J., R. Mora-Rodriguez, P.R. Below, and E.F. Coyle (1995). Dehydration reduces cardiac output and increases systemic and cutaneous vascular resistance during exercise. *J. Appl. Physiol.* 79:1487–1496.

Gopinathan, P.M., G. Pichan and V.M. Sharma (1988). Role of dehydration in heat stress-induced variations in mental performance. *Arch. Environ. Health* 43:15–17.

Hargreaves, M., and C.A. Briggs (1988). Effect of carbohydrate ingestion on exercise metabolism. *J. Appl. Physiol.* 65:1553–1555.

Hargreaves, M., D.L. Costill, A.R. Coggan, W.J. Fink, and I. Nishibata (1984). Effect of carbohydrate feedings on muscle glycogen utilisation and exercise performance. *Med. Sci. Sports Exerc.* 16:219–222.

Havenith, G., V.G.M. Luttikholt, and T.G.M. Vrijkotte (1995). The relative influence of body characteristics on humid heat stress response. *Eur. J. Appl. Physiol.* 70:270–279.

Houmard, J.A., P.C. Egan, R.A. Johns, P.D. Neufer, T.C. Chenier, and R.G. Israel (1991). Gastric emptying during 1 h of cycling and running at 75% VO2max. *Med. Sci. Sports Exerc.* 23:320–325.

Hunt, J.B., A.F.M. Salim, A.V. Thillainayagam, S. Carnaby, E. Elliott, M.L. Clark, and M.J.G. Farthing (1988). Evaluation of a hypotonic oral rehydration solution (ORS) in mammalian models. *Gut* 29:A1470.

Hunt, J.N., J.L. Smith, and C.L. Jiang (1985). Effect of meal volume and energy density on the gastric emptying rate of carbohydrates. *Gastroenterology* 89:1326–1330.

Jones, B.J.M., R.E. Brown, J.S. Loran, D. Edgerton, and J.F. Kennedy (1983). Glucose absorption from starch hydrolysates in the human jejunum. *Gut* 24:1152–1160.

Jones, B.J.M., B.E. Higgins, and D.B.A. Silk (1987). Glucose absorption from maltotriose and glucose oligomers in the human jejunum. *Clin. Sci.* 72:409–414.

Kobayashi, Y., Y. Ando, S. Takeuchi, K. Takemura, and N. Okuda (1980). Effects of heat acclimation of distance runners in a moderately hot environment. *Eur. J. Appl. Physiol.* 45:189–198.

Kozlowski, S., Z. Brzezinska, B. Kruk, H. Kaciuba-Uscilko, J.E. Greenleaf, and K. Nazar (1985). Exercise hyperthermia as a factor limiting physical performance: temperature effect on muscle metabolism. *J. Appl. Physiol.* 59:766–773.

Lamb, D.R., and G.R. Brodowicz (1986). Optimal use of fluids of varying formulations to minimize exercise-induced disturbances in homeostasis. *Sports Med.* 3:247–274.

Lambert, C.P., D.L. Costill, G.K. McConnell, M.A. Benedict, G.P. Lambert, R.A. Robergs, and W.J. Fink (1992). Fluid replacement after dehydration: influence of beverage carbonation and carbohydrate content. *Int. J. Sports Med.* 13:285–292.

Lee, D.T., and E.M. Haymes (1995). Exercise duration and thermoregulatory responses after whole body precooling. *J. Appl. Physiol.* 79:1971–1976.

Leiper, J.B., and R.J. Maughan (1988). Experimental models for the investigation of water and solute transport in man: implications for oral rehydration solutions. *Drugs* 36 Suppl 4: 65–79.

Luetkemeier, M.J. (1995). Dietary sodium intake and changes in plasma volume during short term exercise training. *Int. J. Sports Med.* 16:435–438.

Lyons, T.P., M.L. Riedesel, L.E. Meuli, and T.W. Chick (1990). Effects of glycerol-induced hyperhydration prior to exercise in the heat on sweating and core temperature. *Med. Sci. Sports Exerc.* 22:477–483.

Maughan, R.J. (1991). Effects of CHO-electrolyte solution on prolonged exercise. In: D.R. Lamb and M.H. Williams (eds.) *Perspectives in Exercise Science and Sports Medicine.* Carmel, IN: Benchmark Press, pp. 35–85.

Maughan, R.J. (1994). Fluid and electrolyte loss and replacement in exercise. In: E. Harries, Williams, Stanish and Micheli (eds.) *Oxford Textbook of Sports Medicine.* New York: Oxford University Press, pp. 82–93.

Maughan, R.J. (1985). Thermoregulation and fluid balance in marathon competition at low ambient temperature. *Int. J. Sports Med.* 6:15–19.

Maughan, R.J., and J.B. Leiper (1983). Aerobic capacity and fractional utilisation of aerobic capacity in elite and non-elite male and female marathon runners. *Eur. J. Appl. Physiol.* 52:80–87.

Maughan, R.J., and J.B. Leiper (1995). Sodium intake and post-exercise rehydration in man. *Eur. J. Appl. Physiol.* 75:311–319.

Maughan, R.J., L. Bethell, and J.B. Leiper (1996). Effects of ingested fluids on homeostasis and exercise performance in man. *Exp. Physiol.* In press.

Maughan, R.J., C.E. Fenn, and J.B. Leiper (1987). Effects of fluid, electrolyte and substrate ingestion on endurance capacity. *Eur. J. Appl. Physiol.* 58:481–486.

Maughan, R.J., J.B. Leiper, and B.A. McGaw (1990). Effects of exercise intensity on absorption of ingested fluids in man. *Exp. Physiol.* 75:419–421.

Maughan, R.J., J.H. Owen, S.M. Shirreffs, and J.B. Leiper (1994). Postexercise rehydration in man: effects of electrolyte addition to ingested fluids. *Eur. J. Appl. Physiol.* 69:209–215.

Maw, G.J., S.H. Boutcher, and N.A.S. Taylor (1993). Ratings of perceived exertion and affect in hot and cool environments. *Eur. J. Appl. Physiol.* 67:174–179.

Mitchell, J.B., and K.W. Voss (1991). The influence of volume on gastric emptying and fluid balance during prolonged exercise. *Med. Sci. Sports Exerc.* 23:314–319.

Mitchell, J.B., D.L. Costill, J.A. Houmard, W.J. Fink, R.A. Robergs, and J.A. Davis (1989). Gastric emptying: influence of prolonged exercise and carbohydrate concentration. *Med. Sci. Sports Exerc.* 21:269–274.

Mitchell, J.B., D.L. Costill, J.A. Houmard, M.G. Flynn, W.J. Fink, and J.D. Beltz (1988). Effects on carbohydrate ingestion on gastric emptying and exercise performance. *Med. Sci. Sports Exerc.* 20:110–115.

Mitchell, T.H., A. Gebrehiwot, S. Wing, S.A. Magder, M.G. Cosio, A. Deschamps, and E.B. Marliss (1990). Intravenous bicarbonate and sodium chloride both prolong endurance during intense cycle ergometer exercise. *Am. J. Med. Sci.* 300:88–97.

Mohan, M., J.S. Sethi, T.S. Daral, M. Sharma, S.K. Bhargava, and H.P.S. Sachdev (1986). Controlled trial of rice powder and glucose rehydration solutions as oral therapy for acute dehydrating diarrhea in infants. *J. Pediatr. Gastroenterol. Nutr.* 5:423–427.

Molla, A.M., A. Molla, J. Rhode, and W.B. Greenough (1989). Turning off the diarrhea: The role of food and ORS. *J. Pediatr. Gastroenterol. Nutr.* 8:81–84.

Montain, S.J., and E.F. Coyle (1992). Influence of graded dehydration on hyperthermia and cardiovascular drift during exercise. *J. Appl. Physiol.* 73:1340–1350.

Montain, S.J., W.A. Latzka, and M.N. Sawka (1995). Control of thermoregulatory sweating is altered by hydration level and exercise. *J. Appl. Physiol.* 79:1434–1439.

Montner, P., D.M. Stark, M.L. Riedesel, G. Murata, R. Robergs, M. Timms, and T.W. Chick (1996). Preexercise glycerol hydration improves cycling endurance time. *Int. J. Sports Med.* 17:27–33.

Mota-Hernandes, F., D. Bross-Soriano, M.C. Perez-Ricardez, and L. Velasquez-Jones (1991). Rice solution and World Health Organisation solution by gastric infusion for high stool output diarrhea. *Am. J. Dis. Child.* 145:937–940.

Murray, R. (1987). The effects of consuming carbohydrate-electrolyte beverages on gastric emptying and fluid absorption during and following exercise. *Sports Med.* 4:322–351.

Nadel, E.R. (1980). Circulatory and thermal regulations during exercise. *Fed. Proc.* 39:1491–1497.

Nadel, E.R. (1983). Effects of temperature on muscle metabolism. In: H.G. Knuttgen, et al. (eds.) *Biochemistry of Exercise.* Champaign, IL: Human Kinetics, pp. 134–143.

Nadel, E.R., S.M. Fortney, and C.B. Wenger (1980). Effect of hydration state on circulatory and thermal regulations. *J. Appl. Physiol.* 49:715–721.

Nadel, E.R., G.W. Mack, and H. Nose (1990). Influence of fluid replacement beverages on body fluid homeostasis during exercise and recovery. In: C.V. Gisolfi and D.R. Lamb (eds). *Perspectives in Exercise Science and Sports Medicine. Volume 3: Fluid Homeostasis During Exercise.* Carmel, IN: Benchmark Press, pp. 181–205.

Naveri, H., H. Tikkanen, A.L. Kairento, and M. Harkonen (1989). Gastric emptying and serum insulin levels after intake of glucose-polymer solutions. *Eur. J. Appl. Physiol.* 58:661–665.

Nielsen, B (1994). Heat stress and acclimation. *Ergonomics* 37:49–58.

Nielsen, B., R. Kubica, A. Bonnesen, I.B. Rasmussen, J. Stoklosa, and B. Wilk (1981). Physical work capacity after dehydration and hyperthermia. *Scand. J. Sports Sci.* 3:2–10.

Nielsen, B., G. Sjogaard, J. Ugelvig, B. Knudsen, and B. Dohlmann (1986). Fluid balance in exercise dehydration and rehydration with different glucose-electrolyte drinks. *Eur. J. Appl. Physiol.* 55: 318–325.

Noakes, T.D. (1993). Fluid replacement during exercise. In: J.O. Holloszy (ed.) *Exercise and Sports Science Reviews.* Baltimore, MD: Williams & Wilkins, Vol 21, pp. 297–330.

Noakes, T.D. (1988). Why marathon runners collapse. *S. Afr. Med. J.* 73:569–571.

Noakes, T.D., N. Goodwin, B.L. Rayner, T. Branken, and R.K.N. Taylor (1985). Water intoxication: a possible complication during endurance exercise. *Med. Sci. Sports Exerc.* 17:370–375.

Noakes, T.D., N.J. Rehrer, and R.J. Maughan (1990). The importance of volume in regulating gastric emptying. *Med. Sci. Sports Exerc.* 23:307–313.

Nose, H., G.W. Mack, X. Shi, and E.R. Nadel (1988a). Involvement of sodium retention hormones during rehydration in humans. *J. Appl. Physiol.* 65:332–336.

Nose, H., G.W. Mack, X. Shi, and E.R. Nadel (1988b). Role of osmolality and plasma volume during rehydration in humans. *J. Appl. Physiol.* 65:325–331.

O'Connor, A.M., C.F. Johnston, K.D. Buchanan, C. Boreham, T.R. Trinick, and C.J. Riddoch (1995). Circulating gastrointestinal hormone changes in marathon running. *Int. J. Sports Med.* 16:283–287.

Owen, M.D., K.C. Kregel, P.T. Wall, and C.V. Gisolfi (1986). Effects of ingesting carbohydrate beverages during exercise in the heat. *Med. Sci. Sports Exerc.* 18:568–575.

Peters, H.P.F., L.M.A. Akkermans, E. Bol, and W.L. Mosterd (1995). Gastrointestinal symptoms during exercise. *Sports Med.* 20:65–76.

Rehrer, N.J., E. Beckers, F. Brouns, F. Ten Hoor, and W.H.M. Saris (1989). Exercise and training effects on gastric emptying of carbohydrate beverages. *Med. Sci. Sports Exerc.* 21:540–549.

Rehrer, N.J., F. Brouns, E. Beckers, F. Ten Hoor, and W.H.M. Saris (1990). Gastric emptying with repeated drinking during running and bicycling. *Int. J. Sports Med.* 11:238–243.

Rehrer, N.J., A.J.M. Wagenmakers, and E.J. Beckers (1992). Gastric emptying, intestinal absorption and carbohydrate oxidation during prolonged exercise. *J. Appl. Physiol.* 72:468–475.

Robinson, T.A., J.A. Hawley, G.S. Palmer, G.R. Wilson, D.A. Gray, T.D. Noakes, and S.C. Dennis (1995). Water ingestion does not improve 1-h cycling performance in moderate ambient temperatures. *Eur. J. Appl. Physiol.* 71:153–160.

Rolston, D.D.K., M.M. Borodo, M.J. Kelly, A.M. Dawson, and M.J.G. Farthing (1987). Efficacy of oral rehydration solutions in a rat model of secretory diarrhea. *J. Pediatr. Gastroenterol. Nutr.* 6:624–630.

Rolston, D.D.K., S.N. Zinzuvadia, and V.I. Mathan (1990). Evaluation of the efficacy of oral rehydration solutions using human whole gut perfusion. *Gut* 31:1115–1119.

Rowell, L.B. (1986). *Human Circulation.* New York: Oxford University Press.

Saltin, B., and D.L. Costill (1988). Fluid and electrolyte balance during prolonged exercise. In E.S. Horton and R.L. Terjung (eds.) *Exercise, Nutrition, and Metabolism.* New York: Macmillan, pp. 150–158.

Saltin, B., A.P. Gagge, U. Bergh, and J.A.J. Stolwijk (1972). Body temperatures and sweating during exhaustive exercise. *J. Appl. Physiol.* 32:635–643.

Sawka, M.N., and K.B. Pandolf (1990). Effects of body water loss on physiological function and exercise performance. In: C.V. Gisolfi and D.R. Lamb (eds.) *Fluid Homeostasis During Exercise.* Carmel, IN: Benchmark Press, pp. 1–38.

Sawka, M.N., A.J. Andrew, R.P. Francesconi, S.R. Muza, and K.B. Pandolf (1985). Thermoregulatory and blood responses during exercise at graded hypohydration levels. *J. Appl. Physiol.* 59:1394–1401.

Schedl, H.P., R.J. Maughan, and C.V. Gisolfi (1994). Intestinal absorption during rest and exercise: implications for formulating oral rehydration beverages. *Med. Sci. Sports Exerc.* 26:267–280.

Shi, X., R.W. Summers, H.P. Schedl, S.W. Flanagan, R. Chang, and C.V. Gisolfi (1995). Effects of carbohydrate type and concentration and solution osmolality on water absorption. *Med. Sci. Sports Exerc.* 27:1607–1615.

Shirreffs, S.M., A.J. Taylor, J.B. Leiper, and R.J. Maughan (1996). Postexercise rehydration in man: effects of volume consumed and sodium content of ingested fluids. *Med. Sci. Sports Exerc.* In Press.

Sole, C.C., and Noakes T.D. (1989). Faster gastric emptying for glucose-polymer and fructose solutions than for glucose in humans. *Eur. J. Appl. Physiol.* 58:605–612.

Spiller, R.C., B.J.M. Jones, B.E. Brown, and D.B.A. Silk (1982). Enhancement of carbohydrate absorption by the addition of sucrose to enteric diets. *J. Parent. Enter. Nutr.* 6:321.

Strydom, N.B., C.H. Wyndham, C.H. van Graan, L.D. Holdsworth, and J.F. Morrison (1966). The influence of water restriction on the performance of men during a prolonged march. *S. Afr. Med. J.* 40:539–544.

Sutton, J.R. (1990). Clinical implications of fluid imbalance. In: C.V. Gisolfi and D.R. Lamb (eds.) *Perspectives in Exercise Science and Sports Medicine, Vol 3. Fluid Homeostasis During Exercise.* Carmel, IN: Benchmark Press. pp, 425–448.

Suzuki, Y. (1980). Human physical performance and cardiocirculatory responses to hot environments during sub-maximal upright cycling. *Ergonomics* 23:527–542.

Verde, T., R.J. Shephard, P. Corey, and R. Moore (1982). Sweat composition in exercise and in heat. *J. Appl. Physiol.* 53:1540–1545.

Vist, G.E., and R.J. Maughan (1994). The effect of increasing glucose concentration on the rate of gastric emptying in man. *Med. Sci. Sports Exerc.* 26:1269–1273.

Vist, G.E., and R.J Maughan (1995). The effect of osmolality and carbohydrate content on the rate of gastric emptying of liquids in man. *J. Physiol.* 486:523–531.

Vist, G.E., H.S. Williamson, and R.J. Maughan (1997). Gastric emptying after repeated ingestion of carbohydrate solutions. *Med. Sci. Sports. Exerc.* In Press.

Walker-Smith, J.A. (1992). Recommendations for composition of oral rehydration solutions for children of Europe. *J. Pediatr. Gastroenterol.* 14:113–115.

Walsh, R.M., T.D. Noakes, J.A. Hawley, and S.C. Dennis (1994). Impaired high-intensity cycling performance time at low levels of dehydration. *Int. J. Sports Med.* 15:392–298.

Wapnir, R.A., and F. Lifshitz (1985). Osmolality and solute concentration — their relationship with oral rehydration solution effectiveness: an experimental assessment. *Pediatr. Res.* 19:894–898.

Wyndham, C.H., and N.B. Strydom (1969). The danger of an inadequate water intake during marathon running. *S. Afr. Med. J.* 43:893–896.

Zachwieja, J.J., D.L. Costill, G.C. Beard, R.A. Robergs, D.D Pascoe, and D.E. Anderson (1992). The effect of a carbonated carbohydrate drink on gastric emptying, gastrointestinal distress, and exercise performance. *Int. J. Sports Med.* 2:239–250.

DISCUSSION

BEHNKE: I accept your view that from a scientific standpoint there is no universal carbohydrate-electrolyte solution for every athlete under every condition, but athletic trainers who deal with team sports don't have the luxury of prescribing different sports drinks for different athletes. What formulation would you recommend for a team of 100 university football players in hot weather?

MAUGHAN: If you look at the mainstream sports drinks, it is not just coincidence that the formulation of most of those drinks is very similar. They are typically nearly isotonic with respect to body fluids, and they normally contain about 6–8% carbohydrate and about 20–25 mmol/L sodium, with a little potassium included. Those are probably the key considerations, and the main differences are with respect to taste, although most drinks contain small amounts of other compounds. In that range of composition, these drinks will meet the demands for most people under most circumstances. However, I take the view quite strongly that to maximize water delivery, the solution should be hypotonic, with an osmolality of about 200–250. To achieve this you would probably drop the carbohydrate to about 2%, and possibly increase the sodium concentration to about 60 mmol/L. The problem with this formula is that it does not provide much carbohydrate—only 20 g/L. In a situation requiring more carbohydrate, you would have to increase the carbohydrate concentration to 10–12%, and perhaps even to 15%. Some successful athletes, particularly cross country skiers, have used drink carbohydrate concentrations as high as 40%. With this formulation, though, gastric emptying will be slowed, leading to poor provision of water.

BEHNKE: Do you suggest changing the percentages of electrolytes in a sports drink following a period of acclimatization?

MAUGHAN: I don't think that we know enough to answer that with any conviction. The first place to start is perhaps to say that after a period of acclimatization there is generally an increased sweat loss and therefore a need for an increase in total intake of fluid. Some of our athletes think that part of their acclimatization is to decrease fluid requirements, but of course the opposite is true—an increased volume should be consumed. We know that the sweat electrolyte composition changes with acclimatization so that the sodium concentration of sweat decreases. That might be taken as an indication of a change in the need for sodium; however, during exercise the primary function of added sodium is not to replace sodium lost in the sweat but to stimulate intestinal water absorption and perhaps also to enhance palatability. Only during extreme endurance exercise where sweat losses are very large do you need to replace the electrolyte losses in sweat. I don't think the evidence at this stage would say there is a need for a great change in the formulation in that situation, if only because the variation between individuals is so large. There is no convincing evidence that there is a need to add any electrolytes other than sodium to rehydration solutions intended for use during exercise.

BEHNKE: With regard to gastric emptying, intestinal absorption, and even core temperature, athletic trainers are concerned about the temperature of the sports drink. Whereas some athletes won't touch drinks that are not ice cold, others will drink fluids that are lukewarm or at ambient temperature. What is the influence of the temperature of the drink on physiology?

MAUGHAN: If drinks are ice cold, problems can occur because the volume that athletes can consume is limited. Drink-dispensing machines are usually set at a temperature of 4°C, but it is difficult to drink large volumes of fluid when it is so cold. If people have a free choice of fluids at different temperatures, the optimum temperature seems to be about 14–15°C; above and below that range the voluntary intake tends to decrease. This suggests that drinks should be chilled, but not cold. Of course it depends on the individual's preference, and it also depends on the type of fluid. Many of the sport drinks taste better and feel more refreshing when they are chilled. This is particularly true when one is hot and hypohydrated. In terms of physiology, I don't think there is good evidence of any significant influence of drink temperature. Certainly gastric emptying isn't particularly affected by the temperature at which drinks are ingested. There used to be a belief that cooling drinks accelerated gastric emptying, but this has since been shown to be incorrect. Very cold drinks in large volumes can cause an intestinal dumping syndrome, but within the range we are talking about, chilling or warming drinks doesn't have a large effect on the rate of gastric emptying.

BEHNKE: A team physician I work with has us weigh our athletes in the nude, before and after practice. He will check the weight chart every day. Players who have lost more than 5% body weight will not be allowed to practice again until they have regained 80% of that loss. Is there a general rule of thumb like this that we can imply to assist coaches, athletes, and athletic trainers regarding fluid replacement?

MAUGHAN: The principle of individualizing treatment by monitoring the athlete in this way is extremely sound and should be encouraged, but I would want to think very hard before putting a number on it. When people are hypohydrated they shouldn't be allowed—and certainly not required—to do hard exercise in the heat. If you can monitor their hydration status, which requires a history of body weight, then any dramatic change is almost certainly indicative of hypohydration. There can be some problems, though, because the interpretation of body weight changes requires also some information on food intake and training habits. For example, we encountered some problems with British athletes traveling to Atlanta to gain hot-weather experience in preparation for the Olympic games. There was five-star catering available throughout most of the day in the training camp—all of it free, and some athletes took advantage of this and ate more than normal. Thus, a constant body weight could be the result of an increased food intake, which in turn could mask an underlying hypohydration.

SCOTT: In addition to weighing athletes before and after practice, one way to follow-up on monitoring fluid status is to have the athlete lie down for a couple of minutes, take the pulse, have the athlete stand up for 1 min, and repeat the pulse recording. If there is a difference of 10 or more beats/min, this indicates significant fluid losses, and the athlete should be strongly advised to replenish body fluids.

Also, in my clinical experience, there seem to be differences between blacks and whites regarding salt intake on a daily basis and during exercise. We see many white athletes who are "salt phobics" and who compete in Ironman triathlons and other types of endurance exercise; they end up with convulsions and plasma sodium concentrations depleted below 120 mosmols/L. They say they don't use any salt in their diets at all. This does not seem to occur in black athletes.

MAUGHAN: Changes in body weight during practice will give a good indication of fluid balance, but over a longer period of time, changes in body mass can be misleading if people alter their eating habits, whether consciously or not. Partly because of this concern, particularly in relation to the weight-category sports, we tried out a number of strategies with the British athletes training for the Atlanta Olympics. One example was to have the athletes keep a log of fluid intake and output for about 2 wk while training in the U.K. and again during the training camp in Florida. They measured the urine volume, recorded the time of each urine sample that was passed, and recorded the data in a diary that was provided. That gave us an indication of their urinary habits and their daily urine outputs while training in the U.K. and while training away from home. When the athletes traveled to Florida, they faced a 5 h time shift and a sudden change in the temperature and humidity. The first thing we noticed was a dramatic fall in urine output for the first few days, suggesting that these athletes were acutely hypohydrated, even though they made a conscious effort to increase fluid intake. It was quite easy to convince the athletes that they were not drinking enough until their urine outputs returned to the levels normally seen at home. Also, when they stopped waking in the night to pass urine and returned to their normal patterns, they had some indication that their body clocks had adjusted to local time. This type of self–monitoring is something that people can do quite easily.

Another thing we did was to have some of the squads collect morning urine samples, on which we measured osmolality. We saw some individuals with urine osmolality values in excess of 1,350 mosmol/kg, suggesting a moderately severe level of hypohydration. In some circumstances the athletes themselves did not recognize this, but there were quite clearly some situations where hypohydration was associated with a failure to perform well in training. In many cases, the athletes, and more especially the coaches, were pleased to have an external measure to give them an indication of whether or not they were meeting their fluid needs. The intention of this monitoring was that it should be a part of an educational process wherein the athletes should learn to recognize the symptoms and what to do about it.

Your point about people who are on very low salt intakes is an important one. The health message in recent years has been that we should avoid excessive salt intake, even though it is now recognized that salt intake is only one of the factors associated with hypertension. But of course when you have an excessive salt loss, you need a large salt intake; a high salt intake is not excessive where it is appropriate. If 1 L of sweat with a sodium concentration of 50 mmol/L is replaced with sodium chloride, the amount of salt needed is approximately 3 g; therefore, the athlete training hard in a hot environment and sweating 5–10 L/d may need 15–30 g of salt.

GISOLFI: A point that needs to be emphasized to the coaches and athletic trainers is that athletes typically drink only about 500 mL/h, but they must be encouraged to drink more because during prolonged exercise they are losing 1–2 L/h.

MAUGHAN: You hit the nail right on the head. When we tried to optimize fluid replacement, we gave an initial bolus of 600 mL and then we gave 200 mL about every 15 min. That is what we found was necessary to maintain a high volume in the stomach and to maintain a high rate of fluid delivery for absorption in the intestine, and this seems to work well for dilute solutions.

GISOLFI: Is hypohydration a separate mechanism causing exercise-induced exhaustion, or does hypohydration lead to hyperthermia, which is the ultimate cause of exhaustion?

MAUGHAN: Hypohydration leads to hyperthermia-induced exhaustion, and I certainly didn't mean to imply otherwise. I don't believe hypohydration per se has a primary effect, at least in endurance events. In some other exercise situations, though, it may be a factor. If one begins brief, high intensity exercise in a hypohydrated state, exercise performance will be reduced. That is not a condition in which core temperature is a limiting factor, so in the high-intensity exercise situation, hypohydration may in itself be a factor leading to fatigue.

NADEL: Sodium is the most important cation in a fluid replacement drink, obviously because it is lost from the body in sweat in the greatest amount, but I would like your further comments about replacing other cations lost in sweat.

MAUGHAN: I don't think magnesium is important. Potassium is important, and we just recently completed a study on postexercise rehydration that supports that view. We dehydrated our subjects by 2% of body weight and then gave a volume of fluid equal to the sweat loss in the rehydration period. That is different from the latest studies we have done in which we gave a volume greater than the sweat loss and measured the urine output over the next few hours. We had four drink trials: a glucose solution (90 mmol/L glucose), a sodium chloride drink (60 mmol/L sodium chloride), a potassium chloride drink (25 mmol/L potassium chloride), and also a drink containing glucose, sodium, and the potassium. All the electrolyte-containing drinks reduced urine output relative to the glucose-only drink, but there was no difference in urine output between any of those three electrolyte-containing drinks. Thus, 25 mmol/L potassium was as good as 60 mmol/L sodium, and adding the two together didn't make any difference. The problem with that study was that we only got people back to euhydration at the end of the rehydration period; as soon as urine output began, subjects entered a state of hypohydration. When we looked at urine output over the next 6 h, the volume was pretty close to the minimum obligatory output when the sodium or potassium alone was added, so there wasn't much room for further reducing urine output. Had we given a larger volume of fluid, perhaps twice the volume loss, I think it is quite possible that we would have seen an additive effect of sodium and potassium, and that study is under way now. Yes, adding sodium is important. Adding potassium is probably also important.

NADEL: What is your rationale for adding more potassium than is lost in sweat?

MAUGHAN: It seems to help rehydration by decreasing the loss of water in the urine. Where that fluid is being retained, we don't know; it did not seem to be in the vascular space, presumably because potassium is located primarily in the intracellular space.

SHI: We know that the type of carbohydrate, carbohydrate concentration, and osmolality are very important for water absorption. What is your suggestion for the optimal concentration of sodium in a fluid-replacement drink if we consider factors such as carbohydrate content and osmolality?

MAUGHAN: Sodium can move both ways in the intestine, which is very effective in secreting sodium, which can then be reabsorbed further down the gut. So in one sense one might conclude that extra sodium in a drink is unnecessary, but I take the view that it is disadvantageous to secrete all that sodium and then reabsorb it farther down because sodium absorption in the proximal part of the intestine could better stimulate water absorption. I think the ideal sodium concentration in a drink is a little bit higher than most experts have suggested, but if it is too high, one runs into osmolality problems. Some of the problems associated with a high osmolality can be minimized by adding glucose in polymer form rather than as free glucose or sucrose. Furthermore, if the sodium concentration is too great, many athletes will not find the drink palatable, and if drinks don't taste good, athletes won't drink them. If sodium is in the form of sodium chloride, it can taste unpleasant at concentrations higher than about 30–40 mmol/L, but there are other sodium compounds that don't have that unpleasant salt taste.

KENNEY: Several recent presentations at scientific meetings have shown some positive effects of having very high sodium concentrations in ingested fluids (i.e., higher maintained plasma volumes, lower heart rates, higher sweating rates, etc.). Is there a set of workload/environmental parameters that define situations in which the ability to keep fluid in the vascular space supersedes any problems with gastric emptying or intestinal secretion caused by the high sodium concentrations?

MAUGHAN: Again, there is not enough experimental evidence available to give a definitive answer to that question. The problems of palatability can be overcome, and in the concentrations being used there are no major effects of sodium on gastric emptying. There are certainly benefits from adding more sodium in some situations.

HOUGH: Twenty years ago salt tablets were often recommended by trainers and physicians. I am not an advocate of salt tablets, but what practical advice do you have for trainers and physicians who may be concerned about athletes not obtaining adequate sodium in their diets?

MAUGHAN: I am in favor of using salt tablets only in exceptional circumstances. The main reason for this is that many athletes will reason that if two tablets are good, four will be twice as good, and 10 might make them champions, but it is very easy to take excessive amounts of sodium in tablet form. In most situations, rehydration after exercise is accompanied by food intake that will adequately replace losses of all the important electrolytes. There may be problems when athletes are training hard two or three times a day, particularly in the heat. There may be a suppression of appetite for some time after a hard training session and an excessive reliance on carbohydrate drinks that do not contain enough sodium and that may not be consumed in sufficient volume to replace water losses. In that situation, it is certainly advisable to monitor body weight to ensure that a progressive dehydration is not taking place. Many of these problems have been extensively studied over the years, and some of the answers are to be found in the older literature. Studies from the 1920s on miners and foundry workers in England showed high sweat losses; some of these men were drinking as much as 18–20 pints of fluid in a shift. It was well recognized that failure to replace the sodium as well as the water losses resulted in problems. In most situations, sweat losses are more moderate, and the appetite for salt will increase as people become salt deficient. Individuals who are salt depleted show a definite tendency to put more salt on their food, and this will normally meet their needs. I don't believe that we should return to recommending salt tablets.

KUIPERS: Many athletes report that sports drinks seem to lose their palatability if they keep drinking the same beverage for a long time during an event. They also have the impression that the stomach begins filling up and doesn't empty anymore. Is there anything known about the influence of palatability on gastric emptying?

MAUGHAN: There is no good evidence to help me answer that question, but I do recommend that athletes vary the flavor of the drinks they use rather than sticking with one flavor. If you have to drink 10–15 L of fluid in a day, you are going to get bored with the same flavor. Also, athletes should try out new drinks under the conditions in which they will be used. If one is hypohydrated and hyperthermic, the taste mechanism changes so that a beverage that tastes good in the first couple of miles of a marathon probably doesn't taste good in the last few miles. That may be partly caused by boredom with the taste, but it may also be that the taste mechanism has changed. It comes back to practicing with different drinks and having a well-rehearsed fluid-replacement strategy.

TERJUNG: Following intense exercise, especially in the heat, some individuals can experience frank diarrhea after consuming large volumes of water. This certainly can impact fluid balance, well-being, and recovery in athletes. What can be done to prevent this problem?

MAUGHAN: The first thing is to recognize that diarrhea, whether it is exercise–induced or whether it is traveler's diarrhea, which is rather common when teams travel around the world, will exacerbate any dehydration that is present. The usual recommendation for infectious diarrhea is to increase the intake of fluids, even though this may result in an increased volume of stool production. The main thing is to do everything possible to correct the hypohydration. It is very clear in this situation that dilute glucose-electrolyte solutions are more effective than plain water in restoring fluid balance. Water—and that includes mineral water—will not effectively rehydrate in this situation because of the high electrolyte losses. Oral rehydration solutions designed for treatment of diarrhea generally have a high potassium content because of the large potassium losses that may occur, and this can be important if the diarrhea persists. If it is a one-time occurrence and the recovery is not particularly important, one can afford to be a little more relaxed about the need for recovery. If one must train again in the next day or compete again, one must do everything possible to ensure that the rehydration process is effective.

NADEL: What advice did you give to the British Olympic team in their heat acclimation process?

MAUGHAN: It has often been recommended that athletes travel some-* where hot and live there for several weeks before a major competition that is to take place in a hot environment. However, if you were a marathon runner from the UK used to training at a temperature of about 10°C and you moved to Atlanta 6 wk before the Olympic Games, you probably became heat acclimatized but also detrained before the competition began because it is impossible to do high-intensity, high-volume training in the heat. The sprinters, on the other hand, prefer to train in hot conditions, so there is not one solution for everyone. It is equally clear that endurance-trained people show many of the adaptations that result from heat acclimatization, but training in the heat provides additional benefit and cannot be neglected. One possible approach is to live at home and to do the high-quality training in the morning, and then to train somewhere hot in the afternoon (e.g., in a hot room, sauna or climatic chamber). This is the approach that many of our British athletes took in preparation for the Atlanta Olympics. The intensity of exercise that is necessary for heat adaptation doesn't have to be terribly great, so it should not interfere with the athlete's high-quality training. It is also the case that you don't have to live in the heat to become acclimatized; it is enough to exercise for an hour or so in the heat, and there is no reason not to spend the rest of the day in a cool or air-conditioned environment. It is also not necessary to exercise in the heat every day; 3–4 sessions weekly for 3–4 wk will probably achieve something close to complete adaptation without compromising training. In short, living somewhere hot isn't always a major benefit.

MANDELBAUM: Major League Soccer is a summer soccer league, and the league has no policy or procedures established to ensure that the players do not become excessively dehydrated. Do you agree that it is important that the rehydration message be delivered forcefully to coaches, administrators, and referees?

MAUGHAN: It is absolutely crucial that we direct the educational process towards the administrators as well as the athletes and coaches; everyone must be convinced. When, as in soccer, the rules of the game restrict access to fluids, we have to change the rules of the game to make it a safer and a better game.

5

Ergogenic Aids: Recent Advances and Retreats

LAWRENCE L. SPRIET, PH.D.

INTRODUCTION
CREATINE
    Creatine Function and Theoretical Basis for Ergogenicity
    Creatine Metabolism
    Effects of Creatine Supplementation on Muscle Total Creatine Content
    Exercise Performance and Muscle Metabolism Following Creatine Supplementation
    Additional Effects of Creatine Supplementation
    Practical Implications
CARNITINE
    Carnitine Function and Theoretical Basis for an Ergogenic Effect
    Resting Carnitine Metabolism
    Effects of Exercise and Macronutrient Diet on Muscle Carnitine
    Effects of Supplemental Carnitine on Plasma and Muscle Levels
    Carnitine Supplementation and Exercise Metabolism and Performance
    Practical Implications
CAFFEINE
    Caffeine and Theories of Ergogenicity
    Early Caffeine Research
    Recent Complications in the Study of Caffeine, Metabolism, and Exercise Performance
    Recent Caffeine Studies Examining Endurance Performance and Metabolism
    Mechanisms for Improved Endurance with Caffeine
    Caffeine and Performance During Shorter-Term Exercise
        Graded Exercise Tests
        Intense Aerobic Exercise
        Short-Term Intense Exercise
        Sprint Performance
        Field Studies
    Practical Implications
        Caffeine Dose
        Urinary Caffeine and Doping
        Variability of Caffeine Responses
        Habitual Caffeine Consumption
        Diuretic Effect of Caffeine
        Ethical Considerations

ERYTHROPOIETIN
  Recombinant Human Erythropoietin
  Ergogenic Potential and Safety Concerns of rhEPO
  Hematological and Exercise Responses to rhEPO Administration
  Detection of rhEPO Administration
  Practical Implications
DIRECTIONS FOR FUTURE RESEARCH
  Creatine
  Carnitine
  Caffeine
  Erythropoietin
SUMMARY
BIBLIOGRAPHY
DISCUSSION

INTRODUCTION

The interest in ergogenic aids or "work enhancing" agents has never been greater. Exercise scientists, athletes, coaches, athletic trainers, and team physicians share this interest and are faced with the decision of whether or not a potential ergogenic aid is appropriate for application to sport. Robertson (1991) suggested that the following questions must be considered when deciding if an ergogenic aid is appropriate for sport: Is it safe? Is it legal? Is it effective? How does it work? What is the best mode of application? If the answer to the first two questions is "yes," interest then focuses on the last three questions, and the literature for potential ergogenic aids in this category is usually large. If the answer to one of the first two questions is "no," the body of literature for ergogenic aids in this category is usually limited. Investigations are often considered unethical and are usually directed towards answering basic physiological questions.

This chapter will review the recent advances and retreats that have occurred regarding the efficacy of four ergogenic aids: creatine, carnitine, caffeine, and erythropoietin. This eclectic group is examined in this chapter for the following reasons: 1) all are believed to be widely used in athletic circles, 2) examples of nutritional, pharmacological and physiological ergogenic aids are included, 3) compounds that appear to be ergogenic and others that appear to be non-ergogenic are included, and 4) legal, restricted, and illegal substances, as defined by the International Olympic Committee (IOC), are included.

Creatine and carnitine are nutritional ergogenic aids that have gained widespread popularity. The scientific basis for consuming supplemental creatine to improve the performance of brief intense exercise is reasonably strong. On the other hand, research does not support the suggestion that supplemental carnitine increases fat metabolism and improves aerobic exercise performance. Caffeine is a pharmacological ergogenic aid that has gained acceptance due to its unique position in the diets of many people worldwide. It is often listed as a nutritional ergogenic aid when in fact it contains no nutritional value. The IOC also categorizes caffeine as an acceptable athletic drug because relatively high levels of caffeine are allowed in the body before it is considered illegal. Whereas past research strongly supports caffeine as an ergogenic aid during prolonged aerobic exercise, recent studies have identified some retreats related mainly to the variability that exists among individuals. Lastly, erythropoietin is a physiological substance that is clearly ergogenic when given in pharmacological doses. It is also illegal and can be unsafe if not properly administered.

This chapter will attempt to critically examine the important literature on each of these purported ergogenic aids over the past 10 years. Evidence of improved exercise performance in ergogenic studies is usually defined as a longer time to reach exhaustion at a given power output, production of more total work in a given amount of time, or completion of a given exercise task in a shorter amount of time. These criteria also apply to situations where repeated bouts of brief high-intensity exercise are performed.

In examining the potential ergogenic effect of oral nutritional and pharmacological aids, it is important to remember that these compounds have a chance to be ergogenic only if they reach the blood in significant amounts to increase blood concentrations for some time. The compound must not be degraded in the gut and must be largely absorbed into the portal circulation. It must also escape significant removal and/or metabolic alteration by the liver. It must enter the central circulation and not be immediately excreted by the kidney, resulting in an increased blood concentration that persists for some hours. Lastly, it must be taken up by and/or exert an effect on the organ where it is proposed to have the ergogenic effect (i.e., skeletal muscle, liver, adipose tissue, or brain, etc.) if it is to ultimately improve exercise performance. Although it seems logical to examine these processes first, this is rarely done because the required measurements are invasive. Therefore, if an ergogenic theory for a compound exists, it is easier to initially measure the effect of supplementing with the compound on exercise performance. The more detailed and invasive measurements often follow in an attempt to explain the positive or negative performance findings.

CREATINE

Supplemental dietary consumption of creatine has gained tremendous popularity over the past few years. It is commercially available and believed to improve the performance of brief high-intensity exercise (Maughan, 1995).

Creatine Function and Theoretical Basis for Ergogenicity

Creatine (Cr) is found in large quantities in skeletal muscle and is known to bind a significant amount of phosphate. The phosphocreatine (PCr) content in muscle is about 3–3.5 times that of adenosine triphosphate (ATP), the immediate source of energy in muscle cells (Spriet et al., 1987a). Because ATP is not stored in large amounts in muscle and the entire resting content can be consumed in seconds during exercise, PCr buffers the ATP level by transferring the phosphate group to adenosine diphosphate (ADP) to resynthesize ATP. Although the capacity of PCr to buffer decreases in ATP is low, it does provide time for the activation of aerobic ATP-producing pathways to match the demand for ATP during aerobic exercise. The ability to regenerate ATP during high-intensity exercise is also highly dependent on PCr degradation and glycolysis, a second pathway of anaerobic energy provision. During high-intensity exercise, the required rate of ATP utilization is greater than the rate of ATP synthesis from aerobic pathways and must be supplied anaerobically. However, the capacity of the anaerobic pathways is limited, such that high-intensity exercise can be maintained for only a short period of time.

Therefore, the intent of consuming supplemental Cr is to increase the skeletal muscle Cr content in the hope that some of the extra Cr will bind phosphate, leading to an increased resting PCr content. An increase in the resting PCr store should increase the total amount of ATP resynthesis and possibly improve performance in brief bouts of high-intensity exercise. During maximal exercise lasting 10 s, over 90% of the total ATP provision is derived anaerobically, and PCr degradation and glycolysis contribute equally to provide the necessary ATP (Spriet, 1995a). If high-intensity exercise is continued for 30 s, the PCr store becomes depleted after ~10 s, high power outputs cannot be maintained beyond 10 s, and glycolysis becomes the sole contributor of anaerobic ATP for the final 15–20 s. Over the entire 30 s, anaerobic pathways contribute 75–80% of the total ATP provision. If Cr supplementation increases the concentration of PCr in muscle at rest, high power outputs may be maintained longer, leading to improved performance. In addition, many sports require athletes to perform repeated bouts of high-intensity exercise with varying amounts of recovery time between bouts. As most of the required energy for this type of activity is derived from anaerobic sources, the ability to recover during rest periods is essential for success. Phosphocreatine is resynthesized quickly when exercise stops, and the rate of resynthesis will determine how much PCr is available for the next exercise bout. At the same time, the ability to reactivate the glycolytic pathway during repeated bouts of sprinting is compromised, leaving PCr degradation as the major source of anaerobic ATP during repeated bouts (Putman et al., 1995). Therefore, the rapid resynthesis of PCr back to high resting levels could have a dramatic impact on exercise performance.

An additional positive effect of Cr supplementation may be an increase in cellular buffering of hydrogen ions (H^+). The amount of energy that can be provided from PCr is undoubtedly a function of the size of the PCr store. However, the contribution from anaerobic glycolysis is not limited by glycogen levels but by the accumulation of one of its byproducts, H^+, either through a direct effect on glycolytic enzymes or more likely through inhibition of electrical and contractile processes involved in muscular contraction. Therefore, cellular buffering of H^+ appears to be an important process that delays muscular fatigue. Because PCr degradation during intense exercise consumes H^+ and contributes to cellular buffering, it has been suggested that increased concentrations of PCr in muscles following Cr supplementation may enhance the contribution of this metabolic buffer. This possibility may be important; Spriet et al. (1987b) calculated that PCr degradation buffered ~35% of the total H^+ released during 50 s of intense muscle contractions when muscle blood flow was occluded.

Creatine Metabolism

Creatine (methylguanidine-acetic acid) is found in skeletal, cardiac, and smooth muscle, in brain and kidney tissues, and in spermatozoa, with ~95% of the body's Cr store (120 g) in skeletal muscle (Walker, 1979). Total Cr content in human skeletal muscle averages 125 (115–140, n = 84) mmol/kg dry muscle with ~60–65% of the Cr bound to phosphate (70–90 mmol/kg dry muscle) (Harris et al., 1974). The estimated daily requirement for Cr is ~2 g (Walker, 1979), whereas the dietary intake of Cr from meat and fish is ~1 g/d (Heymsfield et al., 1983). The body synthesizes the remainder of the required Cr in the liver, kidney, and pancreas using the amino acids arginine, glycine, and methionine as precursors. The rate of endogenous synthesis appears to decrease when dietary Cr intake is high. However, people consuming a vegetarian diet appear to have a reduced bodily pool of Cr (blood measurements only), suggesting that removal of Cr from the diet is not adequately compensated for by an increase in endogenous Cr production (Delanghe et al., 1989). Total Cr contents are also slightly higher in females (Forsberg et al., 1991). It is not known what mechanisms are responsible for the normal intrasubject variability in muscle total Cr between individuals of the same gender or between genders. There is also little known about the degradation of creatine once it is transported into muscle, but the decline in total Cr concentration occurs over weeks, not days (Febbraio et al., 1995; Greenhaff, 1995; Hultman et al., 1996; Lemon et al., 1995). For this reason it is not advisable to perform studies with a cross-over design; the washout period following Cr supplementation appears to be long. Older reports in the literature examined the effects of Cr supplementation in humans (Crim et al., 1976; Sipila et al., 1981), but until recently no detailed reports examined measurements of blood and skeletal muscle total Cr content following supplementation.

Effects of Creatine Supplementation on Muscle Total Creatine Content

Harris et al. (1992) provided the first comprehensive examination of oral Cr supplementation in humans. They examined a variety of dietary supplementation regimens and demonstrated that a single 1-g dose increased plasma concentrations of Cr only slightly, from about 50 to 100 μM, whereas a single 5-g dose produced a peak Cr concentration of roughly 800 μM in 1 h (Figure 5-1). The half-life for Cr in plasma appeared to be 1–1.5 h. The goal was to find a dose that produced a plasma concentration above 500 μM for an extended period of time, as this was reported to be the concentration required for 50% of the maximal rate of Cr uptake into rat skeletal muscle (Fitch & Shields, 1966). Even with these large plasma increases, Cr must be transported from plasma against a large concentration gradient into skeletal muscle. Creatine is transported into muscle via a saturable carrier mechanism that is dependent on energy and extracellular sodium (Guimbal & Kilimann, 1993). Repeated doses of 5 g Cr every 2 h elevated plasma Cr concentrations to 0.8–1.0 mM over an 8-h period.

Using this information, Harris et al. (1992) settled on a daily Cr supplementation regimen of 5-g doses, given 4-6 times/d. This regimen produced significant increases in muscle total Cr and PCr contents in young, recreationally active subjects. Muscle total Cr increased from 126.8 ± 11.7 to 148.6 ± 5.0 mmol/kg dry muscle following 2–7 d of supplementation in 17 subjects (5 females, 12 males). Phosphocreatine was also increased from 84.2 ± 7.3 to 90.6 ± 4.8 mmol/kg following Cr sup-

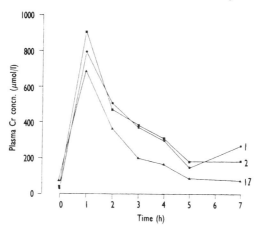

FIGURE 5-1. *Plasma creatine concentrations in three subjects following a single 5-g oral dose of creatine (Cr). Data from Harris et al. (1992).*

plementation, while muscle ATP concentration was unaffected. Supplementation beyond 2–3 d produced no further increases, and the magnitude of the Cr increase was related to the starting total Cr content. For example, all but two of the 17 subjects demonstrated an increase in total Cr, and the two non-responders already had total Cr concentrations above 145 mmol/kg prior to supplementation (Figure 5-2). All subjects appeared to reach an upper total Cr level of 140–160 mmol/kg following supplementation.

In a final experiment, the authors examined the effects of previous intense exercise on the response to Cr supplementation. Five males exercised one leg as hard as possible for 1 h/d for 4–7 d while ingesting 20–30 g of Cr/d (Harris et al., 1992). Total Cr increased from a mean of 118.1 ± 3.0 mmol/kg in both legs before supplementation to 148.5 ± 5.2 in the non-exercised leg and 162.2 ± 12.5 mmol/kg in the exercised leg. Control PCr increased from 81.9 ± 5.6 mmol/kg to 93.8 ± 4.0 and 103.1 ± 6.2 mmol/kg in the non-exercised and exercised legs, respectively, while muscle ATP was again unchanged. This study demonstrated that the increases in muscle total Cr and PCr following supplementation were greatest when coupled with intense daily exercise.

Hultman et al. (1996) recently provided additional information on

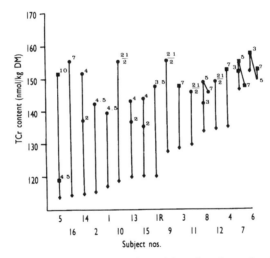

FIGURE 5-2. *Total creatine (TCr) contents in the quadriceps femoris muscles of 17 subjects before (triangles) and after (squares, females; circles, males) creatine supplementation. Data from Harris et al. (1992). Creatine supplementation was: 4 X 5 g/d for 4.5 d (subjects #1, 2), 7 d (#3, 4), and 10 d (#5); 6 X 5 g/d for 7 d (#6-8 with biopsies on days 3, 5 and 7) and on alternate days for 21 d (#9–12). Supplementation results of control legs of five subjects who performed exercise with the contralateral leg are included: 4 X 5 g/d for 3.5 d (#1R); 6 X 5 g/d for 4 d (#13–15 with biopsies on days 2 and 4) and 7 d (#16). Subjects are arranged in order of increasing total Cr content. Numbers on figure denote days of supplementation at the time of biopsy sampling. DM denotes dry mass.*

skeletal muscle loading in healthy men. They reported 20% increases in muscle total Cr with the consumption of 20 g of Cr/d for 6 d (Figure 5-3A & B), similar to the "rapid Cr loading regimen" used by Harris et al. (1992). In one group of subjects, the concentration of total Cr in muscle decreased over the next 28 d, such that it was not significantly different from the pre-supplementation value (Figure 5-3A). However, 28 d after the rapid Cr loading, the absolute total Cr concentration still appeared to be ~10-12 mmol/kg dry muscle higher than the pre-supplementation level. In a second group of subjects, the increase in muscle total Cr following the rapid Cr loading was maintained for 28 d when subjects consumed a maintenance dose of only 2 g Cr/d (Figure 5-3B). In a third group of subjects, ingestion of 3 g Cr/d for 28 d also increased muscle total Cr, from 121.8 ± 3.3 mmol/kg dry muscle on day 0 to 136.5 ± 3.1 and 142.0 ± 3.2 mmol/kg dry muscle on d 14 and 28, respectively. Therefore, this "slow Cr loading regimen" appeared to be as effective as the rapid regimen for increasing muscle total Cr concentration. Changes in muscle PCr concentration generally followed the changes in total Cr with roughly 30% of the increase or decrease in total Cr appearing as PCr and ~70% as free Cr. The exception was the tendency for the concentration of PCr to remain elevated as the concentration of total Cr in muscle decreased over 28 d (Hultman et al., 1996).

Casey et al. (1996) recently measured the effect of ingesting 20 g Cr/d for 5 d on the PCr concentration of type I and II fibers in healthy men. Creatine supplementation increased total muscle Cr by 23 mmol/kg dry muscle and PCr by 8.4 mmol/kg, as reported in previous studies. The increases in PCr contents of type I and II fibers were quantitatively similar following Cr supplementation (type I, 66.6 ± 4.2 to 77.6 ± 3.2 mmol/kg and type II, 79.3 ± 1.5 to 91.0 ± 5.8 mmol/kg). Measurements of free Cr in single fibers were not made.

It should be noted that 20–30 g of Cr/d is a large dose; the total body store is ~120 g. Five grams of Cr is the equivalent of 1.1 kg of fresh, uncooked steak. However, no side effects of Cr supplementation have been reported. Creatine is degraded to creatinine and removed from the body via diffusion in the kidneys. Therefore, ingestion of 20–30 g/d should not present a problem in healthy individuals. However, no information exists regarding potential side effects of consuming supplemental Cr for periods longer than ~35 d.

Exercise Performance and Muscle Metabolism Following Creatine Supplementation

Greenhaff et al. (1993) examined whether the enhanced PCr and total Cr contents following supplementation were associated with im-

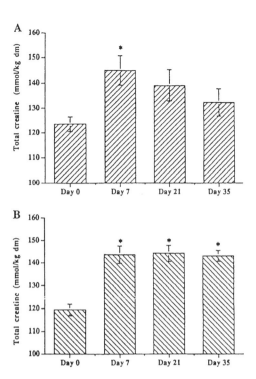

FIGURE 5-3. *Muscle total creatine (Cr) content following creatine supplementation.* Data from Hultman et al. (1996). A: Subjects ingested 20 g Cr for 6 d and no Cr for the next 28 d. Muscle biopsies were sampled before ingestion (day 0) and on days 7, 21, and 35 following the start of supplementation. B: Subjects ingested 20 g Cr for 6 d and then ingested 2 g Cr for the next 28 d. Muscle biopsies were sampled before ingestion (day 0) and on days 7, 21, and 35 following the onset of supplementation. Means ± SE. Dry mass is denoted by dm. *Significantly different from day 0.

proved muscle performance (or delayed fatigue) in high-intensity exercise. Two groups of subjects performed five bouts of 30 maximal voluntary isokinetic knee extensions at 180°/s, with recovery periods of 1 min between bouts, following double-blind placebo and Cr supplementation. No performance changes occurred in the placebo group. After Cr ingestion, muscle peak torque was greater during the final 10 contractions of bout 1, during all contractions of bouts 2, 3, and 4, and during the middle 10 contractions of bout 5. The improvement in performance was believed to be a consequence of greater muscle PCr contents prior to exercise, due to an increased ability to resynthesize PCr during the recovery periods. It was suggested that the increased availability of PCr may help to maintain the required ATP resynthesis rate more easily during exercise. This postulation was supported by lower accumulations of plasma ammonium ions during exercise after Cr ingestion, suggesting a smaller mismatch between ATP demand and provision.

Greenhaff et al. (1994) subsequently examined the effect of Cr ingestion on PCr resynthesis directly in skeletal muscle. They electrically stimulated human vastus lateralis muscles with occluded leg blood flow to
deplete the PCr store before and after Cr supplementation (20 g/d for 5
d). Blood flow was then restored, and PCr resynthesis during 120 s of recovery was measured with needle biopsies at 20, 60, and 120 s. Following
Cr supplementation, PCr was 20% higher in the vastus lateralis after 120 s
of recovery (Figure 5-4). Creatine supplementation caused large increases
in total Cr content (29 ± 3 mmol/kg) and PCr resynthesis during recovery
(19 ± 4 mmol/kg) in five subjects who responded, but had no significant
effect on PCr resynthesis in three subjects who did not respond (total Cr
increases of 8–9 mmol/kg). However, the increase in PCr resynthesis following Cr supplementation occurred mainly in the second minute of recovery.

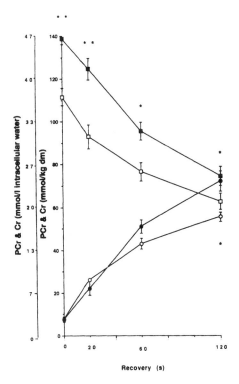

FIGURE 5-4. *Phosphocreatine (PCr, circles) and free creatine (Cr, squares) contents and concentra-*
tions in muscle biopsies sampled after 0, 20, 60, and 120 s of recovery from intense contractions. Data
from Greenhaff et al. (1994). Open symbols represent data obtained before Cr ingestion and
closed symbols following supplementation with 20 g Cr/d for 5 d. Mean ± SE. Dry mass is
denoted by dm. **P< 0.01 vs. data obtained before Cr ingestion. *P< 0.05 vs. data obtained
before Cr ingestion.

At the same time, additional studies examining the ergogenic effect of Cr supplementation on high-intensity exercise began to appear. Balsom et al. (1993a) examined sprint performance before and after supplementation of Cr (20 g Cr/d for 6 d) or placebo using an exercise regimen of ten 6-s bouts of high-intensity cycling (140 rpm, ~880 W) with rest periods of 30 s between bouts. In the placebo group, power output was well maintained during the initial 4 s of each bout, followed by a progressive decline in the final 2 s of bouts 5–10 before and after placebo (Figure 5-5). In the supplementation group the performance results were the same as the placebo group before Cr supplementation. Following Cr ingestion, power output was maintained throughout the final 2 s of bouts 5–10 (Figure 5-5). Concentrations of blood hypoxanthine (a measure of adenine nucleotide degradation) and lactate were lower following supplementation, in spite of a higher power output. These findings supported the postulation that Cr supplementation is associated with better preservation of the energy

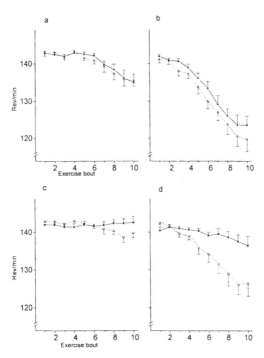

FIGURE 5-5. *Performance of repeated bouts of sprint cycling before and after placebo or creatine (Cr) supplementation.* Subjects performed 10, 6-s bouts of maximal cycling while attempting to maintain a cadence of 140 revolutions/min (rev/min) with rest periods of 30 s between bouts. Data from Balsom et al. (1993a). a and c: Average pedal cadence for the initial 4 s of each exercise bout before (open symbols) and after (closed symbols) either placebo (a) or Cr supplementation (c). b and d: Similar data for the final 2 s of each exercise bout in the placebo (b) and Cr supplemented group (d). Creatine supplementation was 20 g Cr/d for 6 d; placebo group received a similar amount of glucose for 6 d.

state (ATP/ADP ratio) in the muscle cell during high-intensity exercise. They also suggested that Cr supplementation may have decreased the rate of anaerobic glycogenolysis/glycolysis over the entire exercise regimen, although blood lactate is not as good a predictor of muscle glycolytic activity as is blood hypoxanthine for predicting adenine nucleotide degradation.

Birch et al. (1994) reported results similar to those from the study by Balsom et al. (1993a). They examined three, 30-s bouts of maximal isokinetic cycling, separated by 4 min of rest. Creatine supplementation increased peak power output in bout 1 and increased mean power output and total work performed in bouts 1 and 2, but had no effect on performance in bout 3. Peak plasma ammonia accumulation after the three bouts was lower following Cr supplementation, whereas peak blood lactate was unaffected. Placebo ingestion had no effect on sprint performance in any of the bouts or on the post-exercise blood parameters. A similar study was published by Earnest et al. (1995), who reported that Cr supplementation had no effect on peak power output during three 30-s Wingate tests, separated by 5 min rest periods. However, total work performed was higher in all three bouts following Cr ingestion. There were no effects of placebo ingestion on performance in any of the bouts.

A recent investigation by Casey et al. (1996) provided further support for an ergogenic effect of Cr supplementation during sprint exercise. Well-trained male subjects performed two 30-s bouts of maximal isokinetic cycling (80 rpm), separated by 4 min of passive rest, both before and after ingesting 20 g Cr/d for 5 d. Peak work output was not significantly improved by Cr supplementation in either bout, but the total work production was increased in each bout (~4%) following Cr (Figure 5-6). Creatine supplementation increased muscle total Cr and PCr by ~23 and 8 mmol/kg dry muscle, respectively, and the increases in PCr were evident in both type I and type II fibers. Despite an increase in work production following Cr, the cumulative loss of muscle ATP was reduced by 31%. Creatine supplementation also increased the available PCr for degradation during bout 2 in both fiber types (Figure 5-7). In summary, the cumulative increases in peak work and total work were positively correlated with the increases in total muscle total Cr. The increases in PCr in type II fibers before bouts 1 and 2 were positively correlated with exercise PCr degradation in this fiber type and with changes in total work production. The authors suggested that the Cr-induced improvement in performance was due to increased ATP resynthesis resulting from increased PCr availability. It should be noted that in this study no control group was employed, the performance trials were administered in an ordered fashion, and the subjects apparently knew when they received Cr supplementation. Part of the rationale for this approach was probably the invasive nature of the measurements and the amount of work involved in the single-fiber measurements.

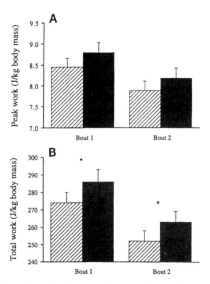

FIGURE 5-6. *Peak and total work production during 2 bouts of maximal intensity, isokinetic (80 revolutions/min) cycling with 4 min of rest between bouts.* Data from Casey et al. (1996). Subjects performed the 2 bouts before receiving creatine (hatched bars) and following 20 g Cr/d for 6 d (filled bars). Means ± SE. *significant difference between pre- and post-creatine supplementation.

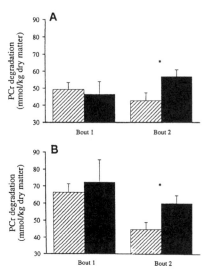

FIGURE 5-7. *Phosphocreatine (PCr) degradation in type I (A) and type II (B) fibers during 2 bouts of maximal intensity, isokinetic (80 revolutions/min) cycling with 4 min of rest between bouts.* Data from Casey et al. (1996). Subjects performed the 2 bouts before receiving creatine (hatched bars) and following 20 g Cr/d for 6 d (filled bars). Means ± SE. *significant difference between pre- and post-creatine supplementation.

Not all studies have reported an increase in exercise performance during high-intensity exercise following Cr supplementation. Cooke et al. (1995) had two groups of untrained men cycle maximally against a constant load of 112 N for 15 s before and following supplementation. One group received a placebo and the other Cr (5 g, 4 times/d for 5 d). Measurements of peak power, time to peak power, total work, and the rate of fatigue during the single bout of sprinting were unaffected by Cr supplementation. The unique aspect of this study was that it examined only one bout of high-intensity exercise, whereas the previous studies examined repeated bouts. These results are reasonably consistent with previous studies (i.e., improvements in total work are not always reported in the first bout of sprinting but become more prominent during repeated bouts) (Balsom, et al., 1993a: Birch et al., 1994; Greenhaff et al., 1993). Febbraio et al. (1995) examined the effects of Cr supplementation on muscle metabolism and exercise performance during repeated sprinting at a power output of 110–125% $\dot{V}O_2$max. Subjects ingested 20 g Cr/d for 5 d and performed four 60-s sprints at a fixed power output, with 60 s of recovery between sprints, followed by a fifth sprint to exhaustion. Total Cr and PCr increased by 19 and 15 mmol/kg dry muscle, respectively, following Cr supplementation, but sprint time during the fifth bout was unaffected (60–70 s). It is possible that the longer sprints employed in this study precluded a positive effect of Cr supplementation on performance because the energy supplied by PCr in a 60-s sprint will represent a much lower percentage of total energy expended than in a sprint lasting 30 s or less. The authors also noted that the concentration of total Cr in muscle had returned to normal 28 d after the Cr supplementation stopped.

In summary, most of the laboratory performance findings, coupled with the PCr resynthesis data of Greenhaff et al. (1993) and Casey et al. (1996), argue that the increases in intramuscular Cr concentrations that occur with Cr supplementation do not always increase the concentration of PCr at rest sufficiently to improve performance during an initial bout of high-intensity exercise. However, an increased concentration of total Cr in muscle does appear to increase the rate of PCr resynthesis during the rest periods between bouts of high-intensity exercise, providing the muscle with a greater PCr store for repeated sprints.

Harris et al. (1993) performed a field study to examine the effects of Cr supplementation on performance during near-maximal brief running. Trained middle-distance runners were randomly placed into a placebo or Cr group in double-blind fashion. All subjects performed 4 x 300 m and 4 x 1,000 m runs with 3–4 min rest periods between repetitions before and after placebo or Cr supplementation. Improvements were noted in the Cr group during the final 300 m and 1,000 m runs of each set of 4 runs, as compared to the placebo group. The best 300 m and

1,000 m times were also 0.3 s and 2.1 s faster, respectively, following Cr supplementation but were unchanged in the placebo group.

From the experiments that measured concentrations of total Cr in muscle, it is clear that not all individuals respond to Cr supplementation. Individuals with high concentrations of total Cr at rest are the least likely to respond. The approximate success of increasing the concentration of total Cr with Cr supplementation was 7/8, 15/17, 5/8, 6/6 and 5/8 subjects in five recent studies (Casey et al., 1996; Febbraio et al., 1995; Gordon et al., 1995; Greenhaff et al., 1993; Harris et al., 1992). There would be no expectation of increases in exercise performance in people who do not respond. The fact that some subjects may not respond may confound the group-performance findings and makes it difficult to cleanly test the effect of increases in the concentration of total Cr in muscle when direct measurements in muscle are not made. One additional study measured the concentration of total Cr in muscle and reported no effect of Cr supplementation in a group of healthy young male subjects (Odland et al., 1997). However, two major problems existed with this study. First, only ratios, and not absolute values, were reported for total Cr, PCr, Cr, and ATP contents, suggesting an analytical problem. Second, the experiment involved a cross-over design with randomly assigned control, placebo, and Cr supplementation trials, each separated by 14 d. This confounded the performance findings because increases in Cr concentration that occurred when supplemental Cr was administered in the first or second trial would not have returned to pre-experiment levels prior to proceeding to the next trial of the study.

Additional Effects of Creatine Supplementation

It has been suggested that PCr plays a central role in the "shuttling" of ATP from the mitochondria to cytoplasmic locations for hydrolysis during predominately aerobic exercise (Bessman & Savabi, 1990). In this scheme, ATP produced in the mitochondria passes its phosphate to free Cr to form PCr at the mitochondrial membrane. The PCr is transported to cytoplasmic ATPase sites where the phosphate is transferred to free ADP, forming ATP for immediate use. The possibility that extra free Cr and PCr in the muscle following Cr supplementation improve this process has been discussed in several papers. However, no conclusive evidence has ever been provided to demonstrate that the PCr shuttle mechanism is functional in skeletal muscle. In fact, energy transduction between the mitochondria and cytoplasm appears to be unaffected in skeletal muscles of rats fed a Cr analog that is a poor substrate for the enzyme, Cr phosphokinase (Meyer et al., 1986). In the end, this argument may be moot because recent studies examining the effect of Cr supplementation on aerobic exercise performance showed no effect during an incremental treadmill test and a cross-country running test over 6 km that lasted ~23 min (Balsom et al., 1993b; Stroud et al., 1994). An interesting finding of Cr supplementation studies has been a small but consistent increase in body mass following Cr supplementation (Balsom et al., 1993a; 1993b; Earnest et al., 1995; Lemon et al., 1995). It has been suggested that this increase is a function of increased muscle water accompanying the increase in muscle Cr and/or may be due to a stimulating effect on protein synthesis that is currently not understood (Bessman & Savabi, 1990). Given the rapidity of the body mass increase with a 5–6 d (20 g/d) Cr supplementation regimen, it seems unlikely that increases in protein synthesis could be responsible. Hultman et al. (1996) reported that urinary volume decreased by 0.6 L/d during the initial days of acute Cr supplementation, suggesting that the increase in body mass was due to water retention. Alternately, increased protein synthesis may be part of the explanation for the 1.7 kg increase in body mass following the more long-term supplementation with 20 g Cr/d for 28 d reported by Earnest et al. (1995).

A recent study examined whether or not caffeine ingestion would further stimulate skeletal muscle Cr uptake above the effect of Cr supplementation alone (Vandenberghe et al., 1996). The authors hypothesized that caffeine-induced elevations in plasma epinephrine concentration would stimulate activity of the sodium-potassium ATPase pump in the membrane of skeletal muscle. This would lead to an increased Na^+ gradient across the membrane and might further stimulate the activity of the Cr transporter, which is known to be sodium dependent (Loike et al., 1986). A double-blind, crossover design was used in which subjects completed three trials separated by 3-wk washout periods. They consumed either placebo (glucose), Cr, or Cr plus caffeine for 6 d during each trial. The Cr dose was ~40 g/d, given in eight equal aliquots throughout the day, and caffeine was given as a morning dose of 5 mg/kg body mass during the last 3 d of the 6-d Cr-loading procedure. Muscle measurements were not made directly but estimated from ^{31}P-magnetic resonance spectroscopy of the gastrocnemius muscle. The ratio of the areas under the PCr and ATP magnetic resonance spectra were estimated. The ß-ATP peaks were unchanged throughout the experiment and assumed equal to 5.5 mmol/kg wet muscle. The muscle PCr contents were then calculated by comparing the PCr and ATP peak spectral areas. Placebo ingestion had no effects on muscle measurements and performance during dynamic knee extension exercise. Creatine supplementation increased muscle PCr content slightly, increased the PCr/ATP ratio, and increased torque production during three sets of dynamic knee extensions with 2-min of rest between sets. Caffeine and Cr ingestion completely abolished the improvement in knee extension torque seen with Cr alone, whereas the increases in the concentration of PCr and the PCr/ATP ratio in muscle were still present.

However, both the muscle and performance data in this paper may be criticized. The fact that the changes in estimated muscle PCr content were very small, coupled with the expected low level of accuracy from this method of estimating muscle compounds, leaves the significance of the findings open to speculation. Also, the use of PCr/ATP spectral ratios for comparing changes assumes a constant relationship between muscle PCr and ATP contents and spectra following Cr supplementation. The performance data may be criticized due to the use of a cross-over experimental design with only three weeks between trials. The counteraction of the Cr ergogenic effect by caffeine is difficult to understand in light of the fact that the last caffeine dose was given ~20 h before the exercise performance test. It is not clear how the presence of caffeine in the body for 3 d would negate the effects of Cr supplementation when the increases in muscle Cr persisted. The authors did not offer any explanations as to how a caffeine-Cr interaction in skeletal muscle cells would negate the effects of Cr alone.

Practical Implications

Creatine is a substance that occurs naturally in the diet and can be synthesized in the body. There do not appear to be any adverse side effects associated with the oral ingestion of supplemental Cr, and this practice is not considered illegal by the IOC. The daily ingestion of 5 g of Cr for 4–6 d ("rapid loading") increases the content of muscle Cr in most people. Engaging in exercise during the days of supplementation appears to increase the effectiveness of muscle Cr loading. Supplementation may be especially effective in individuals who do not consume dietary Cr. People who already have high muscle Cr levels may not respond. The four daily doses of 5 g are usually consumed by dissolving the Cr in ~250 ml of a beverage in early morning, noon, afternoon, and late evening. Muscle Cr levels will return to normal levels in ~30 d, although continuing with a 10-fold lower dose (2 g Cr/d) will maintain the high levels for at least 30 d and probably longer. Consumption of greater doses than described here will be without further effect. It has also been demonstrated that only 3 g Cr/d for 28 d ("slow loading") will produce similar muscle Cr increases. Supplementation-induced increases in muscle Cr content have been shown to improve performance during sprint-like activities and appear most beneficial during sports requiring repeated bouts of high-intensity exercise.

CARNITINE

The use of supplemental carnitine as a potential ergogenic aid is widespread in the athletic world, especially among endurance athletes.

This practice is surprising, given the weak evidence suggesting that supplemental carnitine may improve exercise performance. As reviewed by Kanter and Williams (1995), the usual rationale given for supplementing with carnitine is related to its central role in transporting fat into the mitochondria of skeletal muscle cells. Although other manipulations (e.g., caffeine administration and aerobic training) that increase fat utilization and spare muscle glycogen improve endurance performance during moderate to intense aerobic exercise, the evidence suggesting that carnitine has no intracellular effect in skeletal muscle continues to accumulate. The normal diet appears to provide enough carnitine directly or enough of the amino acids lysine and methionine to synthesize carnitine and maximize carnitine levels in muscle.

Carnitine Function and Theoretical Basis for an Ergogenic Effect

L-carnitine is associated with two primary functions in muscle cells. The main function is to transfer long-chain fatty acids across the inner mitochondrial membrane. Fatty acyl-CoA synthetase activates long-chain fatty acids in the cytoplasm to fatty-acyl CoA (Figure 5-8). Free L-carnitine combines with fatty acyl-CoA to form fatty acylcarnitine and free CoA through the action of carnitine palmitoyl transferase I (CPT I), an enzyme located on the inside of the outer mitochondrial membrane. An acylcarnitine transferase enzyme transports the long-chain fatty acyl carnitine into the mitochondrion in exchange for mitochondrial free carnitine. On the matrix side of the inner mitochondrial membrane, carnitine palmitoyl transferase II (CPT II) removes the carnitine, and the regenerated long-chain fatty acyl-CoA compounds are then available for use in the ß-oxidation pathway.

Therefore, because carnitine plays a critical role in the oxidation of long-chain fatty acids, it has been hypothesized that an increased muscle content of carnitine may improve fatty acid uptake into the mitochondria and may increase fatty acid oxidation. This might increase the percentage of energy coming from fat oxidation and reduce carbohydrate oxidation, thereby "sparing" muscle glycogen and improving endurance performance at power outputs (65–85% $\dot{V}O_2max$) limited by muscle glycogen availability.

A second function of L-carnitine is to buffer increases in mitochondrial acetyl-CoA concentration. When the production of acetyl-CoA is greater than its use in the tricarboxylic acid (TCA) cycle, carnitine acetyltransferase converts acetyl-CoA and L-carnitine to acetylcarnitine and free CoA. The acetylcarnitine is then transported out of the mitochondria and accumulates in the cytoplasm or is reconverted to acetyl-CoA and carnitine via a cytoplasmic version of carnitine acetyltrans-

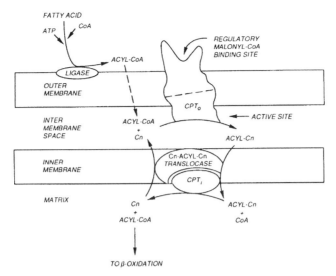

FIGURE 5-8. Schematic representation of the relationship of the key enzymes involved in the transport of long chain fatty acids across the mitochondrial membranes. Diagram from Broquist (1994). CoA, free CoASH; Cn, carnitine; CPT_o and CPT_i, carnitine palmitoyl transferases of the outer (CPT I) and inner (CPT II) mitochondrial membranes.

ferase. The buffering of increases in mitochondrial acetyl-CoA maintains adequate levels of mitochondrial free CoA, a required substrate in many essential reactions associated with energy provision (pyruvate and oxoglutarate dehydrogenases and ß-oxidation enzyme activities). Theoretically, increased mitochondrial carnitine content could enhance this buffering process and maintain a higher free CoA content, thereby stimulating the activity of these key enzymes and increasing energy provision during exercise.

On the other hand, Wagenmakers (1991) proposed an effect of supplemental muscle carnitine that would be detrimental to exercise performance. He argued that increased mitochondrial carnitine may relieve the inhibition of branched-chain 2-oxo acid dehydrogenase and increase the degradation of branched-chain amino acids, leading to a drain of a TCA cycle intermediate, oxoglutarate, a decreased flux through the TCA cycle, and to early fatigue. However, there is no evidence that depletion of TCA cycle intermediates causes fatigue.

Much of the interest in the potential ergogenic effects of carnitine has been generated by in vitro or "test tube" studies examining the energetics of isolated intact muscle mitochondria or muscle homogenates. As reviewed by Wagenmakers (1991), it has been known for some time that the addition of L-carnitine to these preparations stimulates the uptake and oxidation of long-chain fatty acids and the use of carbohydrate-derived substrates and flux through the TCA cycle, most likely by increasing the concentration of free CoA in the mitochondria. Unfortunately, it is a considerable jump from these in vitro studies to whole-body exercise with intact muscles. In mitochondrial preparations, the normal concentration of carnitine outside the mitochondria is artificially low compared to the concentration of carnitine outside the mitochondria in intact muscle cells (~95% of the muscle's total carnitine is believed to be in the cytoplasm). Therefore, adding carnitine to the medium bathing the in vitro intact mitochondria will have the desired effect of stimulating the carnitine related processes cited above.

In vivo, there is no evidence that the cytoplasmic carnitine concentration is ever limiting in healthy individuals. Even during intense exercise, when concentrations of free carnitine in muscles decrease, the remaining levels of cytoplasmic carnitine are sufficient to permit adequate CPT I activity. It is often suggested that the maximal activity of CPT I may be the factor limiting fatty acid uptake into mitochondria, but CPT I activity is not limited by substrate in the form of carnitine. It may be limited by insufficient CPT I protein and/or by a limitation in the second substrate for CPT I, fatty-acyl CoA. Several other sites involved in the release and transport of fatty acids in the blood, across the muscle membrane, and through the cytoplasm to the mitochondria have also been implicated as regulatory sites.

Additional evidence cited to support the use of supplemental carnitine has come from the studies of Dubelaar et al. (1991) using an in situ muscle preparation in dogs. They measured a 34% increase in force production during 8 min of electrical stimulation when the dogs received an intravenous infusion of L-carnitine, as compared to saline. This positive effect of carnitine was not evident in aerobically trained muscle. The positive effect on force was also abolished in the untrained muscle when insulin (and glucose) were infused with carnitine. Plasma carnitine concentration was increased from 23 μM in the saline trial to 322 μM in the carnitine trial, but the infusion had no effect on muscle carnitine levels. Accordingly, the authors suggested that the mechanism underlying the force-enhancing effect of carnitine did not involve the muscle cell. They suggested that the extra carnitine might enhance fatty acid oxidation in the blood vessel walls of muscle capillaries, leading to increased blood flow and enhanced performance. The question again arises as to the applicability of these findings to whole-body human exercise. The major area for concern is the large 14-fold increase in plasma carnitine used to demonstrate the increases in force in this study. As discussed later, plasma carnitine levels following oral supplementation in humans are increased by 75% at the most.

Resting Carnitine Metabolism

As reviewed by Wagenmakers (1991), L-carnitine (ß-hydroxy-γ-trimethylaminobutyrate) is consumed by humans in red meat and dairy products and is absorbed in the small intestine by active transport and passive diffusion. Carnitine can also be synthesized from the amino acids lysine and methionine in the liver and kidneys. The relative amounts of dietary intake and endogenous production of carnitine are not known, but it appears that endogenous production can compensate for reduced intake of dietary Cr, as commonly occurs in vegetarians. Myopathies of carnitine synthesis do occur in humans but are rare. Because skeletal muscle cannot synthesize carnitine, it must be transported to the muscles via the bloodstream. Normal plasma carnitine levels are only 40–60 μM; therefore, because the muscle concentration of carnitine is 4–5 mM, carnitine must be transported into muscle via a saturable active mechanism against a large concentration gradient. As 98% of the body's carnitine store is found in skeletal muscle, a 70 kg person with 28–30 kg of muscle mass has a total body store of approximately 100 mmoles of carnitine. Small amounts of carnitine are also found in heart muscle, plasma, liver, and kidney. The turnover of carnitine is slow (<300 μmol/d, 0.3% of body store), and carnitine is not degraded in the body but is directly excreted in the urine.

Effects of Exercise and Macronutrient Diet on Muscle Carnitine

Early investigations suggested that total muscle carnitine decreased as a result of exercise (Hiatt et al., 1989; Lennon et al., 1983). This suggestion was a consequence of not taking into account the water shifts that occur during exercise. More recent work has demonstrated that exercise at 30–40% $\dot{V}O_2$max has no effect on muscle free carnitine, acetylcarnitine, and total carnitine. Increasing the power output over a range from 60–100% $\dot{V}O_2$max produced sequential and stoichiometric increases in acetylcarnitine and decreases in free carnitine (Constantin-Teodosiu et al., 1991; Sahlin, 1990). Total muscle carnitine was unchanged at all power outputs, and free carnitine decreased from about 16 mmol/kg dry muscle at rest to 5–6 mmol/kg at 90–100% $\dot{V}O_2$ max. Additional studies showed that total muscle carnitine was also unchanged following prolonged exercise at power outputs of 50–80% $\dot{V}O_2$max in the laboratory (Carlin et al., 1986; Constantin-Teodosiu et al., 1992; Spriet et al., 1992), during a marathon run (Janssen et al., 1989), and during a 13.5-h cross-country ski race at altitude (Decombaz et al., 1992). In fact, the increases in acetylcarnitine and decreases in free carnitine that occurred early in exercise were maintained through-out exercise to exhaustion (58–75 min) at 75–80% $\dot{V}O_2$max (Constantin-Teodosiu et al., 1992; Spriet et al., 1992). The point is that free carnitine did not decrease further as exercise was prolonged; it actually may have increased near exhaustion. The findings that total muscle carnitine was not changed during exercise confirmed the earlier work of Soop et al. (1988), demonstrating that no carnitine was released from the exercising muscle of the leg during 120 min of exercise at 50% $\dot{V}O_2$max.

A recent study measured free carnitine and acetylcarnitine in type I and II human skeletal muscle fibers (Constantin-Teodosiu et al., 1996). At rest there were no differences between the fiber types for free and total carnitine, although there was a small but significantly higher acetylcarnitine content in the type I fibers. Following exercise to exhaustion (221 min) at 75% $\dot{V}O_2$ max, total carnitine was not changed in either fiber type. However, free carnitine content decreased and acetylcarnitine increased to a greater extent in type I fibers than in type II fibers. The authors were surprised that the carnitine differences at rest and after exercise were not more pronounced between the fiber types, given the supposed difference in oxidative potential. However, the fact that the subjects were regularly engaging in exercise and were able to cycle for 221 min at 75% $\dot{V}O_2$max suggests that the oxidative potential of their type I and II fibers may have been similar.

Two studies have also reported that prolonged aerobic training had no effect on total muscle carnitine. These studies examined a 2-y span of training in cross-country skiers (Decombaz et al. 1992) and 1 y of marathon preparation in runners (Janssen et al., 1989). However, Arenas et al. (1991) reported small but significant decreases in free and total muscle carnitine following 6 mo of aerobic training in long-distance runners and 6 mo of sprint training in sprinters.

Putman et al. (1993) examined the effect of 2.5–3 d of a high-fat/low-carbohydrate diet followed by the same length of time on a high-carbohydrate/low-fat diet on muscle carnitine responses. The high-carbohydrate diet produced no significant differences in total muscle carnitine at rest and during exercise. However, the high-fat diet altered the proportions of the major forms of carnitine in resting skeletal muscle, increasing acetylcarnitine from about 3 to 11 mmol/kg dry muscle and decreasing free carnitine from about 16 to 8 mmol/kg. During the high-fat diet, exercise at 75% $\dot{V}O_2$max for 48 min resulted in higher concentrations of muscle acetylcarnitine and lower carnitine levels when compared to the high-carbohydrate diet. However, total muscle carnitine contents during exercise were not affected by either diet.

Effects of Supplemental Carnitine on Plasma and Muscle Levels

Another important aspect of determining the potential ergogenic effect of supplemental oral carnitine is its ability to accumulate in the blood in sufficient quantities to promote significant uptake by the muscle cells.

The various carnitine supplementation regimens usually succeed in elevating plasma total carnitine levels by only 35–75%. The supplement dose is usually 2–6 g/d for 5–14 d. A single 2-g dose results in a 32% increase in total plasma carnitine in 1 h (Siliprandi et al., 1990, Vecchiet et al., 1990). However, peak plasma carnitine levels following a 2-g dose are not reached until after 3–9 h (Harper et al., 1988). These modest increases following carnitine supplementation are much less than might be expected. It appears that only 40–60% of ingested carnitine is absorbed in the small intestine, with the remainder excreted (Rebouche, 1991). In addition, the threshold in the kidney for the excretion of free and total carnitine is ~50 μM, which will limit the increase in plasma carnitine following supplementation (Engel & Rebouche, 1984).

Until recently, no attempts have been made to measure the effects of supplemental carnitine administration on carnitine levels in human muscle. Supplementation increases carnitine contents in rat skeletal muscles (Simi et al., 1990), but several lines of evidence suggest that such increases may not occur in humans. This evidence includes the modest increases in plasma carnitine following supplementation and the need to transport carnitine against a large concentration gradient. Lennon et al. (1986) also reported a significant positive relationship between dietary carnitine intake and plasma total carnitine concentration, but no relationship between dietary carnitine and muscle carnitine levels. Lastly, Soop et al. (1988) examined the effects of ingesting 5 g carnitine/d for 5 d and were unable to measure a carnitine uptake across the resting leg muscles, even though arterial carnitine increased from approximately 38 to 68 μM.

Recent investigations have established that acute carnitine supplementation does not change muscle carnitine content at rest or during exercise in humans. Barnett et al. (1994) reported that 14 d of supplementation (4 g/d in two doses, 12 h apart) had no effect on free, short-chain, or total carnitine levels in muscle at rest. Exercise for 4 min at 90% $\dot{V}O_2max$ following control and supplementation conditions produced similar increases in short-chain acylcarnitine and decreases in free carnitine. Not surprisingly, no differences in plasma acidity and lactate were reported between trials. Vukovich et al. (1994) published a study from the same laboratory with similar results. Muscle carnitine levels in resting subjects were unchanged following either 7 d or 14 d of carnitine supplementation (6 g/d, given in three equal doses). Exercise was performed for 60 min at 70% VO_2max before and after 7 d and 14 d of supplementation. Three hours prior to each trial a high-fat meal was consumed to increase the availability of free fatty acids (FFA) during exercise. In addition, half of the subjects received a heparin infusion prior to the day-7 trial and the other half prior to the day-14 trial to further increase concentrations of plasma FFA. During exercise, the muscle carnitine content, respiratory exchange ratio, and lipid oxidation were unaffected by these manipulations, suggesting that there was an adequate amount of carnitine present within the muscle in the normal, non-supplemented condition for sufficient lipid uptake and oxidation to occur.

Arenas et al. (1991) examined the effect of chronic carnitine supplementation on muscle carnitine levels of athletes. Two groups of long-distance runners and two groups of sprinters received either placebo or carnitine supplementation (1 g/d) during a 6-mo training regimen. The training alone (placebo group) produced small but significant decreases in free and total carnitine levels expressed as μmol/g protein over a 6-mo period. However, supplementation prevented this decrease and actually produced small increases in levels of free and total muscle carnitine. These findings are surprising, given the small daily dose of supplemental carnitine. A 1-g dose given once per day would cause very minor increases in plasma carnitine for very brief periods. However, it remains possible that the chronic nature of the supplementation was responsible for the reported increases. It is also not apparent from this study that the small training-induced reductions and increases following supplementation were functionally significant for performance during exercise.

Carnitine Supplementation and Exercise Metabolism and Performance

Given the above information, carnitine supplementation would not be expected to alter exercise metabolism and performance through a skeletal-muscle-dependent mechanism. Surprisingly, there have been reports detailing a shift to increased fat metabolism and improved performance following carnitine supplementation. In an early study, Marconi et al. (1985) reported a 6% increase in VO_2max in six well-trained subjects following carnitine supplementation of 4 g/d for 14 d. Two more recent reports, which appear to be the same investigation, also reported increased total work performed (18%) and VO_2max (7%) during an incremental test to fatigue following ingestion of a single 2-g dose of carnitine 1 h prior to exercise (Siliprandi et al., 1990; Vecchiet et al., 1990). Unfortunately, some subjects were stopped during the exercise test when theoretical maximum heart rates were reached and not when they became exhausted. The authors suggested that the findings with carnitine supplementation were a function of stimulated pyruvate dehydrogenase (PDH) activity, secondary to an increase in mitochondrial free CoA.

The above reports received heavy criticism in a letter to the editor by Hultman et al. (1991), who argued convincingly that the small, single dose had no chance of altering muscle carnitine levels. Recent studies that measured no changes in muscle carnitine following more prolonged supplementation corroborated this criticism. Other studies have reported no effect of carnitine on $\dot{V}O_2$max, although low levels of supplementation were used: 2 g/d for 14–28 d (Greig et al., 1987) and 0.5 g/d for 35 d (Shores et al., 1987). Therefore, the mechanism underlying any carnitine-induced increase in $\dot{V}O_2$max is apparently unrelated to skeletal muscle metabolism. As discussed earlier, large increases in plasma carnitine concentration increased muscle blood flow in an isolated dog muscle preparation, but the small increases in plasma carnitine accompanying supplementation make it highly unlikely that this could be the explanation in maximally exercising humans. However, Soop et al. (1988) reported a non-significant 8% increase in leg blood flow at 50% $\dot{V}O_2$max following carnitine supplementation. It is possible that more carefully controlled studies in the future will reveal that carnitine does not increase $\dot{V}O_2$max.

The effects of carnitine supplementation on the metabolic responses to prolonged exercise at moderate power outputs are also equivocal. Several studies reported no effect of supplementation of 2–6 g carnitine/d for 7–14 d on the respiratory exchange ratio (RER) during prolonged exercise (40-120 min) at 43–70% $\dot{V}O_2$max (Decombaz et al., 1993; Marconi et al., 1985; Otto et al., 1987; Oyono-Enguelle et al., 1988; Vukovich et al., 1994). Others have reported a decreased RER during prolonged submaximal exercise following similar regimens of carnitine supplementation (Gorostiaga et al., 1989; Natali et al., 1993; Wyss et al., 1990). If the increased fat oxidation in these latter studies was a function of increased FFA uptake by muscle, some explanation linking increased plasma carnitine levels and the transport processes thought to be involved with FFA entry into muscle needs to be proposed. However, it is important to note that the only study with direct measurements of glucose and FFA exchange across an exercising limb following carnitine supplementation (5 g/d for 5 d) revealed no differences in substrate exchange during 2 h of exercise at 50% $\dot{V}O_2$max (Soop et al., 1988).

There are few examinations of the effect of carnitine supplementation on endurance performance, and most are reported in abstract form only. Otto et al. (1987) reported no change in the total work performed during a 60-min cycling test designed to achieve maximal work output following supplementation with 0.5 g carnitine/d for 35 d. More recently, Kasper et al. (1994) found no difference in the time required to complete a simulated 5 km run on the treadmill following ingestion of 4 g carnitine/d for 14 d. Stussi et al. (1996) had 12 athletes cycle to exhaustion at 91% $\dot{V}O_2$max on two occasions. Two hours prior to the test, subjects received either 2 g of carnitine or a placebo. Time to exhaustion was unaffected by carnitine supplementation.

Trappe et al. (1994) recently examined the effect of carnitine supplementation (4 g/d for 7 d) on repeated bouts of short-term, high-intensity, intermittent swimming. The authors proposed that supplemental carnitine may increase PDH activity and the concentration of free CoA in the mitochondria during high-intensity exercise. This presumably would result in increased oxidative use of pyruvate, less lactate production, and less H^+ release, thereby improving performance due to reduced acidity. However, no effect of carnitine supplementation on blood acidity or performance was found.

Practical Implications

There is currently no scientific basis for advising healthy athletes to supplement their diets with L-carnitine in an attempt to improve athletic performance. When supplemental carnitine is ingested, only 50% is actually absorbed, and the kidneys allow much of the absorbed carnitine to leave the body. Therefore, blood carnitine levels do not rise much following supplementation, and carnitine levels in skeletal muscles do not increase with this procedure. The best carnitine supplementation studies report no significant changes in muscle metabolism and endurance performance. Athletes should be advised against taking L-carnitine, but if they cannot be convinced, doses of 2–6 g/d for up to 1 mo and 1g/d for 6 mo have been used in experimental studies with no apparent adverse side effects. The use of D-carnitine should be avoided because it may cause a deficiency of L-carnitine and could decrease performance.

CAFFEINE

Caffeine is a drug that is widely consumed throughout the world and is commonly used by athletes in their daily lives and in preparation for athletic competitions. While caffeine is clearly a pharmacological agent, it is often considered a nutritional ergogenic aid, even though it has no nutritional value. This may be due to caffeine's position as an inherent part of the diet in many societies. Caffeine is also a "controlled or restricted drug" in the athletic world; urinary levels greater than 12 μg/ml following competitions are considered illegal by the IOC. However, most athletes who consume caffeine beverages prior to exercise would not approach the illegal limit following a competition. Therefore, caffeine occupies a unique position in the sports world by virtue of the fact that it is a drug that may be a legal ergogenic aid in many exercise situations.

Caffeine and Theories of Ergogenicity

Caffeine may exert a direct effect on some portion of the central nervous system that affects the perception of effort and/or motor-unit recruitment. It may also exert a direct effect on skeletal muscle performance. This may involve 1) ion transport handling (including Ca^{2+}), 2) inhibition of phosphodiesterase, leading to an elevation in cyclic AMP, and 3) direct effects on key regulatory enzymes such as glycogen phosphorylase. Support for the direct effects of caffeine on skeletal muscle is largely derived from in vitro investigations in which pharmacological concentrations of caffeine were used. If these in vitro findings have any relevance during whole-body exercise, the most likely candidates for contributing to an ergogenic effect of caffeine are calcium-handling kinetics and Na^+-K^+ pump activity.

The classic or "metabolic" theory was first used to explain the ergogenic effects of caffeine during aerobic endurance exercise. This theory proposed that caffeine mobilizes FFA from adipose tissue and/or intramuscular fat stores via increases in plasma epinephrine (EPI) and/or by directly antagonizing adipose tissue adenosine receptors. The increased FFA availability would then increase muscle fat oxidation and reduce carbohydrate oxidation from exogenous glucose and muscle glycogen. This "sparing" of carbohydrate, specifically muscle glycogen, in the initial stages of exercise was thought to improve performance during prolonged aerobic exercise, which is presumably limited by carbohydrate availability. Increases in fat availability and oxidation were believed to down regulate carbohydrate metabolism in heart and skeletal muscle, as classically proposed by Randle and colleagues (see Dyck et al., 1993). Increases in muscle citrate and acetyl-CoA were believed to inhibit the enzymes phosphofructokinase and PDH, and the subsequent decrease in glycolytic activity increased glucose 6-phosphate content, which inhibited hexokinase activity and ultimately decreased muscle glucose uptake.

Early Caffeine Research

The metabolic theory for explaining the ergogenic effects of caffeine during endurance exercise was proposed by Costill and colleagues following their pioneering work in the late '70s and early '80s. (See Spriet,

1995b, and Wilcox, 1990, for reviews.) Costill's group reported that caffeine ingestion 1 h prior to exhausting cycling at 80% $\dot{V}O_2$max improved performance from 75 min (placebo) to 96 min in well-trained athletes. A second study demonstrated that caffeine increased the amount of work performed in 2 h of cycling by 20%. These studies reported increased venous concentrations of FFA, decreased RER values, and a 30% increase in fat oxidation in the caffeine trials. A third study reported that caffeine ingestion spared muscle glycogen and increased muscle triglyceride use as a fuel during 30 min of submaximal cycling.

Caffeine research in the '80s was sporadic, and few investigations examined the effects of caffeine on endurance performance. Most studies investigated the effects of caffeine on metabolism and inferred how caffeine affected skeletal muscle metabolism from changes in venous concentrations of FFA and/or decreases in RER. Review articles examining this topic in the early '90s concluded that following the early work, few well-controlled studies had examined the effects of caffeine on endurance performance and that the results were inconsistent (Conlee, 1991; Wilcox, 1990).

Conlee (1991) argued that several factors could confound the results of caffeine studies. Three factors were related to the nature of the experimental design: the exercise modality (cycling vs. running), exercise power output, and caffeine dose. Four factors related to the status of the subjects prior to the experiment: nutritional and training status, previous caffeine use, and individual variation. An additional factor recently suggested was the ability to reliably measure exercise performance (Spriet, 1995b). This factor improves with increased training frequency and intensity and the athletic ability of the subjects. The quality of the investigations has improved as researchers have attempted to control these factors. Since 1990, the volume of research examining caffeine and endurance exercise performance increased significantly. In addition, investigations examining the effects of caffeine on exercise performance during sprinting (<90 s) and intense exercise of short (~5 min) and long duration (~20 min) have recently appeared.

Recent Complications in the Study of Caffeine, Metabolism, and Exercise Performance

Because caffeine appears to be taken up by all of the tissues of the body, it is difficult to independently study the effects of caffeine on specific tissues (e.g., brain, skeletal muscle, and/or adipose tissues) in the exercising human. It has also been realized that several mechanisms may be responsible for performance enhancement in different types of exercise, and those mechanisms may not involve a direct effect of caffeine. For example, caffeine ingestion usually increases plasma epinephrine concentration, which may have widespread effects. Caffeine (a trimethylxanthine) is also rapidly metabolized in the liver to three dimethylxanthine metabolites, paraxanthine, theophylline, and theobromine. These are released into the plasma as the caffeine concentration declines. While the accumulation of the dimethylxanthines in the plasma is not large, paraxanthine and theophylline are believed to be potential adenosine antagonists and metabolic stimuli. Therefore, as caffeine and its metabolites are often present at the same time, it is difficult to resolve which tissues are directly or indirectly affected by which compound.

Another complication that has been magnified recently is the variability of individual responses to caffeine. This problem affects both the metabolic and exercise performance responses to caffeine and becomes more of a problem with less aerobically fit subjects.

Recent Caffeine Studies Examining Endurance Performance and Metabolism

Several well-controlled studies have recently examined the effects of caffeine on exercise performance and metabolism in well-trained athletes accustomed to exhaustive exercise and race conditions. Performance assessments in these laboratory studies were chosen to simulate competitive conditions. This work examined the effects of a caffeine dose of 9 mg/kg body mass on running and cycling times to exhaustion at 80–85% $\dot{V}O_2$max (Graham & Spriet, 1991: Spriet et al., 1992), the effects of varying doses (3–13 mg/kg) of caffeine on cycling performance at 80–85% $\dot{V}O_2$max (Graham & Spriet, 1995; Pasman et al., 1995), and the effects of a moderate caffeine dose (5 mg/kg) on performance of repeated 30 min bouts of cycling (5 min rest between bouts) at 85–90% $\dot{V}O_2$max (Trice & Haymes, 1995). Collectively, this work produced several important findings.

Ingested caffeine is rapidly absorbed into the bloodstream and demonstrates dose-dependent increases in plasma caffeine levels (Figure 5-9). Plasma paraxanthine increases progressively with caffeine doses of 3 and 6 mg/kg but does not increase further with 9 mg/kg (Figure 5-10). Therefore, both caffeine and paraxanthine have the potential to affect all tissues that may be involved in the ergogenic effect of caffeine ingestion. Endurance performance in the caffeine trial was improved by about 20–50% compared to the placebo trial (from 40 min to 77 min) following ingestion of varying doses of caffeine (3–13 mg/kg) in elite and recreationally trained athletes while running (Figure 5-11) or cycling (Figure 5-12) at approximately 80–90% $\dot{V}O_2$max. Without exception, the 3, 5, and 6 mg/kg doses produced an ergogenic effect with urinary caffeine levels that were below the IOC acceptable limit (Figure 5-13). Three of four experiments using a 9 mg/kg dose reported performance increases, while

6/22 athletes tested in these studies had urinary caffeine levels at or above 12 µg/mL. Performance was enhanced with a 13 mg/kg dose, but 6/9 athletes had urinary caffeine levels well above 12 µg/mL (Figure 5-13). The side effects of caffeine ingestion (dizziness, headache, insomnia, and gastrointestinal distress) were rare with doses at or below 6 mg/kg but were prevalent at higher doses (9–13 mg/kg) and associated with decreased performance in some athletes at 9 mg/kg.

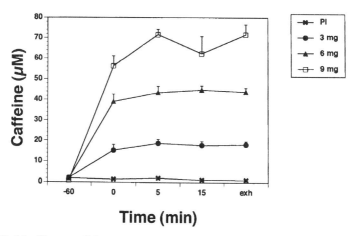

FIGURE 5-9. *Plasma caffeine concentrations during exhaustive (exh) exercise at 80–85% VO₂max following the ingestion of placebo or 3, 6, and 9 mg caffeine/kg body mass 1 h prior to exercise.* Data from Graham and Spriet (1995). Exhaustion occurred between 50–62 min in all trials.

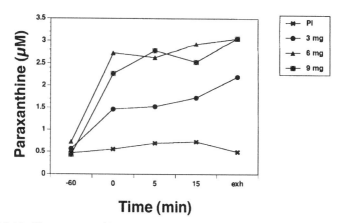

FIGURE 5-10. *Plasma paraxanthine concentrations during exhaustive (exh) exercise at 80–85% VO₂max following the ingestion of placebo or 3, 6, and 9 mg caffeine/kg body mass 1 h prior to exercise.* Data from Graham and Spriet (1995). Exhaustion occurred between 50–62 min in all trials.

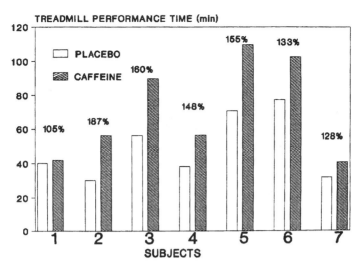

FIGURE 5-11. *Individual treadmill run times to exhaustion at 80–85% $\dot{V}O_2max$ following the ingestion of a placebo or 9 mg caffeine/kg body mass 1 h prior to exercise.* Data from Graham and Spriet (1991). Percentage numbers denote improvement with caffeine ingestion.

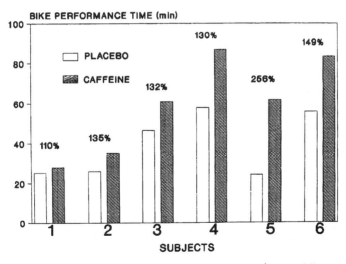

FIGURE 5-12. *Individual cycling times to exhaustion at 80–85% $\dot{V}O_2max$ following the ingestion of a placebo or 9 mg caffeine/kg body mass 1 h prior to exercise.* Data from Graham and Spriet (1991). Percentage numbers denote improvement with caffeine ingestion.

ERGOGENIC AIDS **215**

Caffeine generally produced a two-fold increase in EPI concentrations in venous plasma at rest and during exercise and in venous plasma FFA at rest, but the elevated FFA concentrations with caffeine were no longer apparent after 15–20 min of exercise, suggesting that the working muscles had taken up the FFA. At the lowest caffeine dose (3 mg/kg), performance was increased without significant increases in plasma EPI and FFA, although, the FFA concentration was increased by 70% at rest. Muscle glycogen utilization was reduced by roughly 50% following caffeine ingestion, but this "sparing" was limited to the initial 15 min of exercise at approximately 80% $\dot{V}O_2$max.

Less information is available on the performance and metabolic effects of caffeine in recreationally active or untrained subjects. Performance measures in these groups usually suffer from high test-retest variability. Chesley et al. (1996) reported a variable glycogen-sparing response to a high caffeine dose (9 mg/kg) in untrained males. Only 6/13 subjects demonstrated glycogen sparing (>20% of the muscle glycogen used in the placebo trial) during 15 min of cycling at 80–85% $\dot{V}O_2$max (Figure 5-14). The subjects who spared muscle glycogen experienced smaller decreases in muscle PCr concentrations and smaller increases in free AMP in muscle during exercise in the caffeine vs. placebo trials. There were no differences between trials in the non-sparers. It is not presently clear how caffeine helps to defend the energy state of the cell during this intense exercise, but it may be related to the availability of fat at the onset of exercise. These results demonstrate that the metabolic responses to caffeine ingestion in untrained subjects are more variable than in aerobically trained populations.

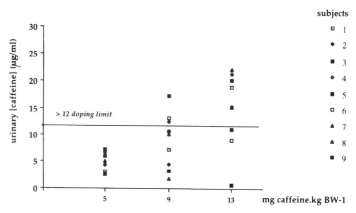

FIGURE 5-13. *Individual caffeine concentrations in urine obtained 15 min following exhaustive exercise and the ingestion of 5, 9, or 13 mg caffeine/kg body weight (BW) 1 h before exercise.* Data from Pasman et al. (1995). Horizontal line depicts the acceptable level of <12 μg caffeine/mL urine, as outlined by the International Olympic Committee.

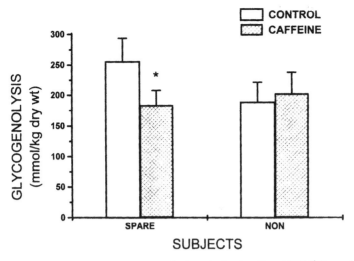

FIGURE 5-14. *Net muscle glycogenolysis during 15 min of cycling at 85% VO₂max in a group of subjects who spared muscle glycogen (SPARE) following caffeine ingestion (9 mg/kg body weight), as compared to control and a group of subjects who did not spare (NON) following caffeine ingestion.* Data from Chesley et al. (1996).

Graham et al. (1995) compared the effects of caffeine (4.5 mg/kg) in "pure" tablet form to the same amount of caffeine in a coffee beverage (about two mugs of strong coffee ingested in 10 min). Caffeine tablets produced the usual metabolic and performance effects, but when ingested as coffee, there was a decreased EPI response and little or no effect on performance, even though the plasma caffeine concentrations were identical. Presumably, the wide variety of chemicals in coffee negated the usual ergogenic benefit.

Mechanisms for Improved Endurance with Caffeine

Presently, it seems likely that a metabolic mechanism is part of the explanation for the improvement in endurance with caffeine, except at the low caffeine doses where this has not been fully examined. The increased plasma FFA concentration at the onset of exercise, the glycogen sparing in the initial 15 min, and the increased intramuscular triglyceride use during the first 30 min of exercise suggest a greater role for fat metabolism early in exercise following caffeine doses of 5 mg/kg and above. However, there have been no definitive measurements of increased exogenous FFA use following caffeine ingestion. Also, these metabolic findings do not preclude other central and peripheral factors that may contribute to enhanced endurance performance. For example, caffeine appears to stimulate Na^+-K^+ pump activity in inactive tissues, leading to an attenuation of the rise in plasma potassium concentration with exercise. It has been postulated that the lower plasma potassium helps maintain the membrane potential in contracting muscle and contributes to the ergogenic effect of caffeine during endurance exercise (Lindinger et al., 1993).

There is growing evidence that EPI does not play a major role in the metabolic changes occurring with caffeine ingestion. Performance can be enhanced with a caffeine dose of 3 mg/kg that does not cause a significant increase in plasma EPI. Also, an infusion of EPI designed to produce resting and exercise concentrations of EPI similar to those induced by caffeine, had no effect on plasma FFA concentration or muscle glycogenolysis during 15 min of cycling at 80% $\dot{V}O_2$max (Chesley et al., 1995). Van Soeren et al. (1996) gave caffeine to spinal-cord injured subjects and reported increased concentrations of FFA in venous plasma with no corresponding changes in EPI.

In summary, the known caffeine-induced alterations in muscle metabolism appear to contribute to an ergogenic effect during endurance exercise at the caffeine doses and exercise intensities that have been studied. Measurements of muscle glycogen and triglyceride use and exogenous FFA turnover are required to determine whether there is a metabolic link to the improved performance at lower caffeine doses and other exercise intensities.

Caffeine and Performance During Shorter-Term Exercise

Several investigations in the past decade have examined the effects of caffeine ingestion on performance (and occasionally metabolism) during exercise lasting less than 20 min. Exercise of this duration will not be limited by muscle glycogen availability, and the focus of explaining an ergogenic effect of caffeine must shift to a direct effect on skeletal muscle and/or the central nervous system.

Graded Exercise Tests. As reviewed by Dodd et al. (1993), several studies reported no effect of moderate caffeine doses on time to exhaustion and $\dot{V}O_2$max during graded exercise protocols lasting 8–20 min. However, two studies from the same laboratory reported prolonged exercise times when high doses of caffeine were given (Flinn et al., 1990; McNaughton, 1987). The initial study used caffeine doses of 10 and 15 mg/kg and reported a small, significant increase in performance. However, although a double-blind design was used, the control trial always preceded the caffeine trials, leading to a potential order effect. The second study used a caffeine dose of 10 mg/kg 3 h before cycling exercise and reported an increased time to exhaustion. The subjects again completed a control trial first, followed by placebo and caffeine trials that were randomized. The high caffeine dose is the most likely explanation for these positive findings, but no mechanistic information presently exists to explain the ergogenic effects.

Intense Aerobic Exercise. Competitive races lasting about 20 min require athletes to exercise at power outputs at or above 90% VO_2max. MacIntosh and Wright (1995) examined the effect of 6 mg caffeine/kg body weight on the performance of 1,500 m swim trials in trained distance swimmers. Caffeine significantly reduced swim trial time from 21:22 ± 0.38 to 20:59 ± 0.36 (min:sec). The authors reported that caffeine lowered plasma concentrations of potassium before the swim trials and raised blood glucose immediately after the swims. They suggested that electrolyte balance and exogenous glucose availability may be related to the ergogenic effects of caffeine.

Short-Term Intense Exercise. In exercise of high intensity (~100% VO_2max) that lasts about 5 min, near-maximal provision of energy from both aerobic and anaerobic sources is required.

Collomp et al. (1991) reported that 250 mg of caffeine increased cycle time to exhaustion at 100% VO_2max from 5:20 with placebo to 5:49, although, the increase was not significant. A third trial, during which subjects received 250 mg caffeine/d for 5 d, also increased time to exhaustion non-significantly (5:40).

Wiles et al. (1992) reported that coffee ingestion (~150–200 mg caffeine) decreased 1,500 m race time on a treadmill in well-trained runners by 4.2 s (4:46.0 vs. placebo, 4:50.2). Subjects were also tested by running for 1,100 m at a predetermined pace, followed by 400 m where they ran as fast as possible, with and without coffee. In the final 400 m, the average speed was 23.5 km/h with coffee and 22.9 km/h without. Following coffee, all subjects ran faster, and the mean VO_2 during the final 400 m was also higher. To more accurately measure such small performance changes, the average response to three trials in both the coffee and placebo conditions was determined.

Jackman et al. (1996) examined the effects of caffeine ingestion (6 mg/kg) on the performance and metabolic responses to repeated bouts of cycling at 100% VO_2max. Three bouts of exercise were performed with intervening rest periods of 6 min. The first two bouts lasted 2 min (constant total work), and the third trial was continued to exhaustion. Cycle time to exhaustion for 14 subjects was significantly improved with caffeine (4.93 ± 0.60 min vs. 4.12 ± 0.36 min for placebo). Muscle and blood lactate measurements throughout the protocol suggested a higher production of lactate in the caffeine trial, even in the initial two bouts when total work was constant. The net glycogenolytic rate was not different during the initial two bouts, and less than 50% of the muscle glycogen store was used in either trial during the protocol. The authors concluded that the ergogenic effect of caffeine during short-term intense exercise was not associated with glycogen sparing and may have been due to either direct action on the muscle or altered central nervous system function related to the sensation of effort and/or motor unit recruitment.

Sprint Performance. Sprint performance is defined here as exercise maintained to fatigue at power outputs 150–300% greater than those required to elicit $\dot{V}O_2$max; in sport, this would be represented by maximal competitive events lasting less than 90 s. The amount of energy derived from anaerobic processes would be ~75–80% of the total in the first 30 s, ~65–70% over 60 s, and ~55–60% over 90 s (Bangsbo et al., 1990).

Williams et al. (1988) reported that caffeine ingestion had no effect on maximal power output or muscular endurance during short, maximal bouts of cycling. The remaining information on sprinting has come from one laboratory with conflicting findings. Collomp et al. (1992) reported that ingestion of 5 mg/kg caffeine did not increase peak power or total work completed during a 30-s Wingate test. However, they later found that 250 mg of caffeine produced a significant 7% improvement in the maximal power output that could be generated during a series of 6-s sprints at varying force-velocity relationships (Anselme et al., 1992). They also examined the effects of 250 mg of caffeine on two 100-m freestyle swims, separated by 20 min (Collomp et al., 1990). In well-trained swimmers, velocity during the first and second swims was improved by 2% and 4%, respectively, but performance times were not reported. Therefore, given the present information, it is not possible to conclude that caffeine has an ergogenic effect on sprint performance. The brief and intense nature of sprint exercise makes it very difficult to study and demonstrate significant differences.

Field Studies. Performance in most laboratory studies examining endurance exercise is measured as the time taken to reach exhaustion at a given power output. However, in the field, performance is measured as the time taken to complete a certain task (e.g., run 10 km, swim 500 m, or complete a 90-min soccer match). Because actual competition involves many additional factors not present in the laboratory, we are always faced with the difficulty of extrapolating laboratory findings to the field. Occasionally, laboratory studies simulate competitive conditions with the subject in control of treadmill speed or cycling cadence and resistance in order to complete a distance or a given amount of work in the shortest possible time. Other studies have measured performance in time trials on the track or in the swimming pool in the absence of actual race conditions, which often make it impossible to employ the controls required to generate conclusive results. Although there is a tremendous need for more field studies examining caffeine and endurance performance, they may be impossible to conduct satisfactorily.

Practical Implications

Caffeine Dose. Athletes are allowed up to 12 µg caffeine/mL urine before it is considered illegal by the IOC. This permits athletes who normally have caffeine in their diets to consume it prior to competition. An athlete can ingest a very large amount of caffeine before reaching the "illegal limit." A 70-kg person could drink 3–4 mugs or 6 regular cups of drip-percolated coffee 1 h before exercise, exercise for 1–1.5 h, and only approach the urinary caffeine limit if tested immediately after the exercise. It is not easy for most people to reach the limit by ingesting coffee. A caffeine level above 12 µg/ml suggests that an individual has deliberately taken caffeine in the form of tablets or suppositories in an attempt to improve performance. Consequently, only a few athletes have been caught with illegal levels of caffeine during competitions, although, formal reports of the frequency of caffeine abuse are usually not made public.

Urinary Caffeine and Doping. The use of urinary caffeine levels to identify caffeine abuse in sport has been criticized. Only 0.5–3% of orally ingested caffeine actually reaches the urine; the majority is metabolized in the liver. Byproducts of caffeine metabolism are not currently measured in doping tests. Body weight, gender, and hydration status of the athlete also affect the amount of caffeine that reaches the urine. The time elapsed between caffeine ingestion and urine sample collection is important and is affected by the exercise duration and environmental conditions. Sport-governing bodies may not regard these concerns as problems because most people with illegal caffeine levels will have used caffeine in a doping manner.

Variability of Caffeine Responses. The variability of most performance and metabolic responses to caffeine is large. This appears to be true for all groups studied, including mild and heavy caffeine users, users withdrawn from caffeine, and non-users, and also appears to be especially prevalent in untrained individuals. Few females have been studied to determine if the variability in response to caffeine ingestion is similar to that in males. Menstrual status needs to be controlled in these studies because estrogen may affect the half-life of caffeine. Therefore, although mean results in a group of athletes may point to an improved athletic performance, predictions that a given individual will improve remain tenuous.

Habitual Caffeine Consumption. Habitual caffeine use may affect an individual's response to acute caffeine ingestion. Caffeine use does not change its metabolism, but the effects of caffeine may be altered via changes in adenosine receptor populations. Several recent studies suggest that chronic caffeine use dampens the EPI response to exercise and caffeine, but does not affect plasma FFA or RER during exercise (Bangsbo et al., 1992; Van Soeren et al., 1993a). However, these changes do not appear to dampen the ergogenic effect of 9 mg/kg caffeine. Endurance performance increased in all subjects in two studies in which both caffeine users and non-users were examined and users abstained from caffeine for 48-72 prior to experiments (Graham & Spriet, 1991; Spriet et al., 1992). However, the performance results were more variable in a subsequent study with more non-users (Graham & Spriet, 1995). In addition, Van Soeren et al. (1993b) recently reported no effect of up to 4 d of caffeine withdrawal on hormonal and metabolic responses to exercise after acute ingestion of 6 or 9 mg/kg doses. Performance times for the recreational cyclists riding to exhaustion at 80–85% VO_2max were improved by caffeine and unaffected by 0–4 d of withdrawal.

Diuretic Effect of Caffeine. It has been suggested that caffeine ingestion may act as a diuretic and lead to poor hydration status prior to and during exercise. However, core temperature, sweat loss, and plasma volume were unaffected during exercise following caffeine ingestion (Falk et al., 1990). Wemple et al. (1997) also reported that urine volumes and body hydration status during exercise were unaffected by caffeine ingested in a fluid replacement drink.

Ethical Considerations. It is possible for endurance athletes to enhance performance "legally" with caffeine because ergogenic effects have been reported with doses of 3–6 mg/kg body weight. It has been suggested that caffeine should be banned prior to competitions in endurance athletes (Graham et al., 1994; Spriet, 1995). This would ensure that no athlete had an unfair advantage on race day but would not prevent caffeine use in training. Athletes would have to abstain from caffeine for 48-72 h prior to competition to achieve this goal. However, in the present climate, what should athletes do? Should they use caffeine in moderate amounts to make sure they are not missing out, or should they avoid this tactic that could be considered doping? The former point of view may be popular because caffeine use is prevalent in society and athletes will not have "illegal" amounts in their urine. Others argue that caffeine use in moderation should not be an issue because other more serious drugs require attention. Although the side effects of caffeine ingestion are not serious, the potential ergogenic effect is impressive. On the other hand, discouraging its use downplays the "doping, win at all costs" mentality and sets the proper example for youth. If young athletes use caffeine, does it become a "gateway" drug for banned and more dangerous substances? The Canadian Center for Drug Free Sport reported in 1993 that more than 25% of youths aged 11–18 reported using caffeine in the last year to help them do better in sports.

ERYTHROPOIETIN

Erythropoietin (EPO) is a naturally occurring hormone that is the prime regulator of red blood cell production in humans. It is released by the kidneys in response to signals from the renal oxygen sensing cells. EPO release increases greatly when kidney oxygenation decreases due to hypoxemia, anemia, and reductions in renal blood flow. Increases in EPO stimulate the production of red blood cells (RBCs) in the bone marrow.

Recombinant Human Erythropoietin

Human EPO was isolated, characterized, and cloned in the mid-1980s, making it possible to genetically engineer EPO using a recombinant DNA technique (Erslev, 1991). The recombinant human EPO (rhEPO) was subsequently used to increase RBC production in patients with renal insufficiency and in autologous blood donors (Eschbach et al., 1987; Goodnough, 1993). It subsequently became commercially available and is now routinely given to kidney failure patients as well as trauma, AIDS, and anemic patients (Erslev, 1991).

Ergogenic Potential and Safety Concerns of rhEPO

It was immediately obvious that the ability of rhEPO to increase RBC mass in humans should produce the same hematological, metabolic, and exercise performance responses that had been well documented for blood doping (see Spriet, 1991, for review). The physiological basis for the ergogenic effect of blood doping is the increase in the number of RBCs/unit volume of blood. This increases the hemoglobin concentration and the oxygen content (CaO_2) or oxygen-carrying capacity of the arterial blood. Maximal cardiac output and blood volume are unchanged following blood doping such that oxygen transport (maximal cardiac output x CaO_2) is increased. Some of this extra transported oxygen is delivered to and taken up by the working muscles, producing increases in VO_2max and endurance performance in active subjects and well-trained endurance athletes (Spriet, 1991).

It also appeared that the administration of rhEPO, which requires three subcutaneous injections weekly for about 6 wk, would be easier than blood doping. Blood doping is a complicated procedure that requires the removal of 2–3 units of blood from an individual, freeze storage of the RBCs for 6–10 wk while normal RBC levels are restored in the subject, and subsequent reinfusion of the reconstituted RBCs. Also, an increased RBC mass should be maintained as long as rhEPO administration is continued. Therefore, the certainty that rhEPO would be ergogenic, coupled with the ease of administration, made it a prime candidate for misuse in endurance sports. Because increases in RBC mass appear to be dependent on the dose of rhEPO (Eschbach et al., 1987), non-supervised administration of high doses might produce dangerously high RBC mass levels. The injection of rhEPO involves the use of a physiological substance given with an abnormal method in pharmacological amounts; consequently, the IOC classified rhEPO as a doping substance and banned its practice in 1990. As with blood doping many years earlier (Wide et al., 1995), this was done even though no methods were available to detect its use through measurements in urine.

Reports in the lay press and scientific journals have suggested that several deaths in endurance cyclists were related to abuse of rhEPO (Adamson & Vapnek, 1991; Cowart, 1989; Deacon & Gains, 1995; Woodland, 1991), although, nothing official has been reported in the medical literature. As outlined recently (American College of Sports Medicine, 1996; Deacon & Gains, 1995), several factors have led to this speculation: (a) the sequence and timing of the availability of commercial rhEPO and the deaths of the cyclists, (b) the history of cyclists using blood doping to improve performance, (c) the similarity between clinical effects of rhEPO and the symptoms associated with the cyclists' deaths, although they were listed as cardiovascular abnormalities, and (d) the rates of improvement in endurance sports since 1990.

Hematological and Exercise Responses to rhEPO Administration

Several studies have demonstrated that rhEPO will increase $\dot{V}O_2max$ and physical work capacity by 10–100% in anemic adults and children with renal disease (Baraldi et al., 1990; Canadian EPO Study Group, 1990; Mayer et al., 1988; Metra et al., 1991; Rosenlof et al., 1989). Furthermore, Ekblom and colleagues examined the effect of rhEPO administration for 6 wk on the metabolic and circulatory responses to submaximal and maximal exercise in healthy, moderate-to-well-trained males (Berglund & Ekblom, 1991; Ekblom & Berglund,1991). Because the rhEPO was expected to increase RBC and hemoglobin levels slowly, the responses were compared to those following rapid elevation of blood variables by reinfusing RBCs. One group (n = 8) received three subcutaneous injections of rhEPO (20 IU/kg body mass/wk) for 6 wk. A second group (n = 7) received the same rhEPO dose for 4 wk, followed by a double dose for the final 2 wk. All subjects received iron supplements during the rhEPO administration period. Prior to the rhEPO study, the second group also participated in a RBC reinfusion study. All subjects had returned to normal hemoglobin levels before the rhEPO study began.

There were no significant differences between groups in any of the measured variables, even though the second group received more rhEPO. The administration of rhEPO for 6 wk increased hemoglobin concentration by 11%, which was greater than that reported in a later study by Casoni et al. (1993), who injected 30 IU of rhEPO/kg body mass every other day into 20 healthy subjects for 6 wk and reported only a 6% increase in hemoglobin concentration. Ekblom and Berglund (1991) found no effect of rhEPO on blood volume and resting blood pressure. During submaximal cycling at 100 and 200 W, $\dot{V}O_2$ was unchanged, and heart rate was lower following rhEPO. Systolic blood pressure was not different at 100 W but was higher following rhEPO at 200 W (191 vs. 177 mm Hg). During an exhaustive incremental treadmill run, maximal heart rate was unchanged, time to exhaustion increased from 500 s to 583 s, and $\dot{V}O_2$max increased from 4.52 to 4.88 L/min following rhEPO. In the subjects who underwent the blood reinfusion and rhEPO administration, hemoglobin concentration increased by 9% following the reinfusion of 3 units of blood and 13% following rhEPO (Figure 5-15). Both procedures had no effect on blood volume, and both produced similar increases in time to exhaustion (13.5–15.5%) and $\dot{V}O_2$max (6.4–7.9%) by the same amounts (Figure 5-15). It should be noted that there were no control groups in this study, although it may be argued that previous work had established that no changes in $\dot{V}O_2$max and performance occurred in control groups. The main conclusion of this study was the similarity in metabolic, circulatory, and exercise performance responses following 6 wk of rhEPO administration and acute RBC reinfusion.

Detection of rhEPO Administration

There is currently no routine testing for rhEPO use among athletes participating in major competitions. However, Wide et al. (1995) re-

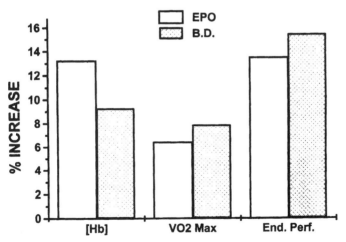

FIGURE 5-15. *Percent increases in hemoglobin (Hb) concentration, $\dot{V}O_2$max and endurance performance (End. Perf.) following erythropoietin (EPO) injection and blood doping (B.D.), as compared to pre-EPO injection and blood doping responses.* Data from Ekblom and Berglund (1991).

ported significant progress towards the development of a reliable test using blood and urine samples to detect rhEPO administration. The basis for the test relates to a difference between the electric charge of rhEPO and naturally occurring EPO. The rhEPO is less negatively charged, and this can be detected as a lower mobility when subjected to electrophoresis in an agarose suspension (Wide & Bengtsson, 1990). The difference in electric charge is a consequence of production of endogenous EPO in the human kidney and synthesis of rhEPO using three different cell lines: hamster ovary and kidney cells and mouse fibroblast cells (Storring & Gaines, 1992).

Wide et al. (1995) injected 15 healthy males with 20 IU of rhEPO three times weekly for 7–9 wk. Blood and urine samples were taken during and for up to 3 wk after the administration of rhEPO. Urinary rhEPO was detected in all blood and urine samples for up to 24 h after rhEPO injection throughout and following the administration period. Urinary rhEPO was detected in 9 of 12 samples 48 h following the last injection but not detected in samples taken 1–3 wk following the last rhEPO injection. Importantly, there were no false positive detections in the study. Unfortunately, this technique loses its ability to detect the use of rhEPO after approximately 2 d, limiting its usefulness for detection during competitions because the physiological effects of rhEPO would still be present (Wide et al., 1995). This points to the need for random testing during training periods because repeated injections of rhEPO are required for some weeks to increase RBC mass and hemoglobin concentration. Wide et al. (1995) also noted that the current analysis for rhEPO is very time consuming; one technician can make only 16 measurements each week.

Other researchers are examining the effectiveness of measuring transferrin receptor levels, an indirect method to identify increases in RBC production (Beguin, 1992). Athletes who use rhEPO apparently have higher than normal levels of transferrin receptors.

Practical Implications

Repeated injections of rhEPO produce an ergogenic effect during submaximal and maximal endurance exercise. However, this practice is illegal as defined by the IOC and has the potential to be dangerous if administration is not supervised. The American College of Sports Medicine (1996) recently published a position statement on this topic and stated that any blood doping procedure (including rhEPO administration) used to improve athletic performance is unethical, unfair, and possibly unhealthy. Therefore, the message for all individuals involved in sport is to stay away from rhEPO.

DIRECTIONS FOR FUTURE RESEARCH

Creatine

The majority of evidence demonstrating that supplemental Cr increases muscle total Cr, Cr, and PCr contents has come from two or three laboratories. Following these findings, most other laboratories have been content to examine only the performance effects of Cr supplementation. Additional attempts to measure muscle changes would be useful to confirm the results and provide more data on the modest increases in PCr content and the response rate to Cr supplementation. Additional studies are required to more carefully study the effects of Cr supplementation on the rate of PCr resynthesis in the rest periods between repeated bouts of sprint activity. It would also be interesting to investigate the relationship between dietary Cr intake and resting muscle total-Cr concentration. This may help determine if some of the variability in resting total-Cr concentration between individuals of the same gender and also between genders is diet related. A thorough investigation of how muscle metabolism and exercise performance of females respond to Cr supplementation is needed. The consistent finding of increased body mass following Cr supplementation needs to be investigated. Is it a function of increased body water, increased protein synthesis, and/or yet unidentified processes? As with most ergogenic aids, additional field studies must be undertaken to more accurately predict the ergogenic effect of Cr in true athletic competitions. Lastly, it will be very important to examine the long-term effects of Cr loading and Cr ingestion during maintenance phases. This includes effects on skeletal muscle and on performance. Also, because studies to date have been limited to ~35 d of Cr ingestion, the potential for side effects from long-term use needs to be investigated.

Carnitine

Given the inability of supplemental carnitine to increase muscle carnitine levels over the short-term (7–28 d), it is not clear why some studies have demonstrated increases in $\dot{V}O_2$max. Additional well-controlled studies from independent laboratories should be conducted to examine the effect of 4–6 g carnitine/d for a period of 7–28 d to confirm or refute previous findings on $\dot{V}O_2$max. It is also not clear why three of eight studies reported increased fat oxidation (based on RER) during prolonged aerobic exercise following carnitine supplementation. Given the small decreases in muscle carnitine reported with training and the small increases in muscle carnitine reported during training in subjects supplemented with carnitine (Arenas et al., 1991), more studies should examine the longer-term effects of carnitine supplementation (>6 mo).

Caffeine

Definitive research into the mechanisms of caffeine's ergogenic effect in exercising humans continues to be hampered by the ability of caffeine, its metabolic byproducts, and EPI to affect both central and peripheral processes during exercise. The metabolic changes associated with endurance improvements following low doses of caffeine and lower exercise intensities have not been adequately studied. Quantitative measurements of exogenous FFA use with and without caffeine ingestion are needed to more definitely link these processes. This will require measurements of blood flow and of arterial-femoral venous FFA differences in the legs of exercising subjects or the use of tracer technology. The effects of caffeine ingestion on metabolic and exercise performance responses in females have not been studied. Experiments to identify the cause of ergogenic effects of caffeine during exercise lasting under 20 min are needed.

Erythropoietin

Most future research will focus on the ability to detect rhEPO use in urine samples of athletes. There is little need to repeat the studies with rhEPO that have been done with the RBC reinfusion technique, as both produce increases in CaO_2. The one existing study is sufficient to convince most scientists that the rhEPO effects are similar to those induced by RBC reinfusion.

SUMMARY

Creatine is normally consumed in the diet and can be synthesized in the body. Supplemental Cr dramatically increases blood plasma levels of Cr for several hours and enhances the uptake of Cr into skeletal muscle. People with low-to-average muscle Cr levels respond to supplemental Cr with significant increases in skeletal muscle Cr levels, whereas, individuals with high initial levels often do not respond to supplementation. The extra muscle Cr following supplementation appears to increase muscle PCr content and promote the rate of PCr resynthesis following exercise. A greater content of PCr in muscle increases the potential for anaerobic energy provision during brief high-intensity exercise. Supplemental Cr and the associated changes in muscle Cr seem to improve performance during repeated brief bouts of sprinting. Creatine supplementation has no effect on aerobic exercise metabolism and performance.

It has been proposed that supplemental carnitine may improve exercise performance by increasing the mitochondrial uptake and oxidation of FFA or by increasing mitochondrial free CoA, thereby, stimulating energy production by activating key enzymes of carbohydrate and fat metabolism. However, it is now clear that ingestion of moderate doses of carnitine that increase plasma carnitine levels by two-fold or less do not increase muscle carnitine levels and that much of the ingested carnitine is either not absorbed in the intestine or is lost via the kidney. Therefore, any ergogenic effects of carnitine supplementation must occur through mechanisms that are non-metabolic, and no evidence currently exists to support this contention. The majority of evidence examining the impact of carnitine on muscle metabolism and exercise performance is negative. The few studies that do report increases in $\dot{V}O_2$max and fat oxidation during aerobic exercise lack data to support a metabolic mechanism. There is presently no substantial scientific basis for advising healthy athletes to supplement their diet with L-carnitine in an attempt to improve athletic performance.

Caffeine ingestion (3–13 mg/kg body weight) prior to exercise increases performance during prolonged endurance cycling and running in the laboratory, and doses below 9 mg/kg generally produce urinary caffeine levels below the IOC-allowable limit of 12 μg/ml. Moderate caffeine doses (5–6 mg/kg) also improve performance of brief intense cycling (~5 min) in the laboratory, decrease swim time for 1500 m (~20 min), and decrease running time for 1,500 m. These results are generally reported in well-trained elite or recreational athletes, but field studies are lacking to confirm the ergogenic effects of caffeine in the athletic world. Caffeine ingestion increases plasma FFA concentrations at rest, increases muscle triglyceride use, and reduces muscle glycogen use early in endurance exercise, suggesting greater fat use and reduced carbohydrate oxidation in the working muscles. However, such a metabolic explanation for the ergogenic effect of caffeine has not been confirmed at low caffeine doses and at all aerobic exercise intensities. Increases in plasma EPI are not important for the metabolic changes induced by caffeine ingestion. Possible mechanisms for improved performance during brief intense exercise include direct effects of caffeine on the central nervous system and/or on excitation-contraction coupling and anaerobic energy provision in muscle.

Erythropoietin is a physiological substance that is ergogenic when given in pharmacological doses as recombinant human erythropoietin (rhEPO). The rhEPO stimulates RBC production in bone marrow, leading to increases in RBC number, hemoglobin concentration, arterial oxygen content, and delivery of oxygen to the working muscles. Consequently, VO_2max is increased, and endurance performance at high aerobic power outputs is improved. The use of rhEPO is illegal as defined by the IOC and can be dangerous if not properly administered. It is also considered unethical and unfair by the American College of Sports Medicine.

BIBLIOGRAPHY

Adamson, J.W., and D. Vapnek (1991). Recombinant erythropietin to improve athletic performance. *New Eng. J. Med.* 324:698–699.

American College of Sports Medicine (1996). Position stand: the use of blood doping as an ergogenic aid. *Med. Sci. Sports Exerc.* 28:i–viii.

Anselme, F., K. Collomp, B. Mercier, S. Ahmaidi, and C. Prefaut (1992). Caffeine increases maximal anaerobic power and blood lactate concentration. *Eur. J. Appl. Physiol.* 65:188–191.

Arenas, J., J.R. Ricoy, A.R. Ecinas, P. Pola, S. D'iddio, M. Zeviani, S. Didonato, and M. Corsi (1991). Carnitine in muscle and urine of nonprofessional athletes: effects of physical exercise, training, and L-carnitine administration. *Muscle and Nerve.* 14:598–604.

Balsom, P.D., B. Ekblom, K. Soderlund, B. Sjodin, and E. Hultman (1993a). Creatine supplementation and dynamic high-intensity exercise. *Scand J. Med. Sci. Sports* 3:143–149.

Balsom, P.D., S.D.R. Harridge, K. Soderlund, B. Sjodin, and B. Ekblom (1993b). Creatine supplementation per se does not enhance endurance exercise performance. *Acta Physiol. Scand.* 149:521–523.

Bangsbo, J., P.D. Gollnick, T.E. Graham, C. Juel, B. Kiens, M. Mizuno, and B. Saltin (1990). Anaerobic energy production and O_2 deficit—debt relationship during exhaustive exercise in humans. *J. Physiol.* 42:539–559.

Bangsbo, J., K. Jacobsen, N. Nordberg, N.J. Christensen, and T. Graham (1992). Acute and habitual caffeine ingestion and metabolic responses to steady-state exercise. *J. Appl. Physiol.* 72:1297–1303.

Baraldi, E., G. Montini, S. Zanconato, G. Zacchello, and F. Zacchello (1990). Exercise tolerance after anemia correction with recombinant erythrpoietin in end-stage renal disease. *Ped. Nephrol.* 4:623–626.

Barnett, C., D.L. Costill, M.D. Vukovich, K.J. Cole, B.H. Goodpaster, S.W. Trappe, and W.J. Fink (1994). Effect of L-carnitine supplementation on muscle and blood carnitine content and lactate accumulation during high-intensity sprint cycling. *Int. J. Sport Nutr.* 4:280–288.

Beguin, Y. (1992). The soluble transferrin receptor: biological aspects and clinical usefulness as quantitative measure of erythropoiesis. *Haematologia* 77:1–10.

Berglund, B., and B. Ekblom (1991). Effect of recombinant human erythrpoietin treatment on blood pressure and some heamatological parameters in healthy males. *J. Int. Med.* 229:125–130.

Bessman, S.P., and F. Savabi (1990). The role of phosphocreatine energy shuttle in exercise and muscle hypertrophy. In: A.W. Taylor, P.D. Gollnick, H.J. Green, C.D. Ianuzzu, E.G. Noble, G. Metivier, and J.R. Sutton (eds.) *Biochemistry of Exercise* International Series on Sport Sciences. Champaign, IL: Human Kinetics, Vol. 21, pp. 109–120.

Birch, R., D. Noble, and P.L. Greenhaff (1994). The influence of dietary creatine supplementation on performance during repeated bouts of maximal isokinetic cycling in man. *Eur. J. Appl. Physiol.* 69:268–270.

Broquist, H.P. (1994). Carnitine. In: M.E. Shils, J.A. Olson and M. Shike (eds.) *Modern Nutrition in Health and Disease.* Philadelphia: Lea & Febiger, pp. 459–465.

Canadian Erythropoietin Study Group (1990). Association between recombinant erythropietin and quality of life and exercise capacity of patients receiving haemodialysis. *Br. Med. J.* 300:573–578.

Carlin, J.I., W.G. Reddan, M. Sanjak, and R. Hodach (1986). Carnitine metabolism during prolonged exercise and recovery in humans. *J. Appl. Physiol.* 61:1275–1278.

Casey, A., D. Constantin-Teodosiu, S. Howell, E. Hultman, and P.L. Greenhaff (1996). Creatine ingestion favourably affects performance and muscle metabolism during maximal exercise in humans. *Am. J. Physiol.* 271:E31–E37.

Casoni, I., G. Ricci, E. Ballarin, C. Borsetto. G. Grazzi, C. Guglielmini, F. Manfredini, G. Mazzoni, M. Patracchini, E. De Paoli Vitali, F. Rigolin, S. Bartalotta, G.P. Franze, M. Masotti, and F. Conconi (1993). Hematological indices of erythropoietin administration in athletes. *Int. J. Sports Med.* 14:307–311.

Chesley, A., R.A. Howlett, G.J.F. Heigenhauser, E. Hultman, and L.L. Spriet (1996). Regulation of muscle glycogen phosphorylase activity during intense aerobic exercise following caffeine ingestion. *Physiologist* 39:In press. (Abstract).

Chesley, A., E. Hultman, and L.L. Spriet (1995). Effects of epinephrine infusion on muscle glycogenolysis during intense aerobic exercise. *Am. J. Physiol.* 268:E127–E134.

Collomp, K., S. Ahmaidi, M. Audran, J.-L. Chanal, and C. Prefaut (1991). Effects of caffeine ingestion on performance and anaerobic metabolism during the Wingate test. *Int. J. Sports Med.* 12:439–443.

Collomp, K., S. Ahmaidi, J.C. Chatard, M. Audran, and C. Prefaut (1992). Benefits of caffeine ingestion on sprint performance in trained and untrained swimmers. *Eur. J. Appl. Physiol.* 64:377–380.

Collomp, K., C. Caillaud, M. Audran, J.-L. Chanal, and C. Prefaut (1990). Influence of acute and chronic bouts of caffeine on performance and catecholamines in the course of maximal exercise. *C.R. Soc. Biol.* 184:87–92.

Conlee, R.K. (1991). Amphetamine, caffeine and cocaine. In: D.R. Lamb and M.H. Williams (eds.) *Perspectives in Exercise Science and Sports Medicine, Vol. 4: Ergogenics: Enhancement of Performance in Exercise and Sport.* Dubuque, IA: Brown and Benchmark, pp. 285–330.

Constantin-Teodosiu, J.I. Carlin, G. Cederblad, R.C. Harris, and E. Hultman (1991). Acetyl group accumulation and pyruvate dehydrogenase activity in human muscle during incremental exercise. *Acta Physiol. Scand.* 143:367–372.

Constantin-Teodosiu, D., G. Cederblad, and E. Hultman (1992). PDC activity and acetyl group accumulation in skeletal muscle during prolonged exercise. *J. Appl. Physiol.* 73:2403–2407.

Constantin-Teodosiu, D., S. Howell, and P.L. Greenhaff (1996). Carnitine metabolism in human muscle fiber types during submaximal dynamic exercise. *J. Appl. Physiol.* 80:1061–1064.

Cooke, W.H., P.W. Grandjean, and W.S. Barnes (1995). Effect of oral creatine supplementation on power output and fatigue during bicycle ergometry. *J. Appl. Physiol.* 78:670–673.

Cowart, V.S. (1989). Erythropoietin: A dangerous new form of blood doping? *Phys. Sports Med.* 17:115–118.

Crim, M.C., D.H. Calloway, and S. Margen (1976). Creatine metabolism in men: creatine pool size and turnover in relation to creatine intake. *J. Nutr.* 106:371–381.

Deacon, J., and P. Gains (1995). A phantom killer. *MacLean's* Nov. 27.

Decombaz, J., O. Deriaz, K. Acheson, B. Gmuender, and E. Jequier (1993). Effect of L-carnitine on submaximal exercise metabolism after depletion of muscle glycogen. *Med. Sci. Sports Exerc.* 25:733–740.

Decombaz, J., B. Gmuender, G. Sierro, and P. Cerretelli (1992). Muscle carnitine after strenuous endurance exercise. *J. Appl. Physiol.* 72:423–427.

Delanghe, J., J.-P. De Slypere, M. Debuyzere, J. Robbrecht, R. Wieme, and A. Ver meulen (1989). Normal reference values for creatine, creatinine and carnitine are lower in vegetarians. *Clin. Chem.* 35:1802–1803.

Dodd, S.L., R.A. Herb, and S.K. Powers (1993). Caffeine and endurance performance: An update. *Sports Med.* 15:14–23.

Dubelaar, M.-L., C.M.H.B. Lucas, and W.C. Hulsmann (1991). Acute effect of L-carnitine on skeletal muscle force tests in dogs. *Am. J. Physiol.* 260:E189–E193.

Dyck, D.J., C.T. Putman, G.J.F. Heihenauser, E. Hultman, and L.L. Spriet (1993). Regulation of fat-carbohydrate interaction in skeletal muscle during intense aerobic cycling. *Am. J. Physiol.* 265:E852–E859.

Earnest, C.P., P.G. Snell, R. Rodriguez, T.L. Mitchell, and A.L. Almeda (1995). The effect of creatine monhydrate ingestion on anaerobic power indices, muscular strength, and body composition. *Acta Physiol. Scand.* 153:207–209.

Ekblom, B., and B. Berglund (1991). Effect of erythropoietin administration on maximal aerobic power. *Scand. J. Med. Sci. Sports.* 1:88–93.

Engel, A.G., and C.J. Rebouche (1984). Carnitine metabolism and inborn errors. *J. Inherited Metab. Dis.* 7 (Suppl. 1):38–43.

Erslev, A.J. (1991). Erythropoietin. *Drug Therapy.* 324:1339–1344.

Eschbach, J.W., J.C. Egrie, M.R. Downing, J.K. Browne, and J.W. Adamson (1987). Correction of the anemia of end-state renal disease with recombinant human erythropoietin. *N. Engl. J. Med.* 316:73–78.

Falk, B., R. Burstein, J. Rosenblum, Y. Shapiro, E. Zylber-Katz, and N. Bashan (1990). Effects of caffeine ingestion on body fluid balance and thermoregulation during exercise. *Can. J. Physiol. Pharmacol.* 68:889–892.

Febbraio, M.A., T.R. Flanagan, R.J. Snow, S. Zhao, and M.F. Carey (1995). Effect of creatine supplementation on intramuscular TCr, metabolism and performance during intermittent, supramaximal exercise in humans. *Acta Physiol. Scand.* 155:387–395.

Fitch, C.D., and R.P. Shields (1966). Creatine metabolism in skeletal muscle. I. Creatine movement across muscle membranes. *J. Biol. Chem.* 241:3611–3614.

Flinn, S., J. Gregory, L.R. McNaughton, S. Tristram, and P. Davies (1990). Caffeine ingestion prior to incremental cycling to exhaustion in recreational cyclists. *Int. J. Sports Med.* 11:188–193.

Forsberg, A.M., E. Nilsson, J. Werneman, J. Bergstrom, and E. Hultman (1991). Muscle composition in relation to age and sex. *Clin. Sci.* 81:249–256.

Goodnough, L.T. (1993). The role of recombinant growth factors in transfusion medicine. *Br. J. Anaesth.* 70:80–86.

Gordon, A., E. Hultman, L. Kaijser, S. Kristjansson, C.J. Rolf, O. Nyquist, and C. Sylven (1995). Creatine supplementation in chronic heart failure increases skeletal muscle creatine phosphate and muscle performance. *Cardiovasc. Res.* 30:413–418.

Gorostiaga, E.M., C.A. Maurer, and J.P. Eclache (1989). Decrease in respiratory quotient during exercise following L-carnitine supplementation. *Int. J. Sports Med.* 10:169–174.

Graham, T.E., and L.L. Spriet (1995). Metabolic, catecholamine and exercise performance responses to varying doses of caffeine. *J. Appl. Physiol.* 78:867–874.

Graham, T.E., and L.L. Spriet (1991). Performance and metabolic responses to a high caffeine dose during prolonged exercise. *J. Appl. Physiol.* 71:2292–2298.

Graham, T.E., E. Hibbert, and P. Sathasivam (1995). Caffeine vs. coffee: coffee isn't an effective ergogenic aid. *Med. Sci. Sports Exerc.* 27:S224. (Abstract).

Graham, T.E., J.W.E. Rush, and M.H. VanSoeren (1994). Caffeine and exercise: metabolism and performance. *Can. J. Appl. Physiol.* 2:111–138.

Greenhaff, P.L. (1995). Creatine and its application as an ergogenic aid. *Int. J. Sports Nutr.* 5:S100–S110.

Greenhaff, P.L., K. Bodin, R.C. Harris, E. Hultman, D.A Jones, D.B. McIntyre, K. Soderlund, and D.L. Turner (1994). The influence of oral creatine supplementation on muscle phosphocreatine resynthesis. *Am. J. Physiol.* 266:E725–E730.

Greenhaff, P.L., A. Casey, A.H. Short, K. Soderlund, and E. Hultman (1993). Influence of oral creatine supplementation of muscle torque during repeated bouts of maximal voluntary exercise in man. *Clin. Sci.* 84:565–571.

Greig, C., K. Finch, D. Jones, M. Cooper, A. Sargeant, and C. Forte (1987). The effect of oral supplementation with L-carnitine on maximum and submaximum exercise capacity. *Eur. J. Appl. Physiol.* 56:457–460.

Guimbal, C., and M.W. Kilimann (1993). A Na^+-dependent creatine transporter in rabbit brain, muscle, heart, and kidney. *J. Biol. Chem.* 268:8418–8421.

Harper, P., C.-E. Elwin, and G. Cederblad (1988). Pharmacokinetics of intravenous and oral bolus doses of L-carnitine in healthy subjects. *Eur. J. Clin. Pharmacol.* 35:555–562.

Harris, R.C., E. Hultman, and L.-O. Nordesjo (1974). Glycogen, glycolytic intermediates and high-energy phosphates determined in biopsy samples of musculus quadriceps femoris of man at rest. Methods and variance of values. *Scand. J. Clin. Lab. Invest.* 33:109–120.

Harris, R.C., K. Soderlund, and E. Hultman (1992). Elevation of creatine in resting and exercised muscle of normal subjects by creatine supplementation. *Clin. Sci.* 83:367–374.

Harris, R.C., M. Viru, P.L. Greenhaff, and E. Hultman (1993). The effect of oral creatine supplementation on running performance during maximal short-term exercise in man. *J. Physiol.* 467:74P. (Abstract).

Heymsfield, S.B., C. Arteaga, C. McManus, J. Smith, and S. Moffitt (1983). Measurement of muscle mass in humans. *Am. J. Clin. Nutr.* 37:478–494.

Hiatt, W.R., J.G. Regensteiner, E.E. Wolfel, L. Ruff, and E.P. Brass (1989). Carnitine and acylcarnitine metabolism during exercise in humans. *J. Clin. Invest.* 84:1167–1173.

Hultman, E., G. Cederblad, and P. Harper (1991). Carnitine administration as a tool of modify energy metabolism during exercise. *Eur. J. Appl. Physiol.* 62:450. (Letter to the Editor).

Hultman, E., K. Soderlund, J.A. Timmons, G. Cederblad, and P.L. Greenhaff (1996). Muscle creatine loading in men. *J. Appl. Physiol.* 81:232–237.

Jackman, M., P. Wendling, D. Friars, and T.E. Graham (1996). Metabolic, catecholamine and endurance responses to caffeine during intense exercise. *J. Appl. Physiol.* 81: In press.

Janssen, G.M.E., H.R. Scholte, M.H.M. Vaandrager-Verduin, and J.D. Ross (1989). Muscle carnitine level in endurance training and running a marathon. *Int. J. Sports Med.* 10(Suppl. 3):S153–S155.

Kanter, M.M., and M.H. Williams (1995). Antioxidants, Carnitine, and Choline as Putative Ergogenic Aids. *Int. J. of Sports Nutr.* 5:S120–S131.

Kasper, C.M., B.D. Reeves, M.G. Flynn, and F.F. Andres (1994). L-carnitine supplementation and running performance. *Med. Sci. Sports Exerc.* 26:S39. (Abstract).

Lemon, P., M. Boska, D. Bredle, M. Rogers, T. Ziegenfuss, and B. Newcomer (1995). Effect of oral creatine supplementation on energetics during repeated maximal muscle contraction. *Med. Sci. Sports Exerc.* 27:S204. (Abstract).

Lennon, D.F.L., E.R. Shrago, M. Madden, F.J. Nagle, and P. Hanson (1986). Dietary carnitine intake related to skeletal muscle and plasma carnitine concentrations in adult men and women. *Am. J. Clin. Nutr.* 43:234–238.

Lennon, D.F.L., F.W. Stratman, E. Shrago, F.J. Nagle, M. Madden, P. Hanson, and A.L. Carter (1983). Effects of acute moderate-intensity exercise on carnitine metabolism in men and women. *J. Appl. Physiol.* 55:489–495.

Lindinger, M.I., T.E. Graham, and L.L. Spriet (1993). Caffeine attenuates the exercise-induced increase in plasma $[K^+]$ in humans. *J. Appl. Physiol.* 74:1149–1155.

Loike, J.D., M. Somes, and S.C. Silverstein (1986). Creatine uptake, metabolism, and efflux in human monocytes and macrophages. *Am. J. Physiol.* 251:C128–C135.

MacIntosh, B.R., and B.M. Wright (1995). Caffeine ingestion and performance of a 1,500-meter swim. *Can. J. Appl. Physiol.* 20:168–177.

Marconi, C., G. Sassi, A. Carpinelli, and P. Cerretelli (1985). Effects of L-carnitine loading on the aerobic and anaerobic performance of endurance athletes. *Eur. J. Appl. Physiol.* 54:131–135.

Maughan, R.J. (1995). Creatine supplementation and exercise performance. *Int. J. Sports Nutr.* 5:94–101.

Mayer, G., J. Thum, and E.M. Cada (1988). Working capacity is increased following recombinant human erythropoietin treatment. *Kidney Int.* 34:525–526.

McNaughton, L. (1987). Two levels of caffeine ingestion on blood lactate and free fatty acid responses during incremental exercise. *Res. Q. Exerc. Sport* 58:255–259.

Metra, M., G. Canella, G. La Canna, T. Guiani, M. Sndrini, M. Gaggiotti, E. Movilli, and L. Dei Cas (1991). Improvement in exercise capacity after correction of anemia in patients with end-state renal failure. *Am. J. Cardiol.* 68:1060–1066.

Meyer, R.A., T.A. Brown, B.L. Kirlowicz, and M.J. Kushmerick (1986). Phosphagen and intracellular pH changes during contraction of creatine-depleted rat muscle. *Am. J. Physiol.* 250:C264–C274.

Natali, A., D. Santoro, L. Brandi, D. Faraggiana, D. Ciociara, and N. Pecori (1993). Effects of acute hypercarnitinemia during increased fatty substrate oxidation in man. *Met.* 42:594–600.

Odland, L.M., J.D. MacDougall, M.A. Tarnopolsky, A. Elorriaga, and A. Borgmann (1997). Effect of oral Cr supplementation on muscle [PCr] and short-term maximum power output. *Med. Sci. Sports Exerc.* 28: In press.

Otto, R.M., K.V.M. Shores, J.W. Wygand, and H.R. Perez (1987). The effect of L-carnitine supplementation on endurance exercise. *Med. Sci. Sports Exerc.* 19:S68. (Abstract).

Oyono-Enguelle, S., H. Freund, C. Ott, M. Gartner, A. Heitz, J. Marbach, A. Frey, H. Bigot, and A Bach (1988). Prolonged submaximal exercise and L-carnitine in humans. *Eur. J. Appl. Physiol.* 58:53–61.

Pasman, W.J., M.A. VanBaak, A.E. Jeukendrup, and A. DeHaan (1995). The effect of different dosages of caffeine on endurance performance time. *Int. J. Sports Med.* 16:225–230.

Putman, C.T., N.L. Jones, L.C. Lands, T.M. Bragg, M.G. Hollidge-Horvat, and G.J.F. Heigenhauser (1995). Skeletal muscle pyruvate dehydrogenase activity during maximal exercise in humans. *Am. J. Physiol.* 269:E458–E468.

Putman, C.T., L.L. Spriet, E. Hultman, M.I. Lindinger, L.C. Lands, R.S. McKelvie, G. Cederblad, N.L. Jones, and G.J.F. Heigenhauser (1993). Pyruvate dehydrogenase activity and acetyl group accumulation during exrcise after different diets. *Am. J. Physiol.* 265:E752–E760.

Rebouche, C.J. (1991). Metabolic fate of dietary carnitine in human adults. *J. Nutr.* 121:539–546.

Robertson, R.J. (1991). Introductory notes on the validation and applications of ergogenics. In: D.R. Lamb and M.H. Williams (eds.) *Perspectives in Exercise Science and Sports Medicine, Vol. 4: Ergogenics: Enhancement of Performance in Exercise and Sport.* Dubuque, IA: Brown & Benchmark, pp. xvii–xxii.

Rosenlof, K., C. Gronhaegen-Riska, and A. Sovijarva (1989). Beneficial effects of erythropoietin on haematological parameters, aerobic capacity, and body fluid composition in patients with hemodialysis. *J. Intern Med.* 226:311–317.

Sahlin, K. (1990). Muscle carnitine meabolism during incremental dynamic exercise in humans. *Acta Physiol. Scand.* 138:259–262.

Shores, K.V., R.M. Otto, J.W. Wygand, and H.R. Perez (1987). Effect of L-carnitine supplementation on maximal oxygen consumption and free fatty acid serum levels. *Med. Sci. Sports. Exerc.* 19:S68. (Abstract).

Siliprandi, N., F. Di LIsa, G. Pieralisi, P. Ripari, F. Maccari, R. Menabo, M.A. Giamberardino, and L. Vecchiet (1990). Metabolic changes induced by maximal exercise in human subjects following L-carnitine administration. *Biochim. Biophys. Acta* 1034:17–21.

Simi, B., M.H. Mayet, B. Sempore, and R.J. Favier (1990). Large variation in skeletal muscle carnitine level fail to modify energy metabolism in exercising rats. *Comp. Biochem. Physiol.* 97A:543–549.

Sipila, I., J. Rapola, O. Simell, and A. Vannas (1981). Supplementary creatine as a treatment for gyrate atrophy of the choroid and retina. *New Eng. J. Med.* 304:867–870.

Soop, M., O. Bjorkman, G. Cederblad, L. Hagenfeldt, and J. Wahren (1988). Influence of carnitine supplementation on muscle substrate and carnitine metabolism during exercise. *J. Appl. Physiol.* 64:2394–2399.

Spriet, L.L. (1995a). Anaerobic metabolism during high-intensity exercise. In: M. Hargreaves (ed.) *Exercise Metabolism.* Champaign, IL: Human Kinetics, pp. 1–40.

Spriet, L.L. (1991). Blood doping and oxygen transport. In: D.R. Lamb and M.H. Williams (eds.). *Perspectives in Exercise Science and Sports Medicine, Vol. 4: Ergogenics: Enhancement of Performance in Exercise and Sport.* Dubuque, IA: Brown & Benchmark, pp. 213–248.

Spriet, L.L. (1995b). Caffeine and Performance. *Int. J. Sports Nutr.* 5:S84–S99.

Spriet, L.L., D.A. MacLean, D.J. Dyck, E. Hultman, G. Cederblad, and T.E. Graham (1992). Caffeine ingestion and muscle metabolism during prolonged exercise in humans. *Am. J. Physiol.* 262:E891–E898.

Spriet, L.L., K. Soderlund, M. Bergstrom, and E. Hultman (1987a). Anaerobic energy release in skeletal muscle during electrical stimulation in men. *J. Appl. Physiol.* 62:610–615.

Spriet, L.L., K. Soderlund, M. Bergstrom, and E. Hultman (1987b). Skeletal muscle glycogenolysis, glycolysis, and pH during electrical stimulation in men. *J. Appl. Physiol.* 62:616–621.

Storring, P.L., and R.E. Gaines (1992). The international standard for recombinant DNA-derived erythropoietin: collaborative study of four recombinant DNS-derived erythropoietins and two highly purified human urinary erythropoietins. *J. Endocrinol.* 134:459–484.

Stroud, M.A., D. Holliman, D. Bell, A.L. Green, I.A. Macdonald, and P.L. Greenhaff (1994). Effect of oral creatine supplementation on respiratory gas exchange and blood lactate accumulation during steady-state incremental treadmill exercise and recovery in man. *Clin. Sci.* 87:707–710.

Stussi, C., P. Hofer, C. Meier, and U. Boutellier (1996). Exhaustive endurance exercise: L-carnitine effect on recovery. *Int. J. Sports Med.* 17:S47. (Abstract).

Trappe, S.W., D.L. Costill, B. Goodpaster, M.D. Vukovich, and W.J. Fink (1994). The effects of L-carnitine supplementation on performance during interval swimming. *Int. J. Sports Med.* 15:181–185.

Trice, I., and E.M. Haymes (1995). Effects of caffeine ingestion on exercise-induced changes during high-intensity, intermittent exercise. *Int. J. Sports. Nutr.* 5:37–44.

Vandenberghe, K., N. Gillis, M. Van Leemputte, P. Van Hecke, F. Vanstapel, and P. Hespel (1996). Caffeine counteracts the ergogenic action of muscle creatine loading. *J. Appl. Physiol.* 80:452–457.

VanSoeren, M.H., T. Mohr, M. Kjaer, and T.E. Graham (1996). Acute effects of caffeine ingestion at rest in humans with impaired epinephrine responses. *J. Appl. Physiol.* 80:999–1005.

VanSoeren, M.H., P. Sathasivam, L.L. Spriet, and T.E. Graham (1993a). Caffeine metabolism and epinephrine responses during exercise in users and non-users. *J. Appl. Physiol.* 75:805–812.

VanSoeren, M.H., P. Sathasivam, L.L. Spriet, and T.E. Graham (1993b). Short term withdrawal does not alter caffeine-induced metabolic changes during intensive exercise. *FASEB J.* 7:A518. (Abstract).

Vecchiet, L., F. Di Lise, G. Pieralisi, R. Ripari, R. Menabo, M.A. Giamberardino, and N. Siliprandi (1990). Influence of L-carnitine administration on maximal physical exercise. *Eur. J. Appl. Physiol.* 61:486–490.

Vukovich, M.D., D.L. Costill, and W.J. Fink (1994). Carnitine supplementation: effect on muscle carnitine and glycogen content during exercise. *Med. Sci. Sports Exerc.* 26:1122–1129.

Wagenmakers, A.J.M. (1991). L-carnitine supplementation and performance in man. In: F. Brouns (ed.) *Advances in Nutrition and Top Sport.* Basel:Karger, pp. 110–127.

Walker, J.B. (1979). Creatine biosynthesis, regulation and function. *Adv.Enzymol.* 50:117–142.

Wemple, R.D., D.R. Lamb, and K.H. McKeever (1997). Caffeine vs. caffeine-free sports drinks: effects on urine production at rest and during prolonged exercise. *Int. J. Sports Med.* 18:40–46.

Wide, L., and C. Bengtsson (1990). Molecular charge heterogeneity of serum erythropoietin. *Br. J. Haematol.* 76:121–127.

Wide, L., C. Bengtsson, B. Berglund, and B. Ekblom (1995). Detection in blood and urine of recombinant erythropoietin administered to healthy men. *Med. Sci. Sports. Exerc.* 27:1569–1576.

Wilcox, A.R. (1990). Caffeine and endurance performance. In: *Sports Science Exchange.* Barringtron, IL: Gatorade Sports Science Institute. 3:1–5.

Wiles, J.D., S.R. Bird, J. Hopkins, and M. Riley (1992). Effect of caffeinated coffee on running speed, respiratory factors, blood lactate and perceived exertion during 1,500-m treadmill running. *Br. J. Sports Med.* 26:166–120.

Williams, J.H., J.F. Signoille, W.S. Barnes, and T.W. Henrich (1988). Caffeine, maximal power output and fatigue. *Br. J. Sports Med.* 229:132–134.

Woodland, L. (1991). Lethal injection. *Bicycling* 32:80–81.

Wyss, V., G. Ganzit, and A. Rienzi (1990). Effects of L-carnitine administration on VO$_2$max and the aerobic-anaerobic threshold in normoxia and acute hypoxia. *Eur. J. Appl. Physiol.* 60:1–6.

DISCUSSION

CLARKSON: Lawrence, will you discuss the role, if any, of creatine supplementation on increasing body weight or possibly muscle mass? This seems to be primarily how creatine is being marketed. Also, is the variability in resting creatine levels in muscle largely due to diet?

SPRIET: Some people claim that protein synthesis would be stimulated by taking creatine supplements, and I suppose you could argue that if it does enhance insulin production, that might be the case, but the rapid increase in weight seems too fast to be attributed to protein synthesis. Others suggest that any weight gain is simply due to bringing more solute into skeletal muscle fibers, which is a big portion of the mass of the body, and that would necessarily retain more water inside the cell. Eric Hultman has told me that he has calculated how much extra water the additional intracellular creatine in skeletal muscle (i.e., 20–25 mmol/kg dry mass) should account for, and it is not enough to explain the 1–1.5 kg increases in mass that have been reported. However, he believes that if creatine stimulates some release of insulin, that may be enough to cause small increases in muscle glycogen, which seems to be associated with increased storage of water.

I don't think anyone knows if the variability among individuals in normal creatine storage at rest is due to diet. My guess is that it's highly unlikely because some studies have used fairly homogeneous populations, and the investigators still observe quite a bit variability in creatine storage. The mean in most studies is about 120-125 mmol/kg dry muscle, but it is not uncommon to find someone with 100 or 145.

MAUGHAN: There is an increasing number of anecdotal reports suggesting that some people using creatine supplements are gaining 5–10 kg of body weight. I don't think that we can disregard those reports; in the lab the total number of people who have been studied amounts to no more than a few hundred, but sales of creatine supplements last year in North America amounted to something like 300,000 kg. There are thousands of people taking creatine, and some of them are experiencing a large gain in body mass. Also, the fact that vegetarians who consume almost no dietary creatine typically have lower values for muscle creatine suggests a relationship between dietary intake and muscle storage of creatine.

SPRIET: I agree that we should not underestimate the validity of the anecdotal reports of large weight gains by some individuals. There are studies that have looked at large groups of vegetarians vs. meat eaters and found that in vegetarians other creatine pools in the body (e.g., the red blood cells, plasma, and urine) also have low creatine concentrations, which would suggest that vegetarians don't have optimal intakes of creatine. This should be a fairly simple question to answer with direct measurements of creatine in the muscles of athletes who are and are not meat eaters.

HORSWILL: Insulin is known to cause the kidney to reabsorb sodium. Perhaps creatine-induced increases in insulin and insulin's effect on sodium could produce retention of water. This might explain the quick gain in body weight that is frequently reported in conjunction with creatine loading.

SPRIET: That is an interesting hypothesis.

HORSWILL: Are there any data on whether creatine supplementation increases plasma volume or blood pressure?

SPRIET: I know of no studies that investigated the effect of creatine on either plasma volume or blood pressure.

HORSWILL: Regarding the mechanism by which creatine loading enhances performance, how important do you think creatine's ability to buffer hydrogen ions might be?

SPRIET: There are two sides to this coin and one could argue either or both sides. On the one side, it is logical to assume that the breakdown of a greater quantity of stored phosphocreatine could help buffer hydrogen ions during a single exercise bout and improve performance of that bout. On the other side, during the recovery period before a subsequent exercise bout, the reduced concentration of hydrogen ions remaining from the first bout could theoretically slow the process of resynthesizing phosphocreatine and impair performance of the subsequent exercise bout. We don't know which, if either, of these scenarios is correct.

KANTER: Does creatine loading affect ATP turnover rate?

SPRIET: Let's assume that performance has been improved in the second or third bout of intermittent exercise separated by recovery intervals of a few minutes each. It appears that the extra phosphocreatine at the beginning of the exercise bout will decrease the insult to the energy status of the cell. This conclusion is based on the lower accumulations of ADP and the attenuation of the decreases in ATP, the increases in ammonia, and the release of hypoxanthine. In other words, the mismatch between energy demand and energy production is diminished, resulting in a more favorable energy state at the end of exercise.

WILLIAMS: The overall impression I have from reading the literature on creatine and exercise performance is that it has a positive effect during repeated brief periods of high-intensity exercise when recovery between each sprint is of the order of 30 s or less. This suggests that creatine supplementation might be of most help to those who participate in the multiple-sprint sports such as soccer, hockey, tennis, and squash. What is your view?

SPRIET: One probably can expect an increase in the second bout of repeated Wingate tests with as much as 4 min of recovery. During sprints separated by only 30 s of rest, which is insufficient to completely resynthesize phosphocreatine, the effect of creatine loading may be maximal, but it appears that even after 4 min of rest there may be increases in total work that can be performed.

SCOTT: Short of a muscle biopsy and/or history of vegetarianism, are there other simple tests we can perform to help us advise our athletes about creatine supplementation?

SPRIET: I don't think we can predict from some sort of noninvasive test which athlete is most likely to benefit from creatine supplementation. Females may have a higher total creatine concentration at rest than males do, and it has been speculated that on average men would thus benefit more than women from creatine supplementation. My bias, of course, is that direct measurements of creatine concentrations in muscle are extremely important because they tell you conclusively whether or not the creatine level has changed.

KANTER: We have been asked by professional athletic trainers if we had an explanation for why players on the team using creatine were getting muscle soreness and cramps in spring training. I suggested that possible increases in muscle water may have accounted for this phenomenon.

SPRIET: We have no idea in those situations of how the creatine supplementation is being controlled. For example, similar symptoms are noted by athletes undergoing glycogen supercompensation regimens in which they seem to have very full muscles that feel very uncomfortable.

HORSWILL: A number of commercial products that contain carnitine with caffeine are marketed with claims that they will decrease body fat by stimulating the oxidation of fat. Are there any data to support these claims?

SPRIET: As far as I'm concerned, there is no systematic evidence to support such claims.

MAUGHAN: Some people take large doses of caffeine four to six times a day, and others are complete abstainers. Has there been any attempt in the studies of the effects of caffeine on exercise performance to distinguish between the habitual user and the non-user of caffeine?

SPRIET: In the first studies we did, where our hypothesis was that we would not see an ergogenic effect with fairly high levels of caffeine, we did not have the luxury of discriminating between users and non-users; we needed to recruit the best endurance athletes we could find. In our first two performance studies, the majority of the individuals were caffeine users. However, in the dose-response study in which we did not see a significant ergogenic effect with the 9 mg/kg, we had more non-users and light caffeine users. The two individuals who did worse at 9 mg than on placebo were non-caffeine users and complained about being disoriented and unable to focus. It is quite likely that this contributed to their poor performances. We need a large center with a tremendous number of people who are interested in these types of studies to study large groups of caffeine abstainers and users. In previous attempts we have made to study the effects of habitual use on the ergogenic effect of caffeine, we had to recruit a lower caliber of athletes. In fact, they were not really athletes, but simply people who liked to engage in regular exercise. I believe we need to do more studies with elite athletes.

MORGAN: I want to emphasize the issue of volunteerism. Eysenck has shown that extroverts, for example, require a greater dose of drugs to get the same sensory response compared with introverts. Extroverts are also far more likely to volunteer for drug experiments than are introverts. So it would be reasonable in studies of ergogenic aids to include measures of personality structure.

SPRIET: Your point is well taken. In his classic studies on caffeine, Costill made it very clear that the performance response is extremely variable. I think this variability probably decreases when subjects are elite athletes. Costill has indicated to me that his lab repeated the classic caffeine studies with less well-trained subjects and discovered that the variability in performance was so great that performance effects could not be detected. We ran into the same type of problem when we used infusion of Intra-Lipid®

and heparin and caused large increases in FFA availability for individuals exercising at 80–85 $\dot{V}O_2$max in a relatively poorly-trained population. Seven subjects seemed able to use that fat and spare muscle glycogen, whereas four others were not.

SCOTT: You commented that a high-carbohydrate diet does not negate the ergogenic effect of caffeine. Will you please expand on that statement?

SPRIET: I am aware of one study that shows that a high-carbohydrate diet negates some of the metabolic effects of caffeine. In the experiment by Pasman et al., and in an experiment published by Emily Haymes' lab, the subjects ate high-carbohydrate diets and experienced the expected ergogenic and metabolic effects of caffeine; there was no evidence to support this adverse effect of a high-carbohydrate diet on the effects of caffeine.

COYLE: Lawrence, isn't it likely that the generally positive effects of caffeine on performance may operate both at the level of the muscle and at the level of the central nervous system? For example, if the caffeine stimulated the central nervous system to recruit additional motor units so that more muscle fibers were sharing a given exercise load, each fiber would not need to contribute as much to the performance. That could reduce glycogenolysis by reducing the AMP levels in the individual fibers.

SPRIET: It is impossible to argue that there are no central effects because obviously it is clear that caffeine gets into the tissues of the central nervous system. We are excited about recent results showing that caffeine responders reduce glycogenolysis and non-responders do not. What we see with respect to caffeine-induced changes in the energy status of the cell, which we believe are important signals for controlling glycogenolysis, is very similar to what we see in short-term aerobic training. It seems that reductions in the accumulations of inorganic phosphate and AMP might be the common mechanism to signal carbohydrate metabolism that less energy is needed than is being produced in glycolysis. I maintain that fat is the default fuel; carbohydrate is the wildcard fuel that can be activated when necessary. Signals related to the energy status of the cell dictate how active the carbohydrate pathway will be. Possibly, one thing that caffeine ingestion, increased FFA delivery, and training-induced increases in triglyceride utilization have in common is that fat somehow manipulates the initial change in energy status at the onset of exercise at intense-aerobic power outputs.

6

Detection of Cardiovascular and Other Health Problems in Athletes

E. Randy Eichner, M.D.

INTRODUCTION
SUDDEN DEATHS OF ATHLETES: SCOPE AND IMPACT
EPIDEMIOLOGICAL INFORMATION ON SUDDEN DEATHS
    Benchmark Studies
    Blunt Chest Trauma
    Other Useful Studies
    Gender Difference?
    Other Lessons
ATHLETE'S HEART
SCREENING ATHLETES FOR CARDIOVASCULAR PROBLEMS
    "Needle-in-Haystack" Dilemma
    Practical Alternative
    Medical History: Questions to Ask
    Physical Exam: Where to Focus
    Heart Murmurs
    Echocardiography: Screening Role?
    Other Routine Laboratory Testing?
LEADING PROBLEMS: DEVELOPMENTS AND IMPLICATIONS
    Hypertrophic Cardiomyopathy
    Marfan Syndrome
    Mitral Valve Prolapse
    Hypertension
    Other Cardiac Problems
CONFLICTS FOR TEAM PHYSICIANS
PRACTICAL IMPLICATIONS
DIRECTIONS FOR FUTURE RESEARCH
SUMMARY
BIBLIOGRAPHY
DISCUSSION

INTRODUCTION

Detecting health problems in athletes is a broad topic. To limit the scope of this review to its most important element, this chapter focuses on health problems that can kill young athletes. In this regard, cardiovascular problems are covered in depth, and other relevant health problems are included. Health problems omitted from this chapter are: 1) covered in other chapters of this text (e.g., overtraining, ergogenic drugs, musculoskeletal and orthopedic problems), 2) covered widely elsewhere (e.g., eating disorders, heat stroke, asthma, anemia), or 3) covered by this author in other publications (e.g., collapse in sickle trait, contagious infections, splenic rupture, Eichner 1993, 1995, 1996).

SUDDEN DEATHS OF ATHLETES: SCOPE AND IMPACT

Exertional sudden death is rare; perhaps only one death per 250,000 per year among all children and young adults (Van Camp, 1993). Yet this year, as every year, the sudden deaths of athletes in action—in the gym, on the field, in the pool, on the rink—shock us once again. The sudden death of any athlete is a tragedy and an irony. Invariably, the public impact is stark and profound. We say to others, surely this can and must be prevented. And we think to ourselves, if the best among us—the fittest of all—collapse and die, what does this imply about the rest of us?

According to Maron (1993a), each time an elite athlete dies in action, provocative questions arise and keen debate ensues on: 1) the screening and disqualifying of athletes, 2) the management of cardiac disease in competitive athletes, and 3) the causes of such sudden deaths. Sudden exertional deaths in young athletes are caused by heart disorders and a few other conditions, some of which are silent until they kill. In one month in 1988, three basketball players died unexpectedly from hypertrophic cardiomyopathy (HCM). The oldest was Don Redden, age 24, who died at home two years after helping his team reach the NCAA Final Four (Cantwell et al., 1989). HCM is the most common cause of such deaths; Maron (1993b) notes that it accounts for half of his series of almost 100 cases of sudden death in young athletes.

In fact, HCM was suspected in the deaths of basketball stars Hank Gathers, who died in 1990 at age 23, and Reggie Lewis, who died in 1993 at age 27. After analysis, the death of Gathers was attributed to myocarditis (Maron, 1993b). That of Lewis, who saw 17 cardiologists in the three months between his first collapse and his fatal one, was ascribed to idiopathic cardiomyopathy (Van Camp, 1993).

Other heart problems also kill young athletes. In 1996 University of Massachusetts swimmer Greg Menton died during a meet at age 20 from anomalous coronary arteries (Noonan, 1996). Anomalous coronaries (no left coronary artery) contributed to the death at age 40 of basketball legend "Pistol Pete" Maravich (Van Camp & Choi, 1988). Volleyball star Flo Hyman died on the court at age 31 of a ruptured aorta from Marfan syndrome (Demak, 1986). Finally, in 1995, Olympic figure skating champion Sergei Grinkov, age 28, collapsed and died on the ice of atherosclerotic coronary heart disease (CHD).

To best prevent these tragedies, we must first review the best epidemiological studies on their settings and causes. As a prelude to this review, here are brief, "nonmedical" definitions. *HCM* is a primary disease of heart muscle that is usually familial, and in time leads to abnormal thickening of the heart's left ventricle ("muscle-bound heart"); *myocarditis* is an inflammation of the heart muscle, often from viral infection; *anomalous coronary arteries* refers to inborn (congenital) abnormalities in the anatomy of the arteries that wrap around the outside of the heart and supply blood to it; *aortic stenosis* is a narrowing of the main heart valve through which blood is pumped into the aorta; and *Marfan syndrome* is a congenital disorder of the connective tissue that leads to weakening, enlargement, and rupture of the aorta. These and other conditions are covered fully below.

EPIDEMIOLOGICAL INFORMATION ON SUDDEN DEATHS

Benchmark Studies

A recent, thorough study of nontraumatic sports deaths in high school and college athletes comes from the National Center for Catastrophic Sports Injury Research (Van Camp et al., 1995). Over a 10-year period ending in 1993, such deaths were reported in 126 high school athletes (115 males) and 34 college athletes (31 males). HCM was the most common cause of death, accounting for 51 (38%) of the 136 deaths studied in detail. Cardiac conditions comprised about 70% of the deaths; after HCM came anomalous coronaries (16 cases), myocarditis (7 cases), and aortic stenosis (6 cases). CHD caused only three deaths. Notable noncardiac causes of death included: 1) rupture of the aorta or of a cerebral vascular malformation, 2) heat stroke, 3)asthma, and 4) fulminant rhabdomyolysis with sickle cell trait. In 5% of deaths, no cause was found despite autopsy and toxicology tests; these deaths were attributed to primary cardiac arrhythmias.

Prior to the Van Camp study (1995), much of the best information on sudden death in athletes came from the National Heart, Lung, and Blood Institute (NHLBI). Before appraising this data, it must be noted that much of it is retrospective and that the NHLBI is a referral center with an abiding interest in HCM. Our knowledge of the natural history of heart disorders in young athletes—and the influence of sports play—is sparse; prospective studies are sorely needed (Maron et al., 1994).

A decade ago, Maron et al. (1986) summarized the NHLBI data and reviewed sudden death in competitive athletes. The gist of this article holds today and accords with that of Van Camp et al. (1995). Maron et al. (1986) reported that in young, competitive athletes (<35 years old), sudden death is usually from congenital or primary cardiovascular disease, often HCM. Most athletes who died had no prior cardiac symptoms. In only about 25% of cases was heart disease found or suspected before participation, and rarely was the correct clinical diagnosis made. In contrast, among older athletes (>35 years old), sudden death is usually due to CHD, and about half of the victims have had known CHD or warning symptoms thereof (Maron et al., 1986). It seems likely that some of these athletes (mainly men) ignore the warning signs.

Blunt Chest Trauma

In 1995, Maron et al. reported on another cause of sudden death in sports, blunt impact to the chest. Each of 25 young victims collapsed in cardiac arrest just after a blow to the chest, usually from a baseball or puck. Despite prompt attempts at resuscitation in many, all died. This tragedy, called cardiac concussion or commotio cordis, is due to ventricular fibrillation triggered by impact over the heart at an electrically vulnerable phase of ventricular excitability. It relates to safety, but not to *detection*, and so will not be considered further.

Other Useful Studies

To probe the causes of sports-related cardiac death, Burke et al. (1991) studied all sudden cardiac deaths in persons aged 14 to 40 during eight years in Maryland. Autopsy data from each person who died during or soon after sports play were compared with those from three persons (matched for age, sex, and race) who died when not exercising. Of 690 cardiac deaths, 34 (5%) were sports-related; all but three were men. Nine of these deaths were from CHD, eight from HCM, four from anomalous coronaries, and two from myocarditis; the rest were from miscellaneous or unclear causes. Compared to control deaths, sports-related deaths were more apt to be from HCM. The trend among the sports-related deaths was that younger black men died of HCM while playing basketball; older white men, of CHD while jogging.

Thomas and Cantwell (1990) have also reported on sudden death during basketball. Media coverage of the deaths of famous basketball players has fueled the notion that basketball confers the greatest risk of death for athletes with hidden heart disease. This notion, however, may not be true; we lack the "denominator" data to prove it. In fact, the reports of Maron et al. (1986) and Van Camp et al. (1995) suggest that deaths during football may be as common as during basketball. Others (Thomas & Cantwell, 1990) note that still unanswered are three vital questions: 1) What is the true incidence of sports-related deaths? 2) Does the incidence vary from sport to sport? and 3) Are athletes on highly competitive teams at greater risk of death than recreational athletes?

Gender Difference?

Another question is whether the incidence of sports-related death varies by gender. The answer may be: male athletes are more apt to die. This gender difference is particularly striking among deaths from HCM. In the report of Van Camp et al. (1995), 50 of the 51 HCM deaths were in males and, in general, after adjusting for gender trends in sports play, estimated death rates in males were fivefold higher than in females. Others agree that sudden exertional death from HCM occurs more often in young males (Liberthson, 1989). The same gender trend is seen in the long Q-T syndrome (Vincent et al., 1992).

Regarding HCM, the roots of this gender difference are elusive, but may involve biological, cultural, or behavioral differences that shape the progression of HCM, choice of sport, or intensity of training and competition. Left ventricular wall thickness in HCM tends to increase during adolescence, but no gender difference has been noted (Maron et al., 1986). Is it plausible that in the presence of HCM, "cardiac stress" during the growth spurt is greater in boys than girls? Or, if no gender difference exists in progression of HCM in adolescence, do young men compete more intensely at their peril? As young women compete and excel in more and more sports, such a behavioral explanation seems insufficient.

Another possibility is that testosterone (endogenous or exogenous) or strength training may accelerate the pathogenesis of HCM in young men. Others speculate that weight lifting by a football player sped the deterioration of a bicuspid aortic valve (Pipe et al., 1988). More research is needed on gender differences in death on the playing field.

Other Lessons

The other lessons in this area can be summarized as follows. The causes of exertional death in children are similar to those in adolescents or young adults; children may be somewhat more apt to die from congenital heart lesions, myocarditis, or primary arrhythmias (Liberthson, 1991; McCaffrey et al., 1991; Rowland, 1992). In Israel, key cardiac causes of sudden death in the young are HCM, myocarditis, and primary arrhythmias (Drory et al., 1991). Common in Italy's Veneto region is right ventricular cardiomyopathy, also known as isolated thinning of the right ventricle or fatty infiltration of the heart (Thiene et al., 1988). This cardiomyopathy, rare in the U.S. (Cantwell, 1995b), may account for 30% of sudden deaths in young competitive athletes in Veneto (Corrado et al., 1990). Why this disease is so common in that part of Italy is unclear. Genetic clustering has been proposed as an explanation, but most cases are sporadic, not familial; case selection and referral bias may be confounders here. Finally, it is worth reemphasizing that not all causes of sudden death in young athletes are cardiac; other conditions can also kill (Table 6-1).

ATHLETE'S HEART

To screen for cardiac problems in athletes, the physician must know the features—the normal adaptations—of "athlete's heart" because many of these features can mimic those of heart disease (Alpert et al., 1989; Mitchell, 1992). In brief physiological terms, regular exercise improves cardiac functional work capacity and reduces heart rate and blood pressure, two major determinants of myocardial oxygen demand. In simple terms, the heart adapts to repeated overload to become a better pump.

TABLE 6-1. *Causes of Sudden Death in Young Athletes.*

Cardiac Causes
More common
    Hypertrophic cardiomyopathy
    Anomalous coronary arteries
    Myocarditis
    Aortic stenosis
    Coronary heart disease
    Aortic rupture (Marfan syndrome)
Less common
    Primary arrhythmia (WPW; long-QT syndrome)
    Commotio cordis (blunt impact to chest)
    Right ventricular cardiomyopathy
    Mitral valve prolapse (rare cause)
    Other
Noncardiac Causes
    Heat stroke
    Fulminant rhabdomyolysis (sickle-cell trait)
    Cerebral hemorrhage (usually ruptured aneurysm)
    Status asthmaticus
    Cerebral or pulmonary embolism
    Hemorrhage (ruptured spleen or ectopic pregnancy; gastrointestinal bleeding)
    Toxic substance abuse
    Infection (meningococcal meningitis; pneumococcemia)

With pressure overload, as occurs in weight lifting, the heart increases in both septal and free-wall thickness to normalize myocardial-wall stress even at high afterload (Law of LaPlace). With volume overload, as occurs in jogging, the heart increases in left ventricular end-diastolic diameter, with a proportional rise in septal and free-wall thickness to normalize wall stress. This increase in left ventricular volume increases the stroke volume. Ejection fraction and myocardial contractility may not change, but the greater stroke volume, along with a thickened ventricular wall and a bradycardia in the trained exerciser, make the heart a more efficient pump.

Bradycardia in exercisers correlates with fitness and relates to increased vagal tone, decreased sympathetic tone, and an intrinsic cardiac adaptation. Also, vagally-mediated arrhythmias and physiologic changes in electrocardiographic (ECG) configuration can occur in dedicated athletes. Strenuous exercise may also enlarge the coronary arteries. Autopsy studies suggest that active men have large coronaries. A crosssectional study (using coronary arteriography) suggests that the coronaries of aerobic athletes are more "expandable" than normal. Eleven middle-aged endurance runners were compared with 11 physically inactive men. Under normal conditions, both groups had similar-sized coronaries. But after nitroglycerin, the runners' coronaries dilated two-fold more than did those of the inactive men (Haskell et al., 1993).

The degree of athlete's heart seems to vary greatly—by type, intensity, duration of training, age, gender, and genetic makeup. Some elite athletes have cardiac dimensions approaching those of HCM, that is, a left-ventricular-wall thickness by echocardiography of 16 mm (Pelliccia et al., 1991). Of course, the beneficial adaptations of athlete's heart (Table 6-2) begin to recede—some faster than others—if training is stopped.

In contrast, prepubertal athletes are less apt to manifest athlete's heart. When prepubertal male swimmers were compared to untrained boys, the swimmers had bradycardia and slight increases in echocardiographic chamber sizes and wall thicknesses, but no clear features on

TABLE 6-2. *Features of Athlete's Heart.*

Resting bradycardia
Enlarged left ventricle
Increased stroke volume
Systolic flow murmur
3rd or 4th heart sound
Increased ECG voltage
Altered ECG repolarization
Vagally-mediated arrhythmias
Enlarged coronary arteries

physical examination or ECG (Rowland et al., 1987). A similar study found no clear signs of athlete's heart in prepubertal distance-runners compared to untrained boys. The practical implication is that, in a child athlete, cardiomegaly or ECG abnormalities suggest not athlete's heart but underlying heart disease (Rowland et al., 1994).

SCREENING ATHLETES FOR CARDIOVASCULAR PROBLEMS

"Needle-in-Haystack" Dilemma

Epstein and Maron (1986) illustrated the practical implications of screening apparently healthy athletes. They assumed that the prevalence of congenital heart disease is 0.5%. They also assumed that, of these cases, about 1% are potentially lethal and actual mortality (sudden cardiac death during sports play) would be about 10% of that one percent. Even with foolproof screening tests, examiners would have to screen 200,000 athletes to find 1,000 with congenital heart disease, 10 with potentially lethal disease, and one who would die during sports play. Screening 200,000 to save one is a "needle-in-a-haystack" enterprise (Ades, 1992).

Screening strategies to prevent exertional cardiac events are limited by the rarity of such events, the poor predictive value of available tests, and the cost of elaborate testing (Thompson, 1993). An echocardiogram, the best test to identify HCM, generally costs $300 to $600. Seven million junior high and high school students take part in interscholastic sports in the U.S.; surely the time and money to do echocardiograms on all of them is prohibitive (Noonan, 1996).

Practical Alternative

The practical alternative is the traditional physical exam and medical history, the latter usually requested in a form to be filled out by the student's parents. Many such forms, however, tend to be deficient. One expert, studying preparticipation forms from the 39 states that require them, says that many forms fail to inquire about a family history of sudden death or of Marfan syndrome, and even fail to ask whether the student has had a heart murmur or a history of fainting (Noonan, 1996). A standardized national form would help. Some experts also call for a paradigm shift, in which informed coaches first teach young athletes about HCM so the athletes will know why the medical screening is important for their health and life, and will more earnestly participate in the medical history.

Medical History: Questions to Ask

General. The medical history should include questions about any family history of heart disease or sudden, premature death, as well as about the athlete's usual level of activity and response to routine exertions, including possible chest pain, syncope, extreme dyspnea, fatigue, or palpitations. Different authors have proposed different forms, asking from 11 to 30 questions (Braden & Strong, 1988; Fields & Delaney, 1990; Pendergrast, 1991). The detailed forms ask about medications, immunizations, allergies (including bee stings), single organs, exercise-induced asthma, relevant chronic illnesses (diabetes mellitus, epilepsy), and history of bone or joint injuries, heat stroke, or concussion. For cardiac screening (Ades, 1992), seven questions are of key importance (Table 6-3).

Chest pain. Chest pain in children and adolescents is usually benign and noncardiac in origin (unlike in adults). In practical terms, the most common cause of chest pain in children is musculoskeletal injury. The causes of chest pain in youngsters are often related to physical activity, including chest wall trauma, exercise-induced asthma, and hyperventilation (Bernhardt & Landry, 1994), or are psychogenic (Stiene, 1992). Adolescents are more likely than children to have psychogenic chest pain. Hergenroeder (1994) offers a practical approach to addressing chest pain in adolescents and a list of common causes. He does not list infections and angina—uncommon causes that must not be dismissed. In children, some experts say the most common cause of chest pain is "idiopathic," a diagnosis of exclusion (Selbst et al., 1988). When followed over the years, such children fare well (Rowland, 1986a; Selbst et al., 1990). Concern should arise, however, if chest pain (or discomfort) is substernal (with or without radiation), tied to exertion, or relieved by rest. This suggests angina, as from HCM (Simons & Moriarity, 1992) or anomalous coronaries. Chest pain may also reflect aortic dissection, as in Marfan syndrome or cocaine use (Cheitlin, 1993).

TABLE 6-3. *Seven Key Questions for Cardiac Screening.*

1. Has it been more than two years since a doctor took your blood pressure and listened to your heart?
2. Did your parents or a doctor ever tell you that you have a heart murmur?
3. Have you had chest pains or fainting in the past two years?
4. Has anyone in your family died suddenly under age 35?
5. Has a doctor diagnosed anyone in your family with a thickened heart or Marfan syndrome?
6. Do you use, or have you ever used, cocaine or anabolic steroids?
7. Has a doctor ever disqualified you from competition?

Syncope. Perhaps the single most vital question to ask in a medical history form is, "Have you ever fainted during exercise?" A "yes" answer suggests underlying heart disease. In a study of sudden death in 44 young Israeli soldiers (mainly of cardiac causes), syncope before death occurred in 23% (Kramer et al., 1988). Yet even syncope is not diagnostic of heart disease. Ades (1992) reports exertional syncope in young skiers and runners (with healthy hearts) who push the limits. Hyperventilation can cause syncope, and some athletes (notably those not performing up to par) suffer "finish-line swoons" that mimic syncope.

Physical Exam: Where to Focus

General. Some view the presports examination as a valuable chance for full health screening. They argue that examinees are "adolescents before they are athletes," and so the examiner must be alert to delayed puberty in the gymnast or runner as well as to signs of drug abuse, eating disorders, depression, sexually transmitted disease, or pregnancy (Brown, 1993). This view has merit, but most examiners key on the main aim, clearing the athlete for sports (Rowland, 1986b).

It is also important for the examiner to realize that athletes rank failure to make the team in some instances worse than failure to pass in school, separation of parents, or death of a close friend (Nelson, 1992). Fortunately, less than one (Magnes et al., 1992) to two percent (Nelson, 1992) of athletes are disqualified from a sport during a preparticipation examination.

Where and how to do the exam is debatable. An office-based physician may know the student better, be aware of psychosocial issues, be best able to examine the heart in a quiet setting, and be ready to provide useful follow-up. Multistation examinations, however, may detect more musculoskeletal problems in athletes and in general are more expedient, sports-directed, and inexpensive (Pendergrast, 1991; Rowland, 1986b). If a multistation format is used, the "heart station" must be partitioned off, and quiet.

Components of the exam. Examiners should record height, weight, and vital signs, noting arrhythmias and hypertension. Noteworthy also are single organs (eye, testis, kidney), skin disease, defective vision, or enlarged liver or spleen (thus vulnerable to trauma and perhaps a clue to underlying disease). The examiner must be alert for features that suggest Marfan syndrome (see below) and, most important, must focus on the cardiovascular examination, including auscultation for murmurs.

Heart Murmurs

Auscultation should be conducted in silence with the athlete initially supine. If a murmur (especially systolic) is heard, it should be evaluated with the athlete in postures other than supine. Soᴉ argue for a set sequence of postures for the examinee for all carᴇ aminations: lying, sitting, standing, squatting, and doing a Valsalva. single maneuver is fail-safe, but the cause of a systolic murmur can ofte be pinpointed by noting the responses to several maneuvers (Lembo et al., 1988).

Hearing a murmur, the physician should ask: 1) Is it normal (functional) or organic (pathologic)? and 2) If it is organic, what is the defect, and how critical is it hemodynamically? "Loud" does not always mean critical. A trifling lesion (e.g., a small ventricular septal defect) may cause a loud murmur, whereas an ominous lesion (e.g., HCM) may cause a soft murmur.

Normal Murmurs. Normal murmurs—caused by turbulent flow through the heart and great arteries—are common. It is said that "all children have a heart murmur at some time, and almost all murmurs are normal" (Pflieger & Strong, 1992). Aside from the continuous murmur of a cervical venous hum, most normal murmurs are systolic ejection murmurs that: 1) begin after the first heart sound, 2) end before the second heart sound, 3) have a crescendo-decrescendo pattern, and 4) are grade 1 or 2 (out of 6 grades) in intensity. When the athlete sits or stands, the fall in ventricular filling and stroke volume makes most normal murmurs decrease or disappear.

Abnormal Murmurs. Organic systolic murmurs are often loud with telltale features, such as the ejection click and carotid thrill of aortic stenosis (Cantwell, 1996) or the holosystolic murmur (with axillary radiation) of mitral regurgitation. The murmur of HCM is discussed below. Any diastolic murmur is almost certainly organic. Two such murmurs are the "sighing" decrescendo blow of aortic regurgitation (Pipe et al., 1988; O'Connor et al., 1995) and the mid-diastolic rumble of mitral stenosis.

Confirmatory Tests. Chest x-ray and ECG are often obtained when a suspicious murmur is heard, on the premise that normal results decrease the odds of a cardiac disorder (Braden & Strong, 1988). Considering what is at stake, however, and the limits of these tests, it seems wise to refer such athletes to a pediatric cardiologist (McCaffrey et al., 1991; Pflieger & Strong, 1992). Debated is the diagnostic role of screening echocardiography. Most experts seem to agree that echocardiography and/or other imaging studies have no cost-effective screening role.

Echocardiography: Screening Role?

Echocardiography is useful to confirm suspected HCM or aortic stenosis, or to gauge aortic root diameter in known or suspected Marfan syndrome. The question is whether screening echocardiography should

lely. Five recent studies address echocardiography.
) screened 501 college athletes. Ninety had an abnor-
screening (history, physical examination, 12-lead ECG)
d an echocardiogram. The latter revealed mild mitral
(VP) in 15% and mild increased septal thickness in 3%.
disqualified from sports. It was concluded that routine
echocardiographic screening is of unproved efficacy
ning a practical, cost-efficient approach to the mass
screening of young athletes is formidable.

Lewis et al. (1989) used echocardiography to screen 265 black college athletes. Eleven percent had mild MVP. Also, 11% had increased septal thickness (13 mm or more); three had maximal septal thickness of 16-18 mm, raising the question of HCM. They were classified, however, as having "athlete's heart" because none had other problems and one had a decline in septal thickness after deconditioning. It was concluded that primary screening with echocardiography is not costeffective. It should be noted here that experts consider a decline in septal thickness after deconditioning to be a sign of athlete's heart, not HCM. Six Olympic rowers who deconditioned for a mean of 13 weeks had a decline in mean maximal septal thickness from 13.8 mm to 10.5 mm (Maron et al., 1992).

Feinstein et al. (1993) used limited echocardiography to screen 1,570 junior and senior high school athletes, found none with HCM, and concluded that routine echocardiographic screening is not practical, cost-efficient, or effective. The last two (of the five) studies reach more optimistic conclusions on a potential screening role for echocardiography. Weidenbener et al. (1995) used limited echocardiography to screen 2,997 high school athletes. No disqualifying lesions were found, but detected were 40 cases (1.3%) of MVP and 10 cases (0.3%) of bicuspid aortic valve. It was concluded that echocardiography can be practical, relatively inexpensive, and helpful.

Finally, Murry et al. (1995) used limited echocardiography to screen 125 college athletes and found that 10% (11 with MVP; two with bicuspid aortic valve) had disorders that merited endocarditis prophylaxis and medical follow-up. They concluded that limited echocardiography may be useful in preparticipation screening. Although more research is needed regarding the diagnostic value of echocardiography in screening large groups of athletes, it seems unlikely that screening echocardiography will soon be used widely or will ever be cost-effective.

Other Routine Laboratory Testing?

Because CHD very rarely causes exertional death in high school or college athletes (Thompson et al., 1994), routine cholesterol screening is not indicated. For early warning in general, however, a family history of premature CHD calls for a lipid profile (Ades, 1992). Scientific consensus finds no rationale for routine preparticipatory urinalysis, blood chemistries, or complete blood count (Fields & Delaney, 1990; Magnes et al., 1992; Rowland, 1986; Taylor & Lombardo, 1990). Finally, more research and debate is needed on the issues of routine screening of female athletes for ferritin status (Harris, 1995) and of young black athletes for sickle cell trait (Eichner, 1993).

LEADING PROBLEMS: DEVELOPMENTS AND IMPLICATIONS

Hypertrophic Cardiomyopathy

General. HCM, the leading killer of young athletes, is a heart-muscle disease ("muscle-bound heart") that is usually familial (autosomal dominant) but may be sporadic in up to 45% of cases. Its prevalence is about one in 500 in young people. The morphologic marker is a thickened left ventricular wall but normal cavity size (hypertrophy without dilatation). Histologic hallmarks are: 1) myofiber disarray, 2) small intramural coronary arteries, and 3) myocardial scarring (Maron, 1987a, 1987b, 1993a).

Symptoms. Symptoms may include exertional dyspnea, fatigue, chest pain, dizziness, and syncope. Too often, however, there is no warning; many athletes who die suddenly of HCM are previously asymptomatic. Also, symptoms correlate poorly with morphologic features. Some patients with mild hypertrophy may have severe symptoms; others, with severe hypertrophy, mild symptoms. Retrospective analysis of deaths suggests a direct relation between the extent of hypertrophy and risk of death (Spirito et al., 1990), but sudden death in HCM has occurred despite normal left ventricular mass, presumably due to myofiber disarray and ventricular fibrillation (Maron et al., 1990; McKenna et al., 1990).

Athletics Despite HCM. Some individuals with HCM have survived years of competitive athletics. Recently reported were 14 persons (13 men, mean age 43) who trained for competition (mostly in swimming, track, marathon, or triathlon) for up to 22 years. Each began training unaware of underlying HCM; none had symptoms during their competitive years. In most, the diagnosis of HCM followed a routine exam, during which a murmur, abnormal ECG, or positive family history was noted. Most had only mild HCM. Even after diagnosis—and after advice to withdraw from competitive sports—one-third of them continued to train and compete (Maron & Klues, 1994). Others argue that the natural history of HCM in the general outpatient population is more benign than suggested by published reports, because most of the literature on HCM comes from only two referral centers that tend to treat patients with moderately severe HCM (Spirito et al., 1989).

Problems in Defining HCM. A practical problem is firmly defining HCM by echocardiogram. Maron (1986) defined the limits of athlete's heart by echocardiogram on more than 1,000 athletes. Pellicia et al. (1991), studied nearly 1,000 elite athletes, set the "upper limit" of left ventricular wall thickness at 16 mm, and concluded that athletes with a wall thickness over 16 mm and a nondilated left ventricle are apt to have HCM. Other studies (Lewis et al., 1989) found that a few healthy black male athletes, for example, have a wall thickness of 16-18 mm. Uncertainties as to the criteria for defining HCM and questions about the natural history of mild HCM make it vexing for team physicians to disqualify an athlete with apparently mild HCM (Simons & Moriarity, 1992).

ECG abnormalities in HCM range from normal to bizarre. The most common include left ventricular hypertrophy, repolarization variations, arrhythmias, and deep Q waves that mimic myocardial infarction (Cantwell, 1995a). No particular ECG abnormality is diagnostic of HCM, and the ECG pattern correlates poorly with prognosis (Maron, 1993b). Also, ECG changes of athlete's heart can be confounders. Experts agree that, despite its limits, the best diagnostic test for HCM is the echocardiogram.

Molecular Discoveries. Recent advances in molecular biology help us begin to understand HCM, but do not yet help physicians in their screening decisions. In half of families (of European descent) with familial HCM, the disease is caused by mutations in the cardiac beta-myosin heavy chain, on chromosome 14 (Curfman, 1992; Watkins et al., 1992). Seven mutations have been found; all are missense mutations (i.e., caused by the substitution of a single amino acid). Patients with different mutations have different prognoses for survival (Watkins et al., 1992).

The myosin heavy chains comprise three functional domains. One confers adenosine triphosphatase activity, allowing ATP to be hydrolyzed to provide energy for muscle contraction. The other two are binding sites for actin and for myosin light chains. Fortunately, the mutations of HCM do not lie in the nucleotide sequences encoding any of these domains because such alterations would likely be lethal. It is thought that mutant heavy chains "poison" or somehow disrupt the structural integrity of sarcomeres or the functional interactions among myofibrils (Curfman, 1992). More research is needed on exactly how mutant chains produce cardiac hypertrophy and impair contractility.

HCM is genetically heterogenous; defects in at least two different genes can cause the disease (Solomon et al., 1990). This complicates genetic testing. Determining a patient's genotype is technically demanding, but once achieved it enables rapid genetic diagnosis of all family members (whether affected or unaffected) and helps predict their risk of premature death (Watkins et al., 1992). Variation in features of HCM within families is as great as variation between families. This suggests that the range of clinical expression of HCM is not explained solely by genes but also by developmental, physiologic, or hormonal factors (Solomon et al., 1990).

Help for Team Physicians. The team physician has scarce science upon which to predict the risk of sudden death for a given athlete with HCM. Signal-averaged ECG, ambulatory ECG monitoring, and thallium stress scans have been proposed to help stratify risk, but we need more research on the utility and cost of such measures (Cantwell, 1995a). For now, the 26th Bethesda Conference of the American College of Sports Medicine and the American College of Cardiology (Maron et al., 1994) advises that athletes with the unequivocal diagnosis of HCM should avoid all competitive sports except possibly those of lowest intensity, or Class IA (Table 6-4).

Marfan Syndrome

General. Flo Hyman, a talented American volleyball player, died suddenly of a ruptured aorta during a 1986 game in Japan. From 1982 to 1984, she had passed three physical exams with the U.S. Olympic program. Her case is a tragic illustration of the fact that the first person to diagnose Marfan syndrome is usually the coroner (Demak, 1986).

Marfan syndrome is a congenital disorder of connective tissue that can lead to aortic rupture from cystic medial necrosis. Perhaps one person in 10,000 has Marfan syndrome; it is transmitted as an autosomal

TABLE 6-4. *Classifying Sports by Static and Dynamic Demands.* Examples of Common Sports from the 26th Bethesda Conference.

	Dynamic Demand		
	Low	*Moderate*	*High*
Static Demand			
I. Low			
	Billiards	Softball	Skiing (X-country)
	Bowling	Doubles tennis	Distance running
	Golf	Volleyball	Singles tennis
II. Moderate			
	Archery	Figure skating	Basketball
	Diving	Football	Ice hockey
	Auto racing	Surfing	Swimming
III. High			
	Gymnastics	Body building	Boxing
	Water skiing	Downhill skiing	Cycling
	Weight lifting	Wrestling	Rowing

dominant, but in 35% of cases no family history is known (Bracker et al., 1988). It is commonly seen in tall, lanky people, which explains why it has been blamed for deaths not only in volleyball but also in basketball.

Features. In Marfan syndrome, the lower half of the body is unusually long. Arm span may exceed height. Other features in the skeletal, ocular, and cardiovascular systems are listed in Table 6-5.

Diagnosis and Management. Clinical suspicion calls for an echocardiogram to check for aortic root dilatation and to gauge the mitral valve prolapse seen in almost all Marfan patients. To forestall aortic root dilatation, patients are told to avoid static exercise and endurance training. Also proscribed are sports that can involve blows to the chest. The 26th Bethesda Conference advises that Marfan athletes with no family history of early death and without aortic root dilatation or mitral regurgitation can play sports with low-to-moderate static demands coupled with low dynamic demands (i.e., sports such as billiards, bowling, golf, archery, diving, and auto racing) (Table 6-4). Echocardiograms should be recorded every six months (Graham et al., 1994).

Mitral Valve Prolapse

General. MVP is one of the most common heart conditions in athletes. It is also one of the most controversial. Debated is how best to diagnose it and how consequential it is clinically (Devereux, 1989). In most young people, MVP seems to be harmless (Washington & Allen, 1990).

Diagnosis. The prevalence of MVP is about 4% in the general population (Marks et al., 1989). Historically, MVP was first recognized by its characteristic click and murmur. Increasingly, MVP is diagnosed by

---

TABLE 6-5. *Telltale Features of Marfan Syndrome.*

Skeletal
> Tall stature (>95th percentile)
> Long limbs (arm span > height)
> Arachnodactyly (spidery-like fingers and toes)
> Joints hyperextensible
> Narrow, high-arched palate
> Pectus excavatum or carinatum
> Scoliosis; loss of thoracic kyphosis

Ocular
> Myopia
> Flat cornea
> Subluxation of lens

Cardiovascular
> Dilatation, ascending aorta
> Aortic regurgitation
> Aortic dissection
> Mitral valve prolapse
> Mitral regurgitation

---

echocardiogram, which can also provide prognostic information on the status of the mitral valve (Devereux, 1989).

Pathogenesis. Primary MVP seems to be an autosomal dominant disorder of collagen synthesis, content, or organization, leading to myxomatous degeneration of valve leaflets and chordae and to weakening of the outer fibroelastic valve tissue. In secondary MVP, the valve has no myxomatous degeneration; it either reflects inflammatory changes or is normal. In very thin athletes, such as ballet dancers or distance runners (and in anorexia nervosa), MVP on echocardiography seems "functional," a mismatch in size between the mitral valve and left ventricle. This mismatch tends to lessen with weight gain (Cantwell & Thomas, 1988).

Clinical Features. The hallmark of MVP is a midsystolic click followed by a mid-to-late apical systolic murmur, best heard when the athlete is standing. Experts disagree on whether just a click (no murmur) means MVP or just "billowing" of leaflets. In a healthy athlete, endocarditis prophylaxis is not given for just a click (Cantwell & Thomas, 1988).

Some adolescents with MVP may have chest pain, palpitations, and/or dizziness—the "MVP syndrome." Unlike angina, the chest pain in these asthenic youngsters is not exertional, is usually sharp and stabbing, and often occurs near the cardiac apex. The exact cause of this pain is unknown, but ischemia does not seem to be a likely cause (McFaul, 1987; Washington & Allen, 1990).

Complications. Complications of MVP are rare but include arrhythmias, embolic stroke, and mitral regurgitation. Chordal rupture with pulmonary edema has occurred in a 26-year-old man during sprinting. This should be considered if an athlete with MVP suddenly has undue dyspnea (Zimmerman & Mogtader, 1987).

Additional Testing. When MVP is diagnosed by physical exam, experts recommend echocardiographic and Doppler assessment of the mitral valve. Here it must be noted that Doppler testing is very sensitive (Douglas, 1989) and may detect trivial regurgitation from all four cardiac valves. Research suggests that thickening and redundancy of the mitral valve leaflets on echocardiography predicts a higher risk of complications, notably infective endocarditis and major mitral regurgitation (Marks et al., 1989). For tall athletes with MVP, the aorta should be scanned to exclude the dilatation seen in Marfan syndrome. Holter monitoring and exercise testing may rarely be recommended for young athletes with MVP who want to take part in high-intensity sports (McFaul, 1987).

Management Tips. Some athletes with MVP have orthostatic hypotension and giddiness during upright exercise. Such persons seem to have poor venous tone (and/or perhaps low blood volume) that exaggerates the normal fall in ventricular filling when upright (Cantwell & Thomas, 1988; Maron et al., 1994). They may tolerate exercise in a sitting position, such as rowing.

The prognosis with MVP is generally benign; the approach to sports, generally permissive (Cantwell & Thomas, 1988; McFaul, 1987; Washington & Allen, 1990). It is crucial to convey the benign nature of MVP to parents and affected youngsters, so as not to create a "cardiac neurosis."

Disqualifiers. Sudden cardiac death is rare in MVP. Only about 12 patients with documented MVP have died during exercise; five were competitive athletes (Maron et al., 1994). The 26th Bethesda Conference bars competitive sports for athletes with MVP (recommends Class IA sports) only if they also have related problems (Table 6-6).

Hypertension

Hypertension is the most common cardiovascular condition in athletes (Kaplan et al., 1994) and the leading reason for failing a preparticipation examination (Magnes et al., 1992), but is not a cause of sudden death in young athletes. It is worth noting that regular exercise can help normalize a mildly elevated blood pressure (Kaplan et al., 1994). Athletes with persistent hypertension are candidates for limited blood testing (creatinine, electrolytes, hemoglobin, cholesterol, and glucose), urinalysis, and ECG. If results are abnormal or if features suggest secondary hypertension, referral for further study is indicated (Kaplan et al., 1994).

Echocardiography and exercise testing are not routinely done because they provide no useful information about eligibility for competition. When an exercise test is done for other reasons, a marked rise in systolic blood pressure (>240 mm Hg) may presage basal hypertension and call for attention (Kaplan et al., 1994).

Moderate hypertension with no target organ damage does not limit eligibility. The 26th Bethesda Conference (Kaplan et al., 1994) bars athletes with severe hypertension and/or target organ damage (eyes, kidneys) from high static sports (Table 6-5).

TABLE 6-6. *Mitral Valve Prolapse: Disqualifiers for Sports.*

Arrhythmogenic syncope
Family history of sudden death
Complex ventricular arrhythmias
Repetitive supraventricular tachyarrhythmias
Mitral regurgitation of moderate-to-marked severity
Prior embolic event

Other Cardiac Problems

Anomalous Coronaries. From case reports and retrospective studies it is known that younger people (<30 years old) with an isolated congenital coronary artery anomaly are at risk of dying suddenly during excitement or during exercise such as running, basketball, soccer, or ice hockey (Liberthson, 1989; Taylor et al., 1992). One such anomaly is a single left coronary artery, with the right coronary artery originating near the left coronary ostium and passing between the aorta and pulmonary artery, where it is "pinched" between these two great arteries (Liberthson, 1989). Because most such athletes are asymptomatic before collapsing, however, and because there are no abnormal physical findings, at present most coronary anomalies probably are not screenable (Rowland, 1992). Fortunately, they are rare.

Arrhythmias. Ventricular preexcitation and long-QT syndrome are cardiac conditions that predispose to arrhythmias.

Ventricular preexcitation. Sudden death in athletes with ventricular preexcitation (Wolff-Parkinson-White syndrome; WPW) is rare (Furlanello et al., 1992; Munger et al., 1993; Widerrmann et al., 1987). Such instances seem to occur mainly in subgroups with short refractory periods in accessory pathways (Zipes & Garson, 1994) or with concurrent cardiac disease, such as HCM (Van Camp, 1995). A protective factor is that over time in some WPW patients, the accessory pathways stop conducting (Klein et al., 1989).

The incidence of WPW ranges from 0.1 to 3 per 1,000 ECGs, but not all WPW patients get tachyarrhythmias (Cantwell & Watson, 1992). All considered, the approach to athletes with WPW tends to be permissive (Cantwell & Watson, 1992). The 26th Bethesda Conference advises that WPW athletes over 20 years of age and without structural heart disease, palpitations, or tachycardia can play all sports. Younger WPW athletes and any WPW athlete with tachyarrhythmias should be referred for in-depth testing before being cleared for sports. The preferred treatment for troublesome WPW is radiofrequency catheter ablation of the accessory pathway (Zipes & Garson, 1994).

Long-QT syndrome. The long-QT syndrome is usually familial (10-15% of cases are sporadic), with affected persons having prolongation of the QT interval, sinus bradycardia, and a propensity to recurrent syncope, ventricular arrhythmias of the torsades-de-pointes type, and sudden death (at the rate of about 0.5% of patients per year), including during exercise or from sudden emotion (Moss, 1992).

In different families, the long-QT syndrome is linked to mutations (on chromosomes 11, 7, 3) of genes encoding different cardiac ion channels (sodium, potassium); a concept similar to that for HCM (different genes, different sarcomeric proteins), suggesting that genetically heterogeneous disorders stem from defects in physiologically similar genes (Towbin, 1995). The discovery of genetic markers (Vincent et al., 1992) has enabled sure diagnosis within families and has shown the vagaries of diagnosing by QT interval (overlap, carriers vs. noncarriers) but has no practical implications for screening athletes. The 26th Bethesda Conference bars athletes with long-QT syndrome from all competitive sports (Zipes & Garson, 1994). Finally, to address the problem of sudden cardiac death in athletes, the team physician may want to have available automated external defibrillators. Such devices can improve cardiac-arrest survival rates (Simons & Berry, 1993).

CONFLICTS FOR TEAM PHYSICIANS

Team physicians face and debate vexing ethical, legal, and practical issues in caring for competitive athletes (Levine & Stray-Gundersen, 1994; Maron et al., 1994). For example, it has been alleged that "eager to hold on to their valuable sideline practices, team doctors all too often strive to help the club, not heal the player" (Nocera, 1995). This charge seems unfair. Surely most—if not all—team physicians have the athletes' best interests at heart. Granted, experts debate *who* should disqualify an athlete, but this debate is needed. For example, the National Collegiate Athletic Association (NCAA) indicates that the team physician is the final authority in matters of medical disqualification (Maron et al., 1994). Others argue that the physician should examine, diagnose, and educate the patient about the risks of his or her medical condition— and recommend one of several possible courses of treatment—but that the decision (to compete or not) should be the patient's responsibility. They argue that such athletes should be allowed to play as long as the responsible institution is satisfied that the athlete is making a reasonable, informed decision (Levine & Stray-Gundersen, 1994). It is thought that the courts will likely uphold any physician who follows professionally determined standards and recommends exclusion from a sport based on reasonable medical judgments.

In the end, surely all can agree with the following heartfelt proposition by an ethicist (Maron et al., 1994): "Doctors are not advocates for the team, the sport, the city, or any other special interest group. There is only one role model that the treating doctor should have and that is to be the benevolent advocate for the health and welfare of the patient."

PRACTICAL IMPLICATIONS

In essence, this entire chapter *is* practical in nature. The challenge is how best to use what we have learned in the past decade to prevent sudden exercise death in young athletes. Each section of the chapter includes implicit or explicit practical tips on how to detect hidden heart problems or other relevant clinical conditions in athletes, and on what to do once they are found.

DIRECTIONS FOR FUTURE RESEARCH

We need more—and better—epidemiological research on the likely settings, causes, and victims of sudden exercise deaths among athletes young and old. We need to improve mass screening of young athletes for hidden heart disease (and consider informed screening for sickle cell trait). A standardized medical history form would help, as would more applied research and education on the best modes of physical examination of athletes. We need more research on a possible screening role for echocardiography and/or other rapid, noninvasive, diagnostic tests. And, if possible, we need to translate molecular advances into practical screening tests.

A recent scientific statement on cardiovascular screening by the American Heart Association offers a timely overview (Maron et al., 1996). It calls for practical research to develop a national standard for preparticipation medical evaluations. It argues that it is *not* prudent to recommend the routine, widespread use of any "noninvasive" test (e.g., 12-lead ECG, echocardiography, or graded exercise test). It concludes that the best available and most practical approach to screening populations of athletes, regardless of age, is a complete and careful personal and family history and physical examination.

SUMMARY

Sudden exercise deaths are rare in young athletes but have a public impact that transcends the numbers and invariably raises questions about the role and value of sports medicine. Most sudden deaths in athletes are caused by heart disease, especially hypertrophic cardiomyopathy; men may be more vulnerable than women in this regard. Other notable causes include anomalous coronaries, myocarditis, aortic rupture (Marfan syndrome), coronary heart disease, and primary arrhythmias.

Screening for hidden heart disease is a "needle-in-a-haystack" enterprise. To screen athletes for cardiac problems, physicians must understand the physiological adaptations of athlete's heart. The value of echocardiography as a screening tool for widespread use is being researched and debated; the practical alternative remains the medical history and physical exam. The history keys on family deaths, chest pain, and syncope; the exam should concentrate on the detection of murmurs.

Echocardiography can confirm hypertrophic cardiomyopathy. At this point in time, the new molecular insights regarding hypertrophic cardiomyopathy (and the long-QT syndrome) have aided understanding of the maladies more than providing useful information for screening athletes.

Marfan syndrome is signaled by habitus; echocardiography should be used to gauge the distention of the aortic root. Mitral valve prolapse is generally benign. Hypertension does not cause death in young athletes, anomalous coronaries may not be screenable, and ominous arrhythmias are rare.

BIBLIOGRAPHY

Ades, P.A. (1992). Preventing sudden death: cardiovascular screening of young athletes. *Phys. Sportsmed.* 20:75–89.

Alpert, J.S., L.A. Page, A. Ward, and J.M. Rippe. (1989). Athletic heart syndrome. *Phys. Sportsmed.* 17:103–107.

Bernhardt, D.T., and G.L. Landry. (1994). Chest pain in active young people: is it cardiac? *Phys. Sportsmed.* 22:70–85.

Bracker, M.D., K.L. Jones, and B.S. Moore. (1988). Suspected Marfan syndrome in a female basketball player. *Phys. Sportsmed.* 16:69–77.

Braden, D.S., and W.B. Strong. (1988). Preparticipation screening for sudden cardiac death in high school and college athletes. *Phys. Sportsmed.* 16:128–140.

Brown, R.T. (1993). Targeting teen health problems: maximizing the preparticipation exam. *Phys. Sportsmed.* 21:77–80.

Burke, A.P., A. Farm, R. Virmani, J. Goodwin, and J.E. Smialek. (1991). Sports-related and non-sports-related sudden cardiac death in young adults. *Am. Heart J.* 121:568–575.

Cantwell, J.D. (1996). Can this college athlete compete? *Phys. Sportsmed.* 24:57–58.

Cantwell, J.D. (1995a). Dyspnea, light-headedness, and palpitations in a young weight lifter. *Phys. Sportsmed.* 23:65–66.

Cantwell, J.D. (1995b). Hypotension in a 10K runner. *Phys. Sportsmed.* 23:43–44.

Cantwell, J.D., and J.G. Spellman. (1989). The athlete's heart. *Your Patient & Fitness* 3:10–15.

Cantwell, J.D., and R.J. Thomas. (1988). Mitral valve prolapse in athletes. *Your Patient & Fitness* 2:18–20.

Cantwell, J.D., and A. Watson. (1992). Does your Wolff-Parkinson-White patient need to slow down? *Phys. Sportsmed.* 20:115–129.

Cantwell, J.D., K.E. Wilson, and R.J. Thomas. (1989). Hypertrophic cardiomyopathy. *Your Patient & Fitness* 3:12–22.

Cheitlin, M.D. (1993). Evaluating athletes who have heart symptoms. *Phys. Sportsmed.* 21:150–162.

Corrado, D., G. Thiene, A. Nava, L. Rossi, and N. Pennelli. (1990). Sudden death in young competitive athletes: clinicopathological correlation in 22 cases. *Am. J. Med.* 89:588–596.

Curfman, G.D. (1992). Molecular insights into hypertrophic cardiomyopathy. *N. Engl. J. Med.* 326:1149–151.

Demak, R. (1986). Marfan syndrome: a silent killer. *Sports Illustrated* 64(7):30–35.

Devereux, R.B. (1989). Diagnosis and prognosis of mitral valve prolapse. *N. Engl. J. Med.* 320:1077–1079.

Douglas, P.S. (1989). Cardiac considerations in the triathlete. *Med. Sci. Sports Exerc.* 21:S214–S218.

Drory, Y., Y. Turetz, Y. Hiss, B. Lev, E.Z. Fisman, A. Pines, and M.R. Kramer (1991). Sudden unexpected death in persons <40 years of age. *Am. J. Cardiol.* 68:1388–1392.

Eichner, E.R. (1993). Sickle cell trait, heroic exercise, and fatal collapse. *Phys. Sportsmed.* 21:51–64.

Eichner, E.R. (1995). Contagious infections in competitive sports. *Gatorade Sports Science Exchange* 8(3):1–4.

Eichner, E.R. (1996). Infectious mononucleosis. Recognizing the condition, reactivating the patient. *Phys. Sportsmed.* 24:49–54.

Epstein, S.E., and B.J. Maron (1986). Sudden death and the competitive athlete: perspectives on preparticipation screening. *J. Am. Coll. Cardiol.* 7:220–230.

Feinstein, R.A., E. Colvin, and M.K. Oh (1993). Echocardiographic screening as part of a preparticipation examination. *Clin. J. Sport Med.* 3:149–152.

Fields, K.B., and M. Delaney (1990). Focusing the preparticipation sports examination. *J. Fam. Pract.* 30:304–312.

Furlanello, F., A. Bertoldi, R. Bettini, M. Dallago, and G. Vergara (1992). Life-threatening tachyarrhythmias in athletes. *Pacing Clin. Electrophysiol.* 15:1403–1411.

Graham, T.P., J.T. Bricker, F.W. James, and W.B. Strong (1994). Congenital heart disease. *Med. Sci. Sports Exerc.* 26:S246–S253.

Harris, S.S. (1995). Helping active women avoid anemia *Phys. Sportsmed.* 23:35–48.

Haskell, W.L., C. Sims, J. Myll, W.M. Bortz, F.G. St. Goar, and E.L. Alderman (1993). Coronary artery size and dilating capacity in ultradistance runners. *Circulation* 87:1076–1082.

Hergenroeder, A.C. (1994). Diagnosing chest pain in adolescents and young adults. *Your Patient & Fitness* 8:6–11.

Kaplan, N.M., R.B. Deveraux, and H.S. Miller Jr. (1994). Systemic hypertension. *Med. Sci. Sports Exerc.* 26:S268–S270.

Klein, G.J., R. Yee, and A.D. Sharma (1989). Longitudinal electrophysiologic assessment of asymptomatic patients with the Wolff-Parkinson-White electrocardiographic pattern. *N. Engl. J. Med.* 320:1229–1233.

Koh, K.K., M.S. Rim, J. Yoon, and S.S. Kim (1994). Torsade de pointes induced by terfenadine in a patient with long QT syndrome. *J. Electrocardiol.* 27:343–346.

Kramer, M.R., Y. Drori, and B. Lev (1988). Sudden death in young soldiers. High incidence of syncope prior to death. *Chest* 93: 345–348.

Lembo, N.J., L.J. Dell'Italia, M.H. Crawford, and R.A. O'Rourke (1988). Bedside diagnosis of systolic murmurs. *N. Engl. J. Med.* 318:1572–1578.

Levine, B.D, and J. Stray-Gundersen (1994). The medical care of competitive athletes: the role of the physician and individual assumption of risk. *Med. Sci. Sports Exerc.* 26:1190–1192.

Lewis, J.F., B.J. Maron, J.A. Diggs, J.E. Spencer, P.P. Mehrota, and C.L. Curry (1989). Preparticipation echocardiographic screening for cardiovascular disease in a large, predominantly black population of college athletes. *Am. J. Cardiol.* 64:1029–1033.

Liberthson, R.R (1989). Sudden exercise death in a 17–year-old girl. *N. Engl. J. Med.* 320:1473–1483.

Magnes, S.A., J.M. Henderson, and S.C. Hunter (1992). What conditions limit sports participation? Experience with 10,540 athletes. *Phys. Sportsmed.* 20:143–160.

Marks, A.R., C.Y. Choong, M.B.B. Chir, A.J. Sanfilippo, M. Ferre, and A.E. Weyman (1989). Identification of high-risk and low-risk subgroups of patients with mitral-valve prolapse. *N. Engl. J. Med.* 1989; 320:1031–1036.

Maron, B.J (1993a). Hypertrophic cardiomyopathy in athletes. Catching a killer. *Phys. Sportsmed.* 21:83–91.

Maron, B.J. (1993b). Sudden death in young athletes. Lessons from the Hank Gathers Affair. *N. Engl. J. Med.* 329:55–57.

Maron, B.J. (1986). Structural features of the athlete heart as defined by echocardiography. *J. Am. Coll. Cardiol.* 7:190–203.

Maron, B.J., and H.G. Klues (1994). Surviving competitive athletics with hypertrophic cardiomyopathy. *Am. J. Cardiol.* 73: 1098–1104.

Maron, B.J., S.A. Bodison, Y.E. Wesley, E. Tucker, and K.J. Green (1987a). Results of screening a large group of intercollegiate competitive athletes for cardiovascular disease. *J. Am. Coll. Cardiol.* 6:1214–1221.

Maron, B.J., R.O. Bonow, R.O. Cannon III, M.B. Leon, and S.E. Epstein (1987b). Hypertrophic cardiomyopathy, parts I and II. *N. Engl. J. Med.* 316:780–789 and 844–852.

Maron, B.J., R.W. Brown, C.A. McGrew, M.J. Mitten, A.L. Caplan, and A.M. Hutter Jr. (1994). Ethical, legal, and practical considerations impacting medical decision-making in competitive athletes. *Med. Sci. Sports Exerc.* 26:S230–S237.

Maron, B.J., S.E. Epstein, and W.C. Roberts (1986). Causes of sudden death in competitive athletes. *J. Am. Coll. Cardiol.* 7:204–214.

Maron, B.J., J.M. Isner, and W.J. McKenna (1994). Hypertrophic cardiomyopathy, myocarditis, and other myopericardial diseases and mitral valve prolapse. *Med. Sci. Sports Exerc.* 26:S261–S267.

Maron, B.J., A.H. Kragel, and W.C. Roberts (1990). Sudden death in hypertrophic cardiomyopathy with normal left ventricular mass. *Br. Heart J.* 63:308–310.

Maron, B.J., A. Pelliccia, A. Spataro, and M. Granata (1993). Reduction in left ventricular wall thickness after deconditioning in highly trained Olympic athletes. *Br. Heart J.* 69:125–128.

Maron, B.J., L.C. Poliac, J.A. Kaplan, and F.O. Mueller (1995). Blunt impact to the chest leading to sudden death from cardiac arrest during sports activities. *N. Engl. J. Med.* 333:347–342.

Maron, B.J., P. Spirito, Y. Wesley, and J. Arce (1986). Development and progression of left ventricular hypertrophy in children with hypertrophic cardiomyopathy. *N. Engl. J. Med.* 315:610–614.

Maron, B.J., P.D. Thompson, J.C. Puffer, C.A. McGrew, W.B. Strong, P.S. Douglas, L.T. Clark, M.J. Mitten, M.H. Crawford, D.L. Atkins, D.J. Driscoll, and A.E. Epstein (1996). Cardiovascular preparticipation screening of competitive athletes. *Med. Sci. Sports Exerc.* 28:1445–1452.

McCaffrey, F.M., D.S. Braden, and W.B. Strong (1991). Sudden cardiac death in young athletes. *Am. J. Dis. Child.* 145:177–183.

CARDIOVASCULAR AND OTHER HEALTH PROBLEMS **261**

McFaul, R.C. (1987). Mitral valve prolapse in young patients. *Phys. Sportsmed.* 15:194–198.
McKenna, W.J., J.T. Stewart, P. Nihoyannopoulos, F. McGinty, and M.J. Davies (1990). Hypertrophic cardiomyopathy without hypertrophy: two families with myocardial disarray in the absence of increased myocardial mass. *Br. Heart J.* 63:287–290.
Mitchell, J.H. (1992). How to recognize athlete's heart. *Phys. Sportsmed.* 20:87–94.
Mitchell, J.H., W.L. Haskell, and P.B. Raven (1994). Classification of sports. *Med. Sci. Sports Exerc.* 26:S242–S245.
Moss, A.J. (1992). Molecular genetics and ventricular arrhythmias. *N. Engl. J. Med.* 327:885–887.
Munger, T.M., D.L. Packer, S.C. Hammill, B.J. Feldman, K.R. Bailey, D.J. Ballard, D.R. Holmes Jr., and B.J. Gersh (1993). A population study of the natural history of Wolff-Parkinson-White syndrome in Olmsted County, Minnesota, 1953–1989. *Circulation* 87:866–873.
Murry, P.M., J.D. Cantwell, D.L. Heath, and J. Shoop (1995). The role of limited echocardiography in screening athletes. *Am. J. Cardiol.* 76:849–850.
Nelson, M.A. (1992). Medical exclusion from participation in sports. *Pediatric Annals* 21:149–155.
Nocera, J. (1995). Bitter medicine. *Sports Illustrated* 83(20):74–88.
Noonan, D. (1996). The heart of the matter. *Sports Illustrated* 84(10):6878.
O'Connor, F.G., W.S. Levy, R.G. Oriscello, and R.P. Wilder (1995). Asymptomatic aortic insufficiency in a runner. *Phys. Sportsmed.* 23:33–42.
Pelliccia, A., B.J. Maron, A. Spataro, M.A. Proschan, and P. Spirito (1991). *N. Engl. J. Med.* 324:295–301.
Pendergrast, R.A. (1991). Use the pre-sports exam to help kids enjoy a healthy season. *Your Patient & Fitness* 3:4–10.
Pflieger, K.L., and W.B. Strong (1992). Screening for heart murmurs. What's normal and what's not. *Phys. Sportsmed.* 20:71–81.
Pipe, A.L., K. Chan, and J.M. Rippe (1988). Asymptomatic heart murmur in a professional football player. *Phys. Sportsmed.* 16: 53–60.
Rosenzweig, A., H. Watkins, D.S. Hwang, M. Miri, W. McKenna, T.A. Traill, J.G. Seidman, and C.E. Seidman (1991). Preclinical diagnosis of familial hypertrophic cardiomyopathy by genetic analysis of blood lymphocytes. *N. Engl. J. Med.* 325:1753–1760.
Rowland, T.W. (1986). Preparticipation sports examination of the child and adolescent athlete: changing views of an old ritual. *Pediatrician* 13:3–9.
Rowland, T.W. (1992). Sudden unexpected death in sports. *Pediatric Annals* 21:189–195.
Rowland, T.W., and M.M. Richards (1986). The natural history of idiopathic chest pain in children. A follow-up study. *Clin. Peds.* 25:612–614.
Rowland, R.W., B.C. Delaney, and S.F. Siconolfi (1987). Athlete's heart in prepubertal children. *Pediatrics* 79:800–804.
Rowland, T.W., V.B. Unnithan, N.G. MacFarlane, N.G. Gibson, and J.Y. Paton (1994). Clinical manifestations of the athlete's heart in prepubertal male runners. *Int. J. Sports Med.* 15:515–519.
Simons, S.M., and J. Berry (1993). Preventing sudden death. The role of automated defibrillators. *Phys. Sportsmed.* 21:53–59.
Simons, S.M., and J. Moriarity (1992). Hypertrophic cardiomyopathy in a collage athlete. *Med. Sci. Sports Exerc.* 24:1321–1324.
Solomon S.D., J.A. Harcho, W. McKenna, A. Geisterfer-Lowrance, R. Germain, R. Salerni, J.G. Seidman, and C.E. Seidman (1990). Familial hypertrophic cardiomyopathy is a genetically heterogenous disease. *J. Clin. Invest.* 86:993–999.
Spirito, P., F. Chiarella, L. Carratino, M.Z. Berisso, P. Pellotti, and C. Vecchio (1989). Clinical course and prognosis of hypertrophic cardiomyopathy in an outpatient population. *N. Engl. J. Med.* 320:749–755.
Spirito, P., and B.J. Maron (1990). Relation between extent of left ventricular hypertrophy and occurrence of sudden cardiac death in hypertrophic cardiomyopathy. *J. Am. Coll. Cardiol.* 15:1521–1526.
Stiene, H.A. (1992). Chest pain and shortness of breath in a collegiate basketball player: case report and literature review. *Med. Sci. Sports Exerc.* 24:504–509.
Taylor, W.C. III, and J.A. Lombardo (1990). Preparticipation screening of college athletes: value of the complete blood cell count. *Phys. Sportsmed.* 18:106–118.
Taylor, A.J., K.M. Rogan, and R. Virmani (1992). Sudden cardiac death associated with isolated congenital coronary artery anomalies. *J. Am. Coll. Cardiol.* 20:640–647.
Thiene, G., A. Nava, D. Corrago, L. Rossi, and N. Pennelli (1988). Right ventricular cardiomyopathy and sudden death in young people. *N. Engl. J. Med.* 318:129–133.
Thomas, R.J., and J.D. Cantwell (1990). Sudden death during basketball games. *Phys. Sportsmed.* 18:75–78.
Thompson, P.D. (1993). Athletes, athletics, and sudden cardiac death. *Med. Sci. Sports Exerc.* 25:981–984.
Thompson, P.D., F.J. Klocke, B.D. Levine, and S.P. Van Camp (1994). Coronary artery disease. *Med. Sci. Sports Exerc.* 26:S271–S275.
Towbin, J.A. (1995). New revelations about the long-QT syndrome. *N. Engl. J. Med.* 333:384–385.
Van Camp, S.P., and J.H. Choi (1988). Exercise and sudden death. *Phys. Sportsmed.* 16:49:52.

Van Camp, S.P., C.M. Bloor, F.O. Mueller, R.C. Cantu, and H.G. Olson (1995). Nontraumatic sports death in high school and college athletes. *Med. Sci. Sports Exerc.* 27:641–647.

Vincent, G.M., K.W. Timothy, M. Leppert, and M. Keating (1992). The spectrum of symptoms and QT intervals in carriers of the gene for the long-QT syndrome. *N. Engl. J. Med.* 327:846–852.

Washington, R.L., and S. Allen (1990). How to manage mitral valve prolapse in children. *Your Patient & Fitness* 2:4–8.

Watkins, H., A. Rosenzweig, D.S. Hwang, T. Levi, W. McKenna, C.E. Seidman, and J.G. Seidman (1992). Characteristics and prognostic implications of myosin missense mutations in familial hypertrophic cardiomyopathy. *N. Engl. J. Med.* 326:1108–1114.

Weidenbener, E.J., M.D. Krauss, B.F. Waller, and C.P. Taliercio (1995). Incorporation of screening echocardiography in the preparticipation exam. *Clin. J. Sport Med.* 5:86–89.

Wiedermann, C.J., A.E. Becker, T. Hopferwieser, V. Muhlberger, and E. Knapp (1987). Sudden death in a young competitive athlete with Wolff-Parkinson-White syndrome. *Eur. Heart J.* 8:651–655.

Zimmerman, F.H., and A.H. Mogtader (1987). Ruptured chordae tendineas and acute pulmonary edema induced by exercise. Occurrence in a young man with mitral valve prolapse. *JAMA* 258:812–813.

Zipes, D.P., and A. Garson, Jr. (1994). Arrhythmias. *Med. Sci. Sports Exerc.* S276–S283.

DISCUSSION

HOUGH: Prepubescent athletes do not generally show the athletic heart syndrome, so evidence of cardiomegaly or abnormal EKG findings in that age group apparently indicates that the patients probably have significant heart disease.

Given the low yield of the EKG, echocardiography, and chest x-rays in evaluating the nature of heart murmurs, how often should these tests be used when a significant murmur is detected? Do they really help guide the diagnosis of the problem and help in the treatment of the young athlete? If there is good outcome-based information that these tests are valid and useful, that information should be used to convince managed health care organizations that the tests need to be done, but to screen seven million young athletes would be tremendously costly, especially if the yield is low.

EICHNER: I think EKG and chest x-ray screening probably have some diagnostic value, but my bias is to refer the athlete to the cardiologist to interpret the results of those tests. As far as I know, there is no wide-scale cost analysis study of echocardiography.

HOUGH: The legal issue is most disconcerting for those of us who provide care at the intercollegiate or interscholastic level, and it makes me wonder what is the best moral and ethical way to screen for problems potentially leading to sudden death.

ROWLAND: The answer to the question of how much testing should be done by a primary care physician depends on the degree of confidence that person has regarding his or her own expertise at cardiac diagnosis. Generally this is not high. There has been a "party line" developed on how to approach screening for cardiac risk, and it is expected that tests such as these should be performed by the cardiologist. As Randy has indicated, the patient's history and physical examination are accepted as the most appropriate screening tools. The use of echocardiography in this setting is not practical. We establish norms for echocardiographic findings as those within the 95th percentile. That means that in any screening situation, by definition 5% are going to be abnormal in a given measurement. Five percent of seven million athletes is far too many to deal with logistically and economically.

I think that it is probably fair to say that all athletes who suffer cardiac-related deaths have underlying heart disease. In most series of such tragedies about 5% are unexplained, but I suspect the absence of explanation is due to inadequate autopsy. If it is true that these people all have underlying disease, theoretically, the abnormalities should be screenable and hence preventable. It seems to be the perception of the public that this is the case and that physicians should be able to prevent all these sports-related deaths. Of course, this is not true. Even though we try our best, we must accept the fact that we don't have the responsibility or even the capability of truly screening all these tragedies and preventing them.

SCOTT: The coaches should institute a teaching session with the team physician teaching the athletes the warning signs of hypertrophic cardiomyopathy, orthostatic hypotension, arrhythmias, and giddiness. If you were to ask high-schoolers what it means if one's cholesterol is too high, they will tell you, but if you ask them what it means if one gets a little dizzy in a game, they might say, "Well, you're a sissy." I think an educational program for the athletes, teaching them how to help the physician get a better history, is very important.

EICHNER: Educating athletes about warning signs is a good idea.

SCOTT: Why are some people able to survive while exercising regularly with hypertrophic cardiomyopathy? What differentiates them? It may be that they have a more benign condition. It has been shown that the cardiac diameter is sports specific and that cyclists can attain greater wall thicknesses than most other sport participants.

EICHNER: As to the survivors with hypertrophic cardiomyopathy, I assume that they had milder lesions or didn't compete as hard early in life. You are right that cyclists are among those with the thickest ventricles in general, although in the Pellicca study of 947 Italian elite athletes, 15 of the 16 thickest septums were in rowers.

GISOLFI: Did the cyclists and rowers who had thick ventricular septums also have high blood pressures?

EICHNER: I don't think so.

GISOLFI: The reason I ask is that about 20 years ago we studied some nationally ranked cyclists and found an unusually high percentage of them with high blood pressure. In fact, several were on drug treatment to lower blood pressure. I wondered if there was an isometric component to cycling that influenced blood pressure. Has anyone in this group observed a correlation between cycling and high blood pressure?

SCOTT: Twenty years ago amphetamine and caffeine abuse could have been involved. Also, with the many aerodynamic positions that cyclists assume, there is an isometric pressure response due to arm and hand-grip position on the handle bars.

SCOTT: There may be a possibility of a computer-read "abbreviated echo" to make the screening of athletes a little better. I know this has been developed for the EKG and for the tilt-table test for determining orthostatic sensitivities. This could be a very simple type of test that may be able to screen out orthostatic changes.

NIEMAN: Randy, will you please elaborate more on myocarditis? I wasn't aware that Hank Gathers had been diagnosed as dying from myocarditis. There are some cardiologists who feel that myocarditis can be triggered by heavy exertion during the course of a systemic illness. Animal data are supportive of this view point.

EICHNER: The final diagnosis on Gathers may vary with who is doing the reporting. Maron's recent report in the *New England Journal of Medicine*, called it myocarditis. Exactly what kind of myocarditis is debated. There is some animal research with new-born mice showing that certain viruses proliferate a thousand-fold greater in the myocardia of mice made to swim versus those allowed to rest, which increases the mortality rate to 50% vs. 5%. So I agree there are some data suggesting that exercise in the face of certain viral infections can increase viral replication in the heart and cause myocarditis and sudden death. This may also apply in humans, but supporting evidence is anecdotal.

ROWLAND: It's always hard to figure out these diagnoses because they are being made in the midst of legal actions. I think there are athletes who die of acute viral myocarditis, but it certainly is a non-screenable condition.

NIEMAN: What about the general recommendation of avoiding heavy exertion during the course of an illness?

EICHNER: I like to use the "neck check." If your symptoms are only "above the neck," at the most a scratchy throat or runny eyes, sneezing, stuffy nose, headache, but no fever, you can begin your workout at a "conversational" pace. Try it for 10 min and if you feel a little better, do your regular workout. If, on the other hand, you feel like you are running through sand or your head pounds with every step, why risk it? Go home and rest. But if you have a fever, or your symptoms are "below the neck" or "body-wide", such as muscle aches, nausea, vomiting, or diarrhea, you have nothing to gain by the workout and should stay home.

KENNEY: My question refers back to Marfan syndrome. I had a recent discussion with a team physician about a 20-year-old college basketball player who has all the classic signs of Marfan syndrome, but the diagnosis is not conclusive. I asked about his aortic root diameter and her answer was, "Well, it is large, but this is a 7–foot guy." Is the aortic-root-diameter criterion for clearly defining Marfan syndrome any more clear or objective than the ventricular septum controversy?

ROWLAND: There are no normative data on large individuals, but I think a good echocardiographer and a cardiologist who is used to seeing patients with Marfan syndrome can detect aortic anomalies by the configuration of the aortic root and its relationship to the size of the other structures such as the left atrium.

SCOTT: Many tall high-school and college-age athletes continue to grow until age 20 or 21. If a physician is suspicious, serial echocardiograms should be recorded every six months in an attempt to detect any change. Obviously, a change over time is a bad sign.

KANTER: Randy, how is it possible that Pete Maravich, who had anomalous coronary arteries, could compete at the level he did all those years without symptoms? What compensatory mechanisms might have occurred that may have helped him to perform at the level that he did?

EICHNER: Perhaps during his playing years a single huge vessel eventually became atherosclerotic and narrowed; sometimes athletes can compete for years with a single coronary.

ROWLAND: This is an outstanding case; here was not just an athlete, not even just a great athlete, but one of the best athletes that has ever lived. Yet he could compete at that level with apparently no symptoms and then suddenly die of markedly abnormal coronary arteries. The autopsy report indicated that his left anterior descending coronary was 2 mm in diameter, so it was congenitally narrowed as well.

KUIPERS: One of the conditions that is a possible cause of sudden death is anaphylactic shock. In Europe in athletic circles it is very popular to give all kinds of injections, such as a "cell-cure," to enhance performance. Some athletes who came to us because they were performing very poorly indicated that the condition started after a "cell-cure." The first injection was given by a doctor, the second and third injections were administered by the athlete. After the second injection there was some local swelling, and after the third injection, the athlete became very sick. I congratulated him because I think he suffered from an anaphylactic shock that could have led to his death. I don't know of any official records of athletes who died from anaphylactic shock. However, based on my personal experience with athletes, I have some suspicion that some of the athletes who died in the resting state may have succumbed to anaphylactic shock.

EICHNER: I have heard rumors about athletes injecting foreign proteins. The concept of exercise-induced urticaria and resultant shock has been overblown as a cause of death in athletes. There has been only one fatal case reported, and that young man also had severe asthma. But if athletes are injecting foreign proteins, they are taking unwise risks.

KUIPERS: I have another comment that may have practical validity. It is well known that most of the attempts at cardiopulmonary resuscitation (CPR) are not successful. When athletes suffer from cardiac arrest during exercise, usually body temperature has increased; perhaps this accounts for a decreased success rate of CPR.

7

The Athlete's Immune System, Intense Exercise, and Overtraining

MARK DAVIS, PH.D. AND LISA HERTLER COLBERT, M.S.

INTRODUCTION
OVERVIEW OF THE IMMUNE SYSTEM
    Innate and Adaptive Immunity
    Neutrophils
    Monocytes/Macrophages
    Natural Killer Cells
    T and B Lymphocytes
    Cytokines
INTENSE EXERCISE AND IMMUNE FUNCTION
    Introduction
    Innate Immunity and Exercise
        Natural Killer Cell Function
        Neutrophil Function
        Monocyte/Macrophage Function
        Cytokines
    Adaptive Immunity
        Lymphocyte Function
EXERCISE TRAINING, COMPETITION, AND INFECTION
    Relationship Between Exercise and Infection
    Epidemiological Studies
    Animal Studies
    Related Study of Psychological Stress
    Summary
OVERTRAINING, IMMUNE FUNCTION, AND INFECTION
    Types of Overtraining Studies
    Induced Overtraining
    Following Athletes Through a Competitive Season
    Focus on Glutamine
    Summary
POTENTIAL MECHANISMS OF OVERTRAINING
    General Theories
    Specific Immunomodulators
    Integrated Psychoneuroimmune Hypothesis
PRACTICAL IMPLICATIONS
SUMMARY
BIBLIOGRAPHY
DISCUSSION

INTRODUCTION

Strenuous physical training is essential for achieving maximal athletic potential, but there is a fine line between optimal training and excessive training. Extensive anecdotal evidence indicates that excessive training can be counterproductive and unhealthy, resulting in reduced exercise capacity and various pathological conditions (Fry et al., 1991; Kuipers & Keizer, 1988). A precise, widely accepted descriptor of this condition has not yet been identified, but terms including *overtraining, excessive training, overreaching, overexertion, staleness, burnout,* and *chronic fatigue* have been used. The symptoms that accompany overtraining include impaired performance, exaggerated fatigue throughout the day, sore muscles, nausea, loss of appetite, mood swings, difficulty in concentration, and increased susceptibility to injuries and infection (Table 7-1). The recurrent infections during periods of maximal training strongly suggest that immune dysfunction plays an important role in the etiology of this syndrome.

Intense training is necessary to provide a stimulus to which the body can eventually adapt (i.e., the overload principle of training). Fatigue and temporarily reduced performance are expected under these circumstances; however, these negative symptoms should subside, and performance should improve within several days of reduced training. Overtraining occurs when the stress of training results in an obvious reduction in performance capacity and the persistence of negative symptoms even after an appropriate period of reduced training (Fry et al., 1991).

The apparent increase in the occurrence and/or severity of infections in athletes in association with intense training and competition is beginning to receive a great deal of attention from both the scientific community and the public. Although research in this area is increasing rapidly, the field is still in its infancy (Figure 7-1). For example, within

TABLE 7-1. *Symptoms reported during acute overtraining.* Adapted from Table 1 in Fry *et al.*(1992).

Category	Symptoms
Central fatigue	Feel lethargic; no interest in everyday tasks; exhausted during the day; ordinary tasks seem difficult
Emotionality	A bit quick-tempered; emotionally unstable; personality change
Concentration difficulties	Difficulty focusing; failure to remember things; unable to narrow concentration
Physical complaints	Sore muscles; dehydrated; stomach complaints and/or nausea; diarrhea
Appetite changes	Loss of appetite

the last 5 y, 343 publications appeared in the scientific literature, compared to only 127 and 53 in the previous two five-year periods (Rainwater et al.,1995). Until recently there was insufficient scientific evidence to establish whether or not overtraining was a valid syndrome and, perhaps more important, what the underlying biological mechanism(s) may be. While it is becoming increasingly clear that various components of the immune system are altered by intense physical training, it is far from certain the extent to which these alterations are related to the various symptoms of overtraining. To date, only about 12 studies have attempted to address the effects of overtraining on the athlete's immune system, and the results from those studies are difficult to interpret. There are fundamental problems with research on overtraining, including a lack of objective diagnostic criteria, widely varying symptoms among individuals said to be overtrained, and the distinct possibility

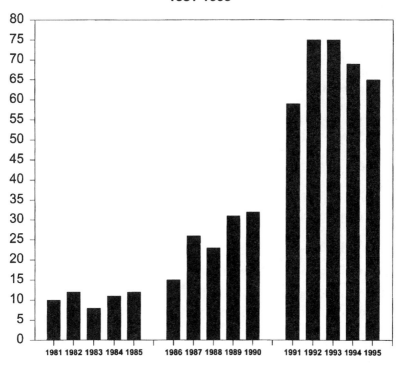

Exercise Immunology Publications
1981-1995

FIGURE 7-1. *Large increase in the number of publications in exercise immunology in the last 15 years.* Data from Rainwater et al., 1995.

that this syndrome is not a single entity but represents a continuum of related symptoms with many different etiologies.

The primary objective of this chapter is to integrate the rather extensive literature concerning immune system alterations that result from intense exercise with the more isolated and controversial reports of overtraining in athletes. The underlying premise here is that overtraining results from excessive repeated bouts of intense exercise/competition and culminates in chronically reduced physical performance. We define intense exercise as that which is particularly stressful to the athlete, usually ends in exhaustion, and elicits substantial increases in plasma concentrations of the stress hormones adreno-corticotropin (ACTH), cortisol, and epinephrine. Concomitant increases in these hormones has long been thought to be a reliable marker of physical and mental stress (Selye, 1983). Exercise at or above about 65% $\dot{V}O_2$max is generally considered the threshold for increases in these hormones. However, substantial increases in stress hormone levels would not be expected unless the exercise is performed at higher relative intensities, to exhaustion, or in stressful environments (Francesconi, 1988; Urhausen et al., 1995). Substantial variability in stress-hormone responses will exist among athletes, depending on such factors as the specificity of training, nutritional condition including hydration status, acclimation level, and the novelty of the exercise (Francesconi, 1988). Ultimately, a case will be made that the influence of intense training on the immune system is best viewed as a subset of the stress response and may be explained, at least in part, on the basis of the stress-hormone responses (Hoffman-Goetz & Pederson, 1994). This chapter will focus primarily on the effects of single and repeated bouts of intense exercise on specific components of the immune system, incidence and severity of infections in athletes, specific evidence of altered immune function in athletes thought to be overtrained, potential physiological/psychological mechanisms to explain the findings, and possible procedures to limit the negative consequences.

OVERVIEW OF THE IMMUNE SYSTEM

Innate and Adaptive Immunity

The immune system is of vital importance for the body's defense against invading microorganisms and viruses and the growth of tumor cells, as well as for the clean-up and repair of injured tissues. This is achieved through two distinct, but interrelated, components of the immune system. These are referred to as innate and adaptive immunity (Roitt et al., 1993). The *innate immune system* (sometimes referred to as non-specific immunity) consists of a variety of physical barriers to pathogens as well as certain leukocytes and circulating proteins of the immune system (Figure 7-2). The skin, mucous secretions, cilia, saliva, pH of body fluids, and gut enzymes are just a few examples of the innate immune system that protect against initial infection by pathogens via the airways and other portals of entry. Additionally, the complement and acute-phase proteins are noncellular, circulating immune components that also provide nonspecific defense against pathogens. Important cells of the innate immune system include natural killer cells (NK), neutrophils, and cells of the monocyte/macrophage lineage.

The characteristics that differentiate cells of the *innate immune system* from those of the *adaptive immune system* are a lack of memory and the ability to recognize foreign particles (antigens) without prior exposure to the antigen. Memory refers to the ability of immune cells to recognize a pathogen to which they have previously been exposed, and to mount a quicker and larger immune response to a second exposure. Although cells from the adaptive system exhibit memory, they can recognize only antigen presented by other host cells in association with certain self-proteins known as the major histocompatibility complexes (MHC-I and II). This means that the "first line of defense" against pathogenic agents lies with the innate immune system. These cells can independently recognize nonself, making them efficient and early responders to infection and/or tumors. By interfering with the early stages of invasion, multiplication, and spread to susceptible organs, the innate system is relatively more important in determining the outcome of an infection. If pathogens evade this first line of defense and a fully established infection occurs, final recovery is, in most instances, determined by the adaptive immune response. The adaptive system is also important in episodes of reinfection. Despite the distinction between these two arms of the immune system, there is considerable interaction among components of both systems, and it is this interaction that affords complete and effective host defense against pathogens (Figure 7-2).

Neutrophils

Neutrophils, monocytes, and macrophages are the primary phagocytic cells of the innate immune system. Neutrophils, the most abundant of the white blood cells (leukocytes), represent over 90% of all circulating granulocytes, a cell type that also includes eosinophils and basophils (Roitt et al., 1993). Neutrophils migrate to sites of inflammation and infection and can phagocytize particulate matter. They are particularly effective against bacterial infections and can destroy ingested bacteria through the release of lysosomal enzymes contained in vacuoles in their interior or via the respiratory burst in which they use oxygen free-radicals such as OH- and H_2O_2, which have potent killing abilities.

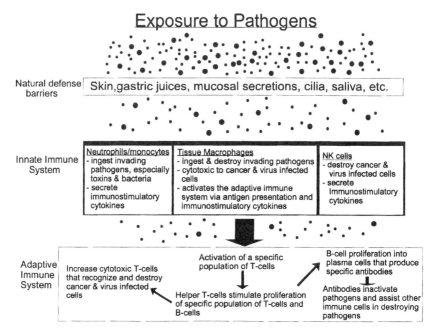

FIGURE 7-2. *Defense against pathogenic agents.* The first line of defense against infections lies with the innate immune system. Natural defense barriers can prevent initial entry of pathogens. Those pathogens that escape are then dealt with by the cells of the innate system, including neutrophils, monocytes/macrophages, and NK cells by mechanisms including phagocytosis and the release of toxic cytokines and enzymes. The T and B cells of the adaptive immune system defend against any remaining pathogenic agents via both cellular- and humoral-mediated processes. Communication throughout these lines of defense create effective immune responses.

Monocytes/Macrophages

Monocytes are mononuclear leukocytes that are produced in the bone marrow, stored briefly, and released into the circulation where they have a half-life of about 2–3 d. In the blood they function as phagocytic cells, producers of cytokines, regulators of blood clotting, and as antigen presenting cells (Roitt et al., 1993). Monocytes are actually immature cells that are in transit to the tissues or fixed sites along specialized vessels. Once they reach these sites, they mature into larger more functional macrophages with half-lives in the order of months (Adams & Hamilton, 1984). Macrophages constitute an important part of the first line of defense against microbial invaders and malignancies. In addition to their function within the innate immune system, they are essential for proper function of the adaptive immune system through presentation of antigen to T-cells via their class I & II MHC surface molecules and production of cytokines that upregulate T-cells and B-cells (Roitt et al., 1993). These cells are also involved in tissue remodeling, inflammation development, and complement production (Adams & Hamilton, 1984). Collectively, these properties indicate a primary role for the macrophage in the functioning of the immune system as a whole.

Natural Killer Cells

The NK cell is a another important part of the innate immune system. This cell is a large granular lymphocyte (distinguished by cell surface markers: $CD56^+$, $CD16^+$, $CD3^-$) that is effective against viral and bacterial infected cells as well as certain tumor cells. It can spontaneously lyse target cells within hours of exposure and requires no MHC expression by the target cell (Robertson & Ritz, 1990). Cytotoxic mechanisms include the puncturing of target cell membranes with perforans and the release of toxic cytokines such as tumor necrosis factor (TNF-a) and interferon(IFN-g).

T and B Lymphocytes

There are two main cells of the adaptive system, the T and B lymphocytes. The T cells are involved in what is known as cell-mediated immunity. Direct cell-to-cell contact is required for these cells to produce an immune response, and T cells can recognize foreign particles only in association with MHC molecules (from antigen presenting cells). There are two subsets of T cells, helper (T_H) and cytotoxic/suppressor (T_C), which are CD4+ and CD8+, respectively. Upon recognition of antigen and stimulation by certain cytokines, both types of T cells proliferate, producing functional clones as well as memory T cells of identical specificity. As referred to earlier, these memory cells allow for a quicker response on future exposure to the same antigen (Roitt et al., 1993).

The T_H cells primarily recognize MHC-II proteins that are displayed on specific antigen presenting cells (APC), which include macrophages and, to a lesser extent, B cells. These antigens are taken into the APC to be displayed. Any foreign particulate matter found in the circulation (e.g., bacteria) may be displayed in this manner. The T_H cells do not directly kill foreign or infected cells but serve to stimulate other T and B cells. Cytokines (discussed below) released by T_H cells not only stimulate T and B lymphocytes, but also activate macrophages and NK cells (Figure 7-3). Without the T_H cell, potent immune responses would not be achieved (Roitt et al., 1993).

The T_C cells primarily recognize MHC-1 proteins that are displayed on all nucleated cell types. The antigen complexed to MHC-1 is produced endogenously; therefore, proteins produced by virus infected cells or tumor cells are displayed in this manner. T_C cells, once bound to the MHC-I antigen complex and stimulated by cytokines, can directly kill the bound cell. Cytotoxic mechanisms are similar to those of the NK cell, including the puncture of the target cell membrane with perforans or the release of cytotoxic cytokines such as TNF-α. The primary difference between the NK and T cells is the MHC restriction requirements of the T cell.

B cells are part of the adaptive immune system and the primary component of humoral immunity. These cells display antibodies, i.e., glycoproteins with antigen binding sites, on their surfaces. Each cell displays an antibody specific for a particular antigen. Binding of that particular antigen with the B cell results in its activation and proliferation. Numerous B cell clones are produced, some that secrete large amounts of that same specific antibody (plasma cells) and others that are maintained in the circulation as memory cells, ready to respond more strongly and more quickly should another encounter with the same antigen occur. As mentioned previously, B cells can serve as APC's for T cells, especially upon reinfection with the same pathogen. In addition, secreted antibodies can bind antigen, effectively preventing it from doing harm until it can be phagocytized (Mackinnon, 1996).

One method that the immune system uses to deal with antigens bound to a B-cell antibody is to destroy them via the complement system. Complement refers to a group of proteins that can be found in the circulation. Once a specific complement protein binds to an antibody-antigen complex on the cell, a cascade of events is initiated involving interactions between the complement proteins. These interactions eventually lead to lysis of the cell itself (Roitt et al., 1993).

Cytokines

It should be apparent that the cells of the innate and adaptive systems do not function alone, but elaborately interact (Rhind et al., 1995). A primary means of interaction is through a group of peptides known as the cytokines. These molecules are signals for stimulation and growth of cells, and for communication between the central nervous system, neuroendocrine system, and immune system (Figure 7-3). This interaction forms the basis of the new, rapidly growing field of psychoneuroimmunology (Ader et al., 1991; Blalock, 1994).

More than 60 cytokines have now been identified (Rhind et al., 1995), although some seem more likely to have a role in exercise immune alterations than others. Of particular interest are cytokines such as interleukin-1 (IL-1), IL-6, and TNF, commonly referred to as *inflammatory cytokines*. These peptides are part of the *acute phase response*, a reaction to infection, inflammation, injury, and/or immunological challenges that has metabolic, neuroendocrine, and immunological effects

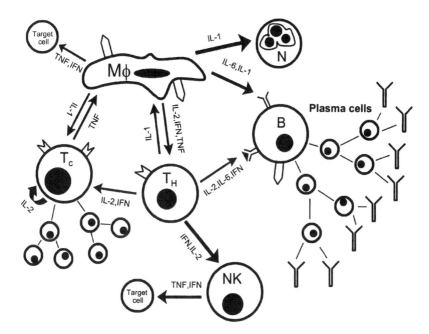

FIGURE 7-3. *Interaction among cells of the immune system.* Cells of both the innate and adaptive systems interact to produce effective immune responses. Cytokines are a primary method of communication for these cells, acting as signals for stimulation and proliferation. Particular cytokines such as IFN and TNF also have direct anti-viral and anti-tumor functions when released by macrophages or NK cells in the vicinity of a target cell. Both macrophages and B cells, which display MHC-II on their cell surface, can present antigen to T_H cells. Also represented is the proliferation of both T and B cells in response to antigen recognition and cytokine stimulation. Outlined are just some of the cell-cytokine interactions that occur and that may be important in studies of exercise effects on immune function. Abbreviations: Mø, macrophage; N, neutrophil; Tc, cytotoxic T cell; T_H, helper T cell; B, B cell; NK, natural killer cell; TNF, tumor necrosis factor; IFN, interferon; IL, interleukin.

(Dinarello, 1984; Evans & Cannon, 1991; Tidball, 1995). Effects attributable to these three cytokines include fever, fatigue, loss of appetite, and nausea in addition to their role in immune cell stimulation (Kent et al., 1992; Schobitz et al., 1994). Because they are expressed in response to injury and inflammation, they are of particular interest in regard to the overtraining syndrome. Interest has also focused on interferon (IFN), which has potent anti-viral effects and may also play a role in the development of fatigue (Adams et al., 1984; Davis, et al., 1995; Rohatimer et al., 1983; Smedley et al., 1983). IL-2 is another important cytokine. Produced by T_H cells, it promotes T-cell differentiation, B-cell growth, and activates macrophages and NK cells (Rhind et al., 1995).

Recently, it has become apparent that cytokines may be part of a larger network of communication within the body that includes the neuroendocrine system. It has been suggested that cytokines, hormones, and neurotransmitters, with their shared receptors throughout the immune and neuroendocrine systems, are part of a common communication circuit (Blalock, 1994; Irwin, 1994; Sheridan et al., 1994). This interaction underlies the importance of psychological stress as well as exercise stress when evaluating the effects of intense exercise and overtraining on the immune system.

INTENSE EXERCISE AND IMMUNE FUNCTION

Introduction

The existing literature on immune responses to acute intense exercise (see definition in the introduction section) contains many references describing alterations in circulating immune cell subsets. Many of these responses are qualitatively summarized in Figure 7-4 and discussed later in this section. The preponderance of studies in this particular area of immunology research is due to the relative ease of taking blood from humans (blood being the most accessible source of immune cells), and because the identification of specific immune cells and their subsets using flow-cytometry techniques is relatively simple to accomplish. However, there are inherent problems with this approach. First, blood actually contains only a small percentage of the total number of lymphocytes, monocytes, and neutrophils residing in the body. Second, most immune reactions occur within the tissues at sites of infection/inflammation or within the lymphatic system. Therefore, it is difficult to determine whether exercise-induced alterations in leukocyte subsets in the blood represent important changes in integrated host-defense or are simply shifts in leukocytes from one compartment to another and back again (Cannon, 1993; Westermann, 1990). For these reasons, and owing to the fact that other excellent reviews on this topic can be found elsewhere (Nieman, 1994; Shinkai et al., 1992), only a small portion of this chapter will focus on exercise-induced changes in circulating immune cell subsets.

A better understanding of the effects of intense exercise on the immune system has been gained through studies involving functional measurements of immunity in humans and by research involving animals where it is possible to assess tissue-specific immune responses. For example, many recent studies commonly include functional assays of lymphocyte mitogenesis; NK cell and macrophage cytotoxicity; neutrophil, monocyte, and macrophage phagocytosis; neutrophil and monocyte bacterial killing (respiratory burst activity); and B-cell immunoglobulin production in vitro (Smith, 1995). Other ways of studying immune function are to measure the concentration of important immunomodulators such as cytokines in the tissue, blood, and urine, and cytokine secretion from stimulated immune cells in vitro. However, there are problems with this approach as well (Smith, 1995; Cannon et al., 1993). While examination of these functional changes may provide a better understanding of possible alterations in host-defense, the physiological and/or clinical significance of (typically smaller) exercise-induced changes in immune function is very difficult to assess in otherwise healthy athletes.

Innate Immunity and Exercise

Components of the innate immune system include natural killer cells (NK), neutrophils, monocytes, and macrophages; soluble factors such as acute phase proteins; complement; and various cytokines, including interferons, interleukins, and tumor necrosis factor (TNF). Exercise studies on this aspect of immunity have lagged far behind those involving the adaptive immune system. This has occurred even though it could be argued that alterations in the function of the innate immune system are relatively more important because it serves as the first line of defense (after structural barriers) against foreign pathogens and malignancies, and is an essential communication link to the adaptive immune system.

Obviously, many factors must be considered when assessing the effects of intense exercise on components of the innate immune system. These include the type, duration, and intensity of exercise, the timing of the immune assessments, differences in initial fitness levels of the subjects, and various environmental and psychological factors. However, despite all these potentially confounding factors, some patterns are beginning to emerge as the number of studies in this area continues to increase (Figure 7-4).

Natural Killer Cell Function. NK cells are a distinct subpopulation of lymphocytes capable of recognizing and killing certain virally-infected cells, many tumor cells, and some microorganisms without prior exposure. Immediately after brief or prolonged maximal exercise there is a transient increase in the absolute concentration and relative proportion of NK cells among other leukocytes which increases the overall NK cell activity (Neiman et al., 1993). This most likely results from an influx of NK cells into the blood from tissues like the spleen and lungs (Muir et al., 1984; Tvede et al., 1994) that is mediated by increases in plasma concentrations of epinephrine (Kappel et al., 1991c; Tonnesen et al., 1987). However, this increase is short-lived and is usually followed by a suppression for the next 2 to 24 h following intense exercise (Gabriel et al., 1991, 1992a, 1992b, 1994a; Kappel et al., 1991c; Neiman, 1993; Strasner et al., 1997). There is considerable debate about whether the decrease in

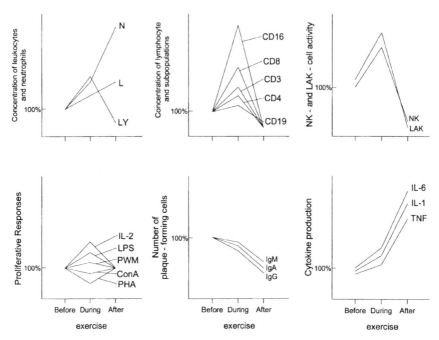

FIGURE 7-4. *Schematic representation of changes in cell concentration and immune function during and after exercise.* Acute exercise results in a leukocytosis both during and after exercise, predominantly due to neutrophilia. Lymphocyte concentrations rise differentially during exercise but drop below baseline levels during recovery. Lymphocyte activity is also affected differentially. NK and LAK activities increase with exercise but then drop below baseline levels afterwards. T⁻ lymphocyte proliferative responses appear to depend on the mitogen used, either increasing or decreasing with exercise. B-cell antibody production tends to decrease both during and after exercise. Production of the inflammatory cytokines increases both during and after exercise. Abbreviations: N, neutrophils; L, leukocytes; LY, lymphocytes; LAK, lymphokine-activated killer cell; NK, natural killer cell; IL, interleukin; LPS, lipopolysaccharide; PWM, pokeweed mitogen; ConA, concanavalin A; PHA, phytohemagglutinin; TNF, tumor necrosis factor. Reproduced with permission from L. Hoffman-Goetz & B.K. Pederson (1994).

NK activity after intense exercise reflects a decrease in the number of NK cells in circulation or a true suppression of function of individual NK cells. The former now appears more likely, given the recent work of Gabriel et al. (1994a) and Nieman et al. (1995). Gabriel et al. (1994a) reported a rapid exit from the circulation of cells expressing a high density of adhesion molecules (e.g., LFA-1) such as NK cells and monocytes after intense exercise. Nieman et al. (1995) showed that NK function actually increases slightly when examined on a per-cell basis following prolonged intense exercise.

Neutrophil Function. Neutrophils (sometimes referred to as polymorphonuclear leukocytes, PMN's) are another part of the "first line of defense" that protects the body against invading microorganisms, especially bacteria (Smith et al., 1990). This protective effect depends on the ability of neutrophils to migrate to inflammatory sites (chemotaxis), to ingest damaged tissues or infective agents (phagocytosis), and to digest these particles (bacterial killing) (Ortega, 1994). Bacterial killing results from the release of proteases and toxic molecules such as hydrogen peroxide and oxygen radicals commonly referred to as the "respiratory burst." The importance of these cells is highlighted by frequent and severe infections seen in patients with neutrophil deficiencies (Johnson et al., 1992).

Several papers now show a substantial increase in neutrophils in circulation immediately, and for 2–4 hours, after acute exercise that is roughly in proportion to the intensity of the exercise (Field et al., 1991; Gray et al., 1993; Hansen et al., 1991). However, only recently has the overall function of these cells been assessed in the blood and tissues. Based on the studies of degranulation, complement receptor expression, and neutrophil size reviewed by Pyne (1994), neutrophils appear to be activated immediately after exercise. However, results are not clear for other important neutrophil functions including phagocytic activity, adherence to endothelium, or respiratory burst activity. These variable results have been based on studies of neutrophils collected from the peripheral blood. Results based on neutrophil function of the upper airways appear clearer, although there aren't many studies of this nature yet (Muns, 1993; Muns et al., 1996).

Muns and colleagues (1993, 1996) evaluated the effects of intense exercise on neutrophils in the upper airway mucosa in humans. These were unique studies in that the focus was on tissue-specific immune cells located at a primary site of entry of various pathogens in human subjects. In the 1993 study, Muns showed that the number of neutrophils in nasal washings increased about threefold following a 20-km race and remained elevated for several days, returning to baseline levels after 1 wk. However, there was a significant decrease in the percentage of these neutrophils that were phagocytic, and the phagocytic activity of each of those cells was reduced approximately two and a half-fold (Figure 7-5).

In a subsequent paper, they found that whereas the initial influx of neutrophils into the nasal mucosa was associated with a similar increase in neutrophil chemotactic activity (NCA) immediately after the competition of a marathon run (Muns et al., 1996), NCA was back to baseline levels after only 1 d while the number of neutrophils, total protein, and albumin remained elevated, suggesting an ongoing inflammatory process. The accumulation of neutrophils and the release of elastase, superoxide anions, and other oxygen free radicals can sustain and prolong the inflammatory process and may increase cell membrane damage and

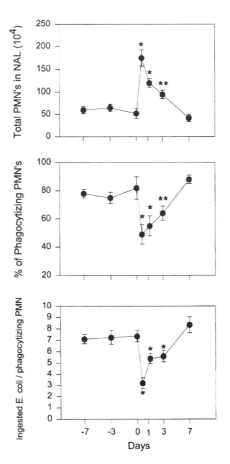

FIGURE 7-5. *Effects of a 20-km race on numbers of polymorphonuclear neutrophils (PMNs) in the upper respiratory tract and their phagocytic function.* PMNs collected from nasal lavage (NAL) 7 and 3 d prior to the race, immediately pre- and post-race, and 1, 3, and 7 d after the race. a) Total PMNs in the nasal lavage, b) % of phagocytizing PMNs, c) bacterial phagocytic ability on a per-cell basis. Significant differences: *p=.01, **p=.05. Data from Muns (1993).

further breakdown the natural mucosal barriers against foreign pathogens (Weiss, 1989).

Evidence of mucosal surface damage has been outlined in another study by Muns et al. (1995). Twelve amateur runners competing in a marathon were compared to healthy, sedentary controls. Nasal mucociliary transit time, cilia beat frequency, and viability of ciliated cells were examined before and after the race. Compared to controls, significant impairments in all three variables were found in runners immediately after the race, with some decreased function lasting for as many as 5 d.

This and the apparent diminished capacity of neutrophils to destroy foreign pathogens that occur following intense exercise may have clinical relevance in terms of resistance to disease in athletes (discussed further in a later section of this review).

Monocyte/Macrophage Function. As mentioned previously, monocytes and macrophages are of critical importance to the innate immune system by virtue of their cytotoxic and phagocytic abilities. They are also important to the adaptive immune system due to their function as antigen presenting cells and their ability to stimulate lymphocytes through the release of cytokines. In fact, it has been suggested that these cells may be the most appropriate immune system component to study when trying to understand the relationship between exercise and susceptibility to disease because of the central role they play in resistance to infection, surveillance against cancer, and regulation of adaptive immunity (Fehr et al., 1989). However, there are relatively few reports involving potential exercise effects on cells of this lineage. This is at least partially due to the relatively small numbers of monocytes in human blood and the inaccessibility of fully differentiated tissue macrophages in humans. Fortunately, most activities of murine tissue macrophages are similar to those of human tissue macrophages (Michna, 1988, 1989).

Transient increases in monocyte numbers in peripheral blood generally occur with intense exercise (Woods & Davis, 1995; Bousquet et al., 1996). This exercise-induced monocytosis is usually short lived, lasting less that an hour, but may last up to 24 h following high-intensity exercise. However, as discussed previously, it is difficult to assess whether these changes in circulating numbers of monocytes represent important changes in integrated host-defense or are simply an inconsequential effect of transient shifts from noncirculating to circulating pools and back again.

There have been several reports of altered function of monocytes and macrophages in response to intense exercise. As with neutrophils, these cells have important functions as phagocytes. The phagocytic process involves several steps including adherence, chemotaxis, attachment, ingestion, and killing, and the influence of intense exercise may vary depending on the specific step that is examined (Rincon, 1994). However, it is generally found that intense exercise increases the capacity of monocytes and macrophages to attach and ingest foreign antigens (Rincon, 1994), although this is not always the case (Bieger et al., 1980).

Important data have also been collected in experiments using monocyte/macrophage infiltration into various tissue compartments as an index of the inflammatory response. Inflammation is defined as the response to infectious agents and/or tissue damage characterized by increased blood supply and capillary permeability, subsequent migration of neutrophils and monocytes/macrophages into the affected area, and cytokine release (Michna, 1989; Bousquet et al., 1996). We recently reasoned that the ability to mount an inflammatory response to a particular stimulus may be a better indicator of changes in monocyte/macrophage function than is simple quantification of monocyte numbers in blood. We measured the number and function of monocytes and macrophages infiltrating the peritoneal cavity following intraperitoneal injection of a heat-killed bacteria suspension (P. Acnes) the day before 7 d of either moderate (30 min, 18 m/min, 5% grade) or exhaustive (2–4 h, 18-35 m/min, 5% grade) treadmill exercise in mice (Woods et al., 1994). We found that exhaustive exercise dramatically reduced the influx of these cells by greater than 50% in comparison to the moderate exercise and control groups. The potential clinical significance of this in terms of host defense against infection, malignancy, or tissue damage has not been addressed.

Studies examining the effects of intense exercise on fully differentiated tissue macrophages have generally reported a stimulating effect. For example, human connective tissue macrophages collected from a group of trained subjects exhibited increased phagocytic function in response to an exhaustive 15-km run (Fehr et al., 1989). This has also been confirmed in old mice (de La Fuenta et al., 1990) and guinea pigs (Ortega et al., 1992). We have likewise found substantial increases in macrophage anti-tumor cytotoxicity in the peritoneal cavity (Woods et al., 1993, 1994) and lungs (Davis et al., 1994) of mice following prolonged running to fatigue. However, when we tested the effect of prolonged running to fatigue on anti-viral function of lung macrophages, we found the opposite. Alveolar macrophages were more susceptible to viral infection following prolonged intense exercise (Davis et al., 1997), and this was associated with an increased susceptibility to infection following nasal inoculation with the same virus in mice (Davis et al., 1997). This further illustrates the danger of assuming that an exercise-induced change in one function of one component of the immune system must reflect a change in the overall function of that component or of overall integrated host defense.

The effect of intense exercise on cytokine production by macrophages has not been directly studied. There is good evidence that intense exercise is associated with increases in the concentration of various cytokines in the blood, urine, and muscles. It is important to note that the most well-documented increases involve cytokines primarily released by monocytes and macrophages, especially the inflammatory cytokines, including IL-1, IL-6, INF α/β, and TNF-α. It has been suggested that these cytokines may be secreted by tissue macrophages in response to exercise-induced tissue damage (Bousquet et al., 1996; Evans & Cannon, 1991; Rhind et al., 1995; Tidball, 1995) and/or in response to systemic endotoxemia (Bosenberg et al., 1988).

Cytokines. As previously mentioned, cytokines play an essential role in communication within the immune system and between the immune and neuroendocrine systems. Many of the cytokines, including IL-1, IL-6, and TNF-α, are also important mediators of inflammation and the related acute-phase response. Defense against infection and malignancies, as well as the tissue repair processes are all regulated by cytokines (Roitt et al., 1993).

Intense exercise can alter the production of numerous cytokines and modulate receptor number, as reviewed recently by Rhind et al. (1995) and by Northoff et al. (1994). Reported changes in cytokine concentrations are conflicting. This may be due to the variety of methods used to measure cytokine production, including bioassays, radioimmunoassays, and enzyme-linked immunoassays. Alternately, the fact that most cytokines are found in picogram concentrations in plasma may make small changes due to exercise difficult to detect. A third consideration is that changes in cytokine concentrations are probably most important within the tissues and at sites of infection/inflammation, making changes in absolute concentrations in plasma, as with changes in immune cell number, hard to interpret.

In general, however, these recent reviews (Bousquet et al., 1996; Northoff et al., 1994; Rhind et al., 1995) have concluded that exercise can increase plasma and urinary cytokines, particularly IL-1 and IL-6. Effects on TNF-α and IFN are less clear, and it appears that IFN levels may actually decrease with intense exercise. It is possible that the increased appearance of cytokines, especially the inflammatory cytokines, reflects an acute inflammatory response to strenuous exercise (Drenth et al., 1995). Indeed, some have likened the elevation of these inflammatory cytokines in the serum following strenuous exercise to an acute-phase response (Evans & Cannon, 1991; Northoff et al., 1994; Rhind et al., 1995; Tidball, 1995). Furthermore, it may be hypothesized that repeated bouts of intense exercise, as occurs with heavy training in athletes, may be deleterious. Repeated elevations of these cytokines could potentially result in some of the negative signs and symptoms associated with overtraining, including fatigue, sleepiness, anorexia, apathy, and irritability —symptoms that have been attributed to pro-inflammatory cytokines and interferon (Dantzer & Kelley, 1989; Davis et al., 1995; Rohatimer et al., 1983; Schobitz et al., 1994; Smedley et al., 1983).

Adaptive Immunity

Lymphocyte Function. The number and function of T- and B-lymphocytes are known to change following intense exercise. These responses appear to be transient and variable depending on the intensity and duration of exercise and the timing of the observation (Cannon, 1993; Gabriel et al., 1991; Neiman, 1994; Shinkai et al., 1992). An increase in the number of lymphocytes (lymphocytosis) usually occurs for a short period during intense exercise but returns to baseline levels rapidly when exercise ends and then usually decreases to below baseline levels (lymphocytopenia) for 6-24 h following prolonged intense exercise. The lymphocytosis is comprised mainly of NK cells and to a lesser extent T_C cells (CD8$^+$), which results in a small decrease in the CD4/CD8 ratio during and following intense exercise. However, it can be argued that this is not clinically significant because the total number of these cells is actually increased during this time, even though the ratio of the two may be slightly lower. These alterations in lymphocyte subsets are thought to reflect changes of blood volume and transient shifts between various tissues and blood. It is also possible that many of the changes that have been attributed to strenuous exercise may be related to natural circadian rhythms, a confounding factor not adequately addressed in many studies (Cannon, 1993; Strasner et al., 1997). And, once again, there is the unresolved issue of relating any of these changes to overall integrated host defense.

A potentially better measure of altered host defense involving the adaptive immune system may be derived from experiments that examine functional capacities of T- and B- lymphocytes. One of the most important and most studied functions of lymphocytes is their ability to proliferate (clone themselves) following an antigenic challenge. The literature suggests that the proliferative response of T-cells depends on the specific challenge. For example, the ability of lymphocytes to proliferate following stimulation with T-cell-dependent mitogens such as concanavalin A (con A) and phytohemagglutinin (PHA) decreases following intense exercise (Hoffman-Goetz & Pedersen, 1994)(see Figure 7-4). This effect may be due to the altered composition of the lymphocyte subpopulation in the blood sample. For example, the decreased response to PHA may result from a decrease in the CD4/CD8 ratio (Tvede et al., 1989). However, recent work by Nieman et al. (1994) suggests that the suppression is more likely due to decreased function of the individual T-cells themselves.

Much less is known about the effects of intense exercise on B-lymphocyte function. It has generally been observed that the percentage of B-cells (CD19$^+$) changes little in response to intense exercise (Hoffman-Goetz & Pedersen, 1994). However, the fraction of antibody-producing cells following stimulation with pokeweed mitogen (PWM), IL-2, or Epstein-Barr virus (EBV) is significantly suppressed both during and 2 h after intense bicycle exercise and does not return to baseline for 24 h

(Tvede et al., 1989). Only a few studies have measured the effects of acute intense exercise on serum antibody (IgG) concentrations. These studies show little (<20%) if any increase after intense exercise, especially when the concentrations are corrected for changes in plasma volume (Mackinnon, 1996).

Conversely, the concentration of salivary IgA, commonly used as a marker of secretory immunoglobulin, decreases in response to intense exercise. It appears that exercise intensity may be the most important factor in determining the IgA response to exercise (Mackinnon, 1996). For example, Mackinnon and Jenkins (1993) found that the salivary IgA secretion rate was more than 50% lower after supramaximal interval exercise that took only 5 min, whereas other studies show that moderate exercise up to 90 min duration does not appear to alter IgA concentration or secretion rate (Mackinnon & Hooper, 1994; McDowell et al., 1991). This has been suggested to have clinical relevance because this aspect of the immune system protects the body's mucosal surfaces exposed to the environment (e.g., eyes, nose, mouth, upper and lower respiratory tracts, as well as the gastrointestinal, urinary and genital tracts) (Mackinnon & Hooper, 1994). A recent report involving elite hockey and squash players showed that intense training induced a decrease in the concentration of salivary IgA that was associated with the subsequent appearance of an upper respiratory infection (Mackinnon et al., 1993). Another study, available only in abstract form, reported that intramuscular injections of immunoglobulin at 4-wk intervals for 6 mo decreased the duration of infection in athletes, when compared to placebo injections (Frohlich et al., 1987). Finally, a third study used thymodulin administration over 3 mo of intense training in athletes and noted an apparent decrease in both the incidence of infectious illness and number of days of symptoms, changes that were attributed to the ability of the drug to counteract some of the immunosuppressive effects of the prolonged intense training (Garagiola et al., 1995).

EXERCISE TRAINING, COMPETITION, AND INFECTION

Relationship Between Exercise and Infection

Given the known changes in various immune parameters following strenuous exercise, it would seem likely that regular, intense training might be associated with an increased risk of infection. This increased risk has indeed been noted in numerous reviews on the topic of exercise and infection (Brenner et al., 1994; Eichner, 1995; Fitzgerald, 1991; Nieman, 1992, 1994; Nieman & Nehlsen-Cannarella, 1992). Such evidence for an increased risk of infection with strenuous exercise comes from both epidemiological and experimental studies.

Nieman and Nehlsen-Canarrella (1992) suggest that a "J" shaped curve can be used to illustrate the relationship between risk of an upper-respiratory-tract infection (URTI) and exercise. This model suggests that while sedentary individuals have an average risk of URTI, those who engage in excessive exercise may have a higher risk, and those who exercise moderately may actually have a decreased risk of infection. While the decreased risk in those who exercise moderately has not been shown conclusively, there is growing evidence that excessive and/or strenuous exercise does indeed increase the risk of an URTI.

Epidemiological Studies

Perhaps the best evidence in support of this theory comes from surveys conducted in marathon and ultramarathon runners (Nieman et al., 1990; Peters & Bateman, 1983). Nieman et al. (1990) used a questionnaire to survey 2,311 runners from the 1987 Los Angeles Marathon. Information regarding infectious episodes and training regimens was requested for the 2 mo prior to, and 1 wk following, the marathon. The incidence of infection in the week following the marathon was 12.9% among the runners, but only 2.2% in a matched group of runners who did not participate. This indicates an odds ratio of 6 to 1 in favor of the runners experiencing illness vs. the controls. Additionally, information regarding training habits during the 2 mo period prior to the marathon indicated that those runners training more than 60 mi/wk were twice as likely to be sick compared to those running less than 20 mi/wk. It was concluded that both heavy training and/or participation in the marathon increased the likelihood of URTI. Peters and Bateman (1983) also looked at the incidence of URTI in runners after a 56-km race. Compared to 15.3% of matched controls, 33.3% of the runners had symptoms of URTI in the 2-wk period following the race. Additionally, the faster runners tended to have a greater incidence of symptoms than did the slower runners. Peters et al. (1993) also looked at URTI following a 90-km race. In accordance with the study by Nieman et al. (1990), those runners training the hardest prior to the race had a higher incidence of URTI (85%) compared to those who trained less (45%).

Other studies have looked at the incidence of infection in trained persons over time. Heath et al. (1991) had a cohort of 530 runners record URTI symptoms and running mileage for 1 y. Those runners training less than 10 mi/wk had the lowest odds ratio for URTI, while those who trained more than 17 mi/wk had twice the odds ratio for infection. Although other variables such as a low body mass index and living alone were also found to be significantly related to infection, increased training mileage was a significant risk factor for URTI. A similar study was done in 42 Danish elite orienteers compared to 41 matched controls

(Linde, 1987). The orienteers experienced 2.5 episodes of URTI in 1 y, compared to only 1.7 episodes in the nonathletes (P<0.05). Collectively, epidemiological studies seem to support the belief that strenuous exercise is associated with an increased risk of infection.

Animal Studies

Although the epidemiological studies are informative, controlled experimental studies in which specific doses of both exercise and virus can be given, and other forms of stress and immunomodulatory factors controlled for, are necessary to determine if a link between exercise and infection truly exists. To date, no studies of this kind have been done in humans, although there are animal studies of this design, as reviewed by Cannon (1993). One study in humans was done to correlate infection with psychological, but not exercise, stress (Cohen et al., 1991). The results of this work will be examined later.

As reviewed by Cannon (1993), most animal studies of exercise and infection have used swimming by mice as the exercise intervention. Swimming as an exercise modality is controversial as it is not a natural activity in rodents, and may be more of a psychological than physical stress. Replication of the virus and overall mortality in response to exercise varied greatly in these studies, with exercise proving to be beneficial, harmful, or having no effect. In these studies, the exercise was given after infection with the virus, not allowing for conclusions regarding resistance to infection with exercise training. Additionally, the studies all used different pathogens, such as Coxsackie virus, Influenza, and Trypanosoma cruzi, and it is unlikely that the immune response to one can be easily compared to the others. Studies in our laboratory (Davis et al., 1997) have shown that an acute bout of exhaustive exercise prior to inoculation with the herpes simplex virus results in both increased morbidity and mortality in mice compared to a control group of animals. Due to the variety of viruses used, modes of exercise, timing of exercise in relation to inoculation, and species of animal, it is too early to draw conclusions regarding these types of experiments.

Related Study of Psychological Stress

While controlled exercise studies are not available, exercise is a form of stress; therefore, it may be important to consider the work by Cohen et al. (1991) in which infection rates were compared to levels of psychological stress in subjects. Questionnaires designed to evaluate the level of psychological stress of the 394 subjects were administered prior to inoculation with one of five different respiratory viruses. Subjects were kept quarantined 2 d before and 6 d after inoculation, and were monitored daily by clinicians for detection and evaluation of symptoms.

Infection rates were assessed by presence of virus and virus-specific antibodies of nasal-wash samples taken daily after inoculation. Results showed that rates of infection were increased with increasing categories of stress level that were adjusted for control variables such as age, allergic status, season, and number of subjects housed together. Although it is not yet clear how exercise stress relates to other forms of stress on the body, results from this study are intriguing. The overtraining syndrome includes psychological stress, and so this study, despite the absence of exercise, may be relevant to the overtrained population.

Summary

Although the authors of the reviews mentioned earlier (Brenner et al., 1994; Nieman, 1992) tend to support the idea that people who exercise strenuously are more susceptible to infection, particularly in the period immediately following intense competition, Cannon (1993) has pointed out that probably the best evidence still comes from epidemiological-type studies and that the results from controlled experimental studies are not yet conclusive. Although it is recognized that the intensity and duration of exercise are important in determining risk, perhaps more important to remember is the fact that exercise may differentially effect those components of the immune system responsible for defense against specific pathogens. While exhaustive exercise may increase the risk of URTI by certain viruses, it may not affect the risk of other viral or bacterial infections. More studies are needed in this regard.

OVERTRAINING, IMMUNE FUNCTION, AND INFECTION

Types of Overtraining Studies

There are few studies on athletes that are specifically characterized as being "overtrained." However, experiments have attempted to simulate an overtraining state by increasing the workload of athletes for a period of 1–4 wk. Other studies have examined athletes during periods of intense training within their normal season. Both types of studies will be included in this review as they may offer some insights regarding the progression into the overtrained state; however, it should be remembered that these athletes may not actually fit the definition of overtrained (Table 7-2).

Both resting and postexercise immune measures have been examined in many of these studies and will be reviewed here. We have chosen to focus primarily on resting measures of immune function in overtrained athletes or at least athletes who are being overtrained versus athletes in general. For a thorough review of immune function in athletes, the reader is referred to a recent article by Nieman (1996).

TABLE 7-2. *Studies of overtraining, immune function, and infection.*

Author	Subjects	Treatment	Immune Measures	Clinical
Lehmann et al. 1991	male runners (n=8)	33% training vol/ 4 wk	↓ leuk, ↑ ex norepi, ↓ rest catechol/cort	↑ symptoms
Verde et al. 1992	male runners (n=10)	38% training vol/ 3 wk	↑ rest/↓ ex lymph fxn, ↓ rest/↑ ex T_H/T_S, ↓ rest/↑ ex IgG, ex cort	↑ symptoms URTI, 2/10
Fry et al. 1992, 1994	soldiers (n=5)	2x/day interval training/10 days	↑ lymph fxn, lymph ↓ NK	↓ performance ↑ symptoms
Baj et al. 1994	male cyclists (n=15)	reg training season	↓ leuk, ↓lymph, ↓ T_H/T_S, ↑ lymph fxn, ↓ neutr	___
Hack et al. 1994	male runners (n=7)	reg training season	↓ neutr ↓ neutr fxn	___
Pyne et al. 1995	Swimmers (n=12)	reg training season	↓ neutr fxn ↔ neutr	URTI
Hooper et al. 1995; Mackinnon 1994	male/female swimmers (n=14)	reg training season OT(n=3)	↓ IgA, leuk, ↑ neutr (in taper), ↑ norepi (in taper)	↓ performance ↑ symptoms
Rowbottom et al. 1995	male/female athletes (n=10)	diagnosed OT	↔ leuk ↔ lymph ↔ cort, glutamine	overtraining syndrome
Parry-Billings et al. 1992	athletes (n=40)	diagnosed OT	↔ lymph fxn ↔ IL-1, IL-6 ↓ glutamine	overtraining syndrome
Mackinnon & Hooper,1996	male/female swimmers (n=24)	reg training season OT(n=8)	↔/↓ glutamine	↓ performance ↑ symptoms ↓ URTI in OT

Abbreviations: **catechol**, catecholamines; **cort**, cortisol; **ex**, exercise; **fxn**, function; **IL-1**, interleukin 1; **IL-6**, interleukin 6; **leuk**, leukocyte; **lymph**, lymphocyte; **neutr**, neutrophil; **NK**, natural killer cell; **norepi**, norepinephrine; **OT**, overtrained; T_H/T_S, $T_{helper}/T_{supressor}$ ratio; **URTI**, upper respiratory tract infection; **vol**, volume; ↔, no change.

Induced Overtraining

A prospective study of middle- and long-distance runners (Lehman et al., 1991) attempted to induce the overtraining syndrome by increasing the volume of training done over the course of 4 wk. The average increase in running distance for the 8 subjects was 33%, the distance run increased from a mean of 85.9 km to 174.6 km across the 4-wk period. A battery of tests was conducted at various points throughout the study, including substrate and hormone concentrations, leukocyte counts, and performance measures during a maximal treadmill test. A non-significant decrease in maximal treadmill run time and increases in athletes' complaint indices including words such as "burnt out" and "exhausted" suggested that some of these subjects may have been suffering from overtraining. Of the large number of measures examined, the only ones relating to immune function were total resting leukocyte count and measures of catecholamines and cortisol concentrations in plasma. Total leukocyte count was significantly lower at rest on day 28 compared to day 1. The norepinephrine response to a submaximal workload was increased, while nocturnal norepinephrine excretion decreased. The authors suggested that these hormonal changes may represent an overexertion-related exhaustion of the sympathetic nervous system.

A second study increased the training volume of a group of distance runners by 38% and then had them try to maintain that increase for 3 wk (Verde et al., 1992). No change in run time to fatigue was noted; however, based on subject reports of fatigue and on an inability to maintain a normal training volume during the recovery period, it was concluded that 6 of the 10 subjects were undergoing excessive training. Two of the 10 subjects developed an URTI following the increased training. In contrast to the previous study, multiple measures of immune function both at rest and in response to acute exercise were made. The increased training resulted in a decreased T-helper/T-suppressor cell ratio, increased lymphocyte proliferation, and a blunted response of IgG and IgM to pokeweed mitogen stimulation at rest. In response to a 30-min acute exercise bout, the cortisol response was blunted, lymphocyte proliferation was suppressed, T-lymphocyte percentage was decreased, and the decrease in the T-helper/T-suppressor ratio and IgG synthesis normally seen with acute exercise was eliminated. Despite these changes for the group as a whole, there was wide variation in inter- and intra-individual responses, and, therefore, these types of measures may not provide a practical indicator of overtraining on an individual basis. Subjective measures of fatigue, vigor, and other mood states were evaluated with the Profile of Mood States (POMS) score. Increased ratings of fatigue and decreased ratings of vigor were the most consistent indicators among athletes that the training was too heavy.

Another group (Fry et al., 1992; 1994) has used twice daily interval training for 10 d in an attempt to induce an acute overtraining syndrome. Five members of the Australian army underwent the 10 d of training, followed by 5 d of active recovery. Subjects were tested on specific days for various immunological, psychological, and physiological parameters. Performance decreased in this group, including a decreased total run time in a maximal treadmill test. In addition, there was also a significant change in the POMS score: increased fatigue and mood disturbance, and decreased vigor were noted. Immune changes included an increase in resting lymphocyte activation with the training, as measured by an increase in HLA-DR+ and CD25+ antigens. Associated with the lymphocyte activation with training was an increase in the lymphocyte-activating cytokine IL-2, which remained elevated through the recovery period. The total number of peripheral NK cells was decreased by the training and remained significantly lower through the recovery period.

Following Athletes Through a Competitive Season

Three studies (Baj et al., 1994; Hack et al., 1994; Pyne et al., 1995) have followed athletes through different parts of their regular training seasons and examined immune changes, primarily of neutrophils. Fifteen male cyclists were examined both at the start of training and following a period of intense training and racing (Baj et al., 1994). As seen previously, total leukocyte count dropped significantly over the course of training, as did the lymphocyte count and T-helper/T-suppressor ratio. Lymphocyte proliferation following stimulation with PHA was increased; however, lymphocyte IL-2 generation was decreased. The difference between this lower IL-2 generation and the increased production in the study by Fry et al. (1994) may be that a different stimulating agent (ConA vs. PHA) was used in the assay. Leukocyte aggregation was decreased as were stimulated and nonstimulated chemoluminescence of neutrophils, all of which indicate that neutrophil activity was depressed with training. The authors noted that these changes in resting immune measures may reflect adaptation or exhaustion of the athletes' immune systems and that the meaning of these changes remains unclear until they are related to negative clinical outcomes. Absent from these studies, but highly needed, are correlations between decreased immune function and incidence of infection.

Hack et al. (1994) primarily looked at neutrophil function. Runners were examined before and after maximal treadmill tests conducted during periods of moderate and intense training and were compared to an untrained control group. There was no effect of moderate training on neutrophil counts or phagocytic activity either at rest or after acute exercise. Both of these variables were significantly (p<.05) decreased with intense training, compared to either moderate training or to the controls. These changes in neutrophil count and function are consistent with the changes seen by Baj et al. (1994). However, whereas the former group suggested that the neutrophil changes may have been adaptive, Hack and colleagues clearly indicate that this represents an "exhaustion" of neutrophils. Unfortunately, neither study examined concurrent incidence of infection.

One study that did examine both neutrophil function and incidence of URTI was published recently by Pyne et al. (1995). Twelve well-trained swimmers were studied throughout a 12-wk intensive training program. As in the study of runners by Hack et al. (1994), neutrophil function (oxidative activity) assessed by a flow cytometric assay was significantly lower compared to non-training controls across the training period. This assay, which allowed enumeration of neutrophils that produced H_2O_2 in response to stimulation, demonstrated that the number of cells that responded positively decreased throughout the training period. Total neutrophil count did not decrease across the 12 wk and was only significantly lower than controls early in the training. This study highlights the importance of assessing function, and not just cell number, in response to exercise training. An important measure that distinguishes this study is that of URTI incidence during the training period. Medical reviews by physicians revealed that despite the decrease in neutrophil function, there was no difference between swimmers and controls in incidence of infection. As has been consistently noted, perhaps these small changes in immune function do not have bearing on clinical outcomes such as URTI. Alternatively, since there was no evidence that the subjects in this study were overtrained, it may be that these athletes easily handled the heavy training load.

A group of Australian researchers has followed athletes through their seasons and looked at signs of overtraining (Hooper et al., 1995; Mackinnon & Hooper, 1994). Their studies, however, have focused on defining overtraining and on comparing markers in overtrained or "stale" athletes to those in the non-stale athletes. Fourteen elite swimmers were examined periodically throughout their 6-mo competitive season. Having met several criteria, including decreased performance and persistent fatigue as recorded in log books, three of the swimmers were defined as stale. The 1994 study (Mackinnon & Hooper, 1994) compared salivary IgA concentrations between the two groups of swimmers and found that the stale athletes had 18–32% lower levels throughout the 6-mo period, compared to the well-trained athletes. In a second experiment within that study, three consecutive days of treadmill running (90 min/d at 75% $\dot{V}O_2$max) resulted in progressively decreased postexercise salivary IgA. As IgA is an important first line of defense against pathogens taken in through the airways, these studies suggest that decreased IgA may be one mechanism by which increased infection follows strenuous exercise or training. The 1995 study (Hooper et al., 1995) also examined leukocyte counts and found that the only significant difference between the two groups was an increased neutrophil count in the stale swimmers during the taper part of the training. The conclusion from this study, which focused on identifying markers to distinguish stale athletes, was that athlete self-reports of well-being are probably the most efficient markers.

Focus on Glutamine

A recent study (Rowbottom et al., 1995) compared 10 athletes suffering from the overtraining syndrome and age-matched controls with respect to numerous hematological, biochemical, and immunological indicators. Subjects were chosen only if: (1) they met the definition for chronic fatigue syndrome (CFS), including debilitating fatigue and lack of vigor, and (2) they reported less than acceptable levels of performance in their respective sports. Of all the variables measured, including leukocyte counts and lymphocyte subsets, none was significantly different from the corresponding value for the control group, except for the plasma concentration of glutamine, considered a key substrate for cells of the immune system. Some subjects had deficits in certain cell counts, but no variable was significantly changed in a majority of the athletes. This reinforces the idea that individuals probably respond to overtraining in a highly variable manner and that this syndrome may not be characterized by a strict set of physiological or immunological changes. An important caveat to the interpretation of results in this study is that the subjects were so severely fatigued that only 3 of the 10 were still training at the time of data collection, and this training was at a reduced level. Therefore, changes that might have been caused by repeated bouts of acute exercise may have been obscured.

This study also reemphasizes the importance of examining immune cell function rather than just number. Given the fact that glutamine levels were low in these overtrained individuals, we might expect immune cell function to be decreased. Functional measures would have been a valuable addition to this study.

Parry-Billings et al. (1992) also reported decreased plasma glutamine in a group of 40 overtrained athletes, compared to controls. Measures of immune function were examined, and no differences found between the two groups. Immune variables examined were T-lymphocyte proliferation and plasma IL-1 and IL-6 levels; however, these were measured in only 4–6 subjects/group. Nor did this study address incidence of infection or illness in the overtrained group.

A recent study directly addressed the question of decreased glutamine levels and their relation to incidence of URTI (Mackinnon & Hooper, 1996). Twenty-four elite swimmers underwent 4 wk of increased training consisting of a 36.5% increase in swim volume (km/wk) and an additional increase in time spent in on-land training. Eight of the swimmers were identified as overtrained (OT), the rest as well-trained (WT). Plasma glutamine levels tended to increase across the 4 wk for the WT group, while levels remained relatively unchanged in the OT group; however, statistically significant differences between the two groups were identified only at the 2-wk time point. Interestingly, URTI was self-reported by only 12.5% of OT swimmers compared to 56% of WT swimmers, suggesting that plasma glutamine level is not related to URTI. This evidence, coupled with the data of Pyne et al.(1995) revealing no change in URTI incidence with decreased neutrophil function in overtrained athletes, suggests that small changes in glutamine levels or leukocyte function may not translate into increased infection rates. As noted by Mackinnon and Hooper (1996), URTI may not be related to the overtraining syndrome but to intense exercise and competition by athletes in general.

Related to this line of research is a study that was conducted on changes in immune function and risk of viral infection in U.S. Air Force Academy cadets undergoing 6 wk of Basic Cadet Training (BCT) (Lee et al., 1992). Although the study design does not allow for the subjects to be considered overtrained, it is worthy of comparison against some of the studies reviewed here in which periods of intense training were imposed on athletes. Ninety-six cadets were evaluated for levels of stress, mononuclear cell proliferation, reactivation of latent Epstein-Barr virus (EBV) infections, and illness during an orientation period and then again during the BCT. Reports of well-being decreased significantly from orientation to BCT while perceived stress was increased (p<.05). PHAstimulated leukocyte proliferation significantly decreased during BCT; however, reactivation of EBV, as measured by specific antibody titers, was unchanged. An aim of this research was to correlate immune cell function with the incidence of infection, but neither of the two immune measures was associated with illness in the cadets. Perhaps the one relationship that would have been most interesting to examine in terms of this review is that of stress level (perceived) and resultant infections. This, however, was not done and cannot be deduced from the data presented.

Summary

Collectively, the studies reviewed here reaffirm the notion that overtraining is a complex syndrome comprised of many variables, some of which may be changed in some athletes but not in others undergoing the same physical and psychological stressors. Additionally, most of the studies either failed to address or did not find relationships between decreased immune function and increased incidence of infection/illness. Those studies that did not see an association may have suffered from too small a sample size or too short a period of intensified training through which to examine these athletes. Given the relatively strong epidemiological evidence linking intense exercise with immunosuppression and increased infection, it is likely that there are important relationships that have not yet firmly been identified due to both a lack of overtraining studies and limitations in study design.

POTENTIAL MECHANISMS OF OVERTRAINING

General Theories

In recent years, research has focused on unraveling the etiology of the overtraining syndrome. However, for a number of reasons, little progress has been made. A fundamental problem involves the difficulty in the objective diagnosis of overtraining, and because of this, there is a lack of good overtraining studies in the literature. There are still no objective parameters that can be used for diagnosis of the overtraining syndrome. Rather, diagnosis of overtraining has been based largely on identifying the multitude of physiological and psychological symptoms that may accompany overtraining. The most important of these symptoms appears to be a decrease in performance following a reasonable recovery period. The decrease in the level of performance may or may not be associated with physiological and immunological problems and may differ widely among individuals. In fact, there is increasing support for the position that the overtraining syndrome is not a distinct entity but a continuum of related symptoms that may have different etiologies. It has even been suggested that most athletes diagnosed with the overtraining syndrome are actually suffering from chronic fatigue syndrome (Dyment, 1993; Fry et al., 1991, 1994; Parker & Brukner, 1994)

For these reasons, it has been difficult to elucidate the mechanisms by which overtraining may effect the athlete's immune system. Assuming that overtraining results from the accumulation of the negative effects of excessive physical and psychological stress associated with intense exercise and training, there are three general models that have been proposed to explain at least part of this relationship: the Open Window Hypothesis (Pederson and Ullum, 1994) and two similar models involving neuroendocrine/immune interactions (Fry et al., 1991; Smith & Weidemann, 1990). The Open Window Hypothesis was originally developed to explain the apparent negative effects of strenuous exercise on natural killer cell activity (Pederson & Ullum, 1994). This hypothesis suggests that intense exercise causes a brief initial enhancement of immune function followed by a more prolonged period of immune suppression lasting for several hours. It follows then that an "open window" of opportunity exists for several hours after intense exercise that increases the risk of illness. The models developed by Fry et al. (1991) and Smith and Weidemann (1990) proposed that intense exercise causes the release of various stress hormones that combine to exert either immunostimulation or suppression, depending on the stress of the exercise experience. While it is clear that these models were developed to explain different aspects of the relationship between exercise, immune function, and illness, they are not mutually exclusive and may, in fact, be woven into a single integrated model as will be discussed later.

Specific Immunomodulators

In addition to the more global models proposed above, others have proposed more discrete mechanisms to explain various aspects of the apparent immunosuppression that occurs in many athletes. They include theories related to the very high respiratory flow rates that may damage the mucosal surfaces and suppress mucosal immune mechanisms (Mackinnon, 1996), hyperthermia (Brenner et al., 1995; Pederson et al., 1994), depletion of important nutrients required for optimal function of immune cells, including glutamine and vitamin C (Newsholme, 1994; Keast et al., 1995; Peters et al., 1993; Shephard & Shek, 1995), and negative aspects of the inflammatory response that occur as a result of muscle damage and infection (Bousquet et al., 1996; Tidball, 1995). While it is likely that each of these could contribute separately to altered immune function with intense training/competition, it is also possible that the physiological/psychological stress associated with these perturbations may exert their effects through a more generalized pathway involving neuroendocrine-immune interactions.

Mackinnon (1996) speculated that high respiratory flow rates and the subsequent release of soluble factors and/or structural changes to the epithelium may alter mucosal immune function during intense exercise bouts. These more localized mechanisms seems likely given the fact that serum levels of immunoglobulins do not change much, but mucosal secretion of IgA and IgM is inhibited with intense exercise. She also suggested that these high flow rates may affect a secretory component, transepithelial IgA transporter, whose inhibition could result in a lower secretion of IgA into the mucosal fluids. However, this mechanism remains untested.

Hyperthermia can have numerous effects on the immune system, some of which have been examined by Kappel et al.(1991a, 1991b). These investigators immersed healthy volunteers in either a hot water bath that increased rectal temperature to 39.5°C or a thermoneutral water bath and found that immune alterations that resembled those that occur during intense exercise were associated with the exposure to the hot bath. These responses included an increase in NK cell function and total lymphocyte concentration during the hyperthermia and increases in monocyte and neutrophil concentrations along with a drop in lymphocyte concentration afterwards. However, at least in the case of monocytes and neutrophils, there was not an apparent effect on cell function when assessed on a per cell basis (Kappel et al., 1994). Interestingly, these effects were not associated with large increases in plasma epinephrine and norepinephrine that have been used, at least in part, to explain similar changes that occur during intense exercise.

It has also been hypothesized that depletion of important nutrients that are essential for optimal functioning of immune cells might contribute to immune suppression with intense exercise and overtraining (Keast et al., 1995; Parry-Billings et al., 1992; Peters et al., 1993; Shephard & Shek, 1995). One such hypothesis that has gained the most attention involves glutamine, an important fuel for most immune cells (Keast et al., 1995; Parry-Billings et al., 1992). Decreases in glutamine concentration can impair a number of key functions of T- and B-lymphocytes and macrophages when studied *in vitro*, and substantial decreases in plasma glutamine occur as a result of physical stressors such as trauma, sepsis, and surgery that appear to induce immune suppression. It is also apparent that supplementation with branched-chain amino acids, glutamine-containing dipeptides, and free glutamine designed to maintain plasma glutamine concentration following severe injury may improve macrophage function and general immunity (Parry-Billings et al., 1992).

The evidence that glutamine deficiencies in overtrained athletes are associated with immune function is not strong. In support of the hypothesis, investigators have shown that plasma glutamine levels are low in marathon runners after a race and in athletes who are said to be overtrained (Parry-Billings et al., 1992; Keast, et al., 1995). Keast et al. (1995) also provided evidence that plasma glutamine decreases as exercise intensity increases from 30% $\dot{V}O_2$max to 120% $\dot{V}O_2$max and that plasma glutamine was depressed by the sixth day of a 10-day intensive interval training program and was not back to baseline levels until 5 d after the training. From this and other results, some investigators have begun to suggest that plasma glutamine concentrations may represent an objective, measurable difference between overtrained subjects and their normal controls (Rowbottom et al., 1995).

Although these authors argue that the suppression in plasma glutamine is sufficient to reduce immunological reactivity and place subjects at risk of infection, this has not yet been established. It remains to be shown that there is any correlation between the apparently low glutamine concentrations in some athletes and other clinical symptoms of overtraining, such as impaired performance and immunosuppression. In fact, evidence from the studies reviewed in the overtraining portion of this review tend to suggest that small decreases in plasma glutamine are not related to increased URTI or to changes in immune function in overtrained athletes. Furthermore, it has also not been demonstrated that glutamine supplementation can enhance the immune system and decrease susceptibility to infection in athletes as it has been shown to do in seriously ill patients after surgery, burns, and trauma. At the present time it is not known if glutamine supplementation is beneficial in the treatment of athletes affected by exercise-induced stress and overtraining.

It is well known that athletes sometimes modify their diets in strange ways, hoping that these changes will enhance their athletic performances and perhaps their physical appearances. In a recent review article, Shephard and Shek (1995) pointed out several ways in which an athlete's diet may negatively affect immune function. Athletes often overconsume one food product or macronutrient such as carbohydrates, protein, and amino acids at the expense of other nutrients. This obviously alters the normal balance of nutrients within the body and may lead to shortages of individual nutrients. It is also common for athletes to take megadoses of some minerals and vitamins and yet be deficient in other micronutrients. For example, antioxidants are often taken in megadoses to limit the damaging effects of oxygen radicals that result from increased oxidative metabolism and muscle injury. However, in theory, the overconsumption of antioxidants could potentially impair immune function by inhibiting the oxidative burst activity that is an important function of many immune cells.

There are reports that supplementation with iron (Kluger et al., 1993), zinc (Singh et al., 1994), and vitamin C (Peters et al., 1993) may enhance immune function in athletes. However, except perhaps in the case of vitamin-C supplementation (600 mg daily for 21 d) prior to an ultramarathon race, after which there was a significant reduction in upper respiratory infection for 14 d, there has been no compelling evidence to recommend vitamin and mineral supplements to athletes during intense exercise and training (Shephard & Shek, 1995). In theory, immunosuppression may also occur when athletes undergo intense training combined with caloric restriction. This is often done to offset weight gain, to enhance physical appearance, or as a result of simply not knowing how much food is actually necessary to meet increased energy requirements. These practices could easily lead to depletion of glycogen reserves that would impair athletic performance and lead to increased injuries (Costill et al., 1988; Kirwan et al., 1988; Sherman & Maglischo, 1995) and might also impair immune function (Chandra, 1977). Under these circumstances, immunosuppression could occur through (1) increased competition between muscle and immune cells for key amino acids such as glutamine, (2) overconsumption or underconsumption of vitamins and minerals, and (3) activation of the hypothalamic-pituitary-adrenal axis (HPA) and the sympathoadrenal system resulting from the metabolic and psychological stress associated with these alterations in homeostasis.

Integrated Psychoneuroimmune Hypothesis

The potential mechanisms described above may explain specific decreases in various components of the immune system that may exist, at least in part, from intense exercise and overtraining. However, it is likely that more than one of these responses occur simultaneously and are responsible for various symptoms. These alterations in homeostasis may combine to increase the perceived stress of the intense exercise/training. The effects of these stressors on immune function are now known to be controlled by an elaborate network involving the central nervous system, endocrine system, and immune system. We hypothesize that this interaction may best explain many of the negative changes seen with intense exercise and overtraining (Figure 7-6). This *Psychoneuroimmune Hypothesis* is an extension of the proposals by Fry et al. (1991) and Smith and Weideman (1990). It is suggested that intense (i.e., stressful) exercise would activate the HPA and the sympathoadrenal system with a subsequent release of stress hormones such as epinephrine, ACTH, and cortisol, all of which are known to have potent immunosuppressive properties (Irwin, 1994; Sheridan et al., 1994). Important aspects of the Psychoneuroimmune Hypothesis involve 1) the emergence of corticotrophin releasing hormone (CRH) in the hypothalamus as an important controller of an elaborate neuroendocrine-immune network involved in the integrated response to stress (Irwin, 1994; Sheridan et al., 1994; Blalock, 1994) and 2) an increased importance of various cytokines in eliciting sickness behavior (Hart, 1988; Kent et al., 1992). These interactions are the hallmark of a new field of study called psychoneuroimmunology (PNI) (Blalock, 1994; Dantzer & Kelley, 1989). We believe that these new ideas may help to explain, diagnose, and prevent the various symptoms that many overtrained (overstressed) athletes experience.

Activation of hypothalamic CRH through a combination of physiological/psychological stresses associated with intense training and competition, fluid and carbohydrate depletion, and perhaps hyperthermia would stimulate both the HPA and the sympathoadrenal system to increase the release of the stress hormones epinephrine and cortisol (Irwin, 1994; Sheridan et al., 1994). Increased concentrations of these hormones are likely to explain the immunosuppression that occurs for several hours after an intense bout of exercise (i.e., Open Window Hypothesis). It is further hypothesized that this may occur in addition to the more chronic, albeit lesser in magnitude, stimulation of CRH due to psychological stress, overall nutritional inadequacies, inflammatory cytokine release resulting from muscle damage, and perhaps low-level endotoxemia. It is important to note that the increase in cortisol concentration that normally follows acute periods of stress has important

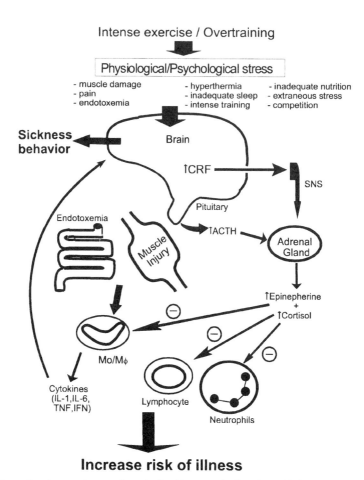

Intense exercise / Overtraining

Physiological/Psychological stress
- muscle damage
- pain
- endotoxemia

- hyperthermia
- inadequate sleep
- intense training

- inadequate nutrition
- extraneous stress
- competition

Sickness behavior

Brain

↑CRF

SNS

Pituitary

Endotoxemia

Muscle Injury

↑ACTH

Adrenal Gland

↑Epinepherine + ↑Cortisol

⊖

⊖

⊖

Mo/Mφ

Lymphocyte

Neutrophils

Cytokines (IL-1,IL-6, TNF,IFN)

Increase risk of illness

FIGURE 7-6. *Psychoneuroimmune hypothesis of immune dysfunction with intense exercise and overtraining.* This model suggests that the increased risk of illness and other symptoms of overtraining (decreased performance and sickness behavior) may be at least partially explained by immune system alterations. Repeated periods of intense exercise and other stresses would stimulate hypothalamic CRH activity. This would increase plasma concentrations of both cortisol and epinephrine, causing an inhibition of neutrophil, lymphocyte, and monocyte/macrophage function and an increased risk of illness. The increase in cortisol would also suppress the release of pro-inflammatory cytokines and exacerbate the associated symptoms that may result from muscle/tissue damage. On a more chronic basis, a down-regulation of the HPA axis might lessen the immune suppression but increase the inflammatory response to new or existing injury and infection. The resulting increase in inflammatory cytokines would exaggerate and prolong the negative symptoms (inflammation, sickness behavior, and decreased performance) that occur with overtraining.

functions with respect to suppressing the inflammatory response and associated symptoms, and protecting against excessive tissue damage following infection and injury. It would therefore seem that a normal response to intense exercise might be a short-lived immunosuppression that might leave one slightly more susceptible to infection but that helps to dampen the potentially more destructive influence of the inflammatory response. Unfortunately, in the case of overtraining, the more chronic stress may downregulate the HPA and sympathoadrenal axis (Kuipers & Keizer, 1988; Barron et al., 1985) such that disinhibition of the immune system may lead to an exaggerated inflammatory response. This would include inflammatory cytokine release (perhaps in the tissues and not readily detectable in plasma), exaggerated tissue damage, and increased symptoms of sickness behavior that would remain for extended periods and require a long time to recover (Dantzer & Kelley, 1989; Kent et al., 1992; Rohatimer et al., 1983; Schobitz et al., 1994; Smedley et al., 1983) (Figure 7-6). Clearly, however, a systematic investigation of the primary tenants of this hypothesis is required before any or all of its components can be validated. In the interim, the psychoneuroimmune hypothesis may serve a theoretical framework from which to design much needed research in this area.

PRACTICAL IMPLICATIONS

Exercise of high intensity and volume is both necessary and irreplaceable in training for many competitive sports. As reviewed here, this type of work is associated with a variety of detrimental effects on immune function. Although scarce data are available to directly link this immunosuppression to increased rates of infection, the association is logical. Therefore, added measures should be taken to protect the athlete against infection, as well as to prevent the overtraining syndrome from occurring in the first place (Table 7-3).

Based on the overtraining studies reviewed in this chapter, the most consistent as well as easiest way to identify an overtrained athlete is through a subjective evaluation of performance and fatigue. We recommend that athletes maintain log books that, in addition to the training records kept by many athletes already, contain ratings of fatigue and stress levels. A specific tool to identify training-induced distress in athletes is being developed by Raglin and Morgan (1994) and may prove useful in the near future. This scale uses seven items from the Profile of Mood States (POMS) questionnaire, items designed to evaluate depression and/or anger. The prediction rate for distress was 69% in the swimmers on whom it was developed, and a 67% prediction rate in a cross-validation study of track-and-field athletes. Before recommending further use, the authors are verifying and testing the seven-item scale. Coaches and athletes alike should be looking for decreased/stale performance accompanied by increased levels of stress and fatigue. These variables should be monitored in athletes and their training schedules should be adjusted accordingly in an effort to avoid the overtrained state. Even before signs of overtraining occur, it should be recognized that adequate rest is necessary between competitions and hard days of training.

Guidelines for decreasing risk of infections have already been suggested by Nieman (1994). These suggestions include keeping other stresses to a minimum, obtaining adequate sleep, not losing weight too rapidly, and eating a well-balanced diet. Because stimulation of the HPA axis and the resultant release of the glucocorticoids and catecholamines can be immunosuppressive, it may be that the strategies outlined by Nieman can decrease the activation of this axis, perhaps by decreasing metabolic, psychological, or physical stress. It may be a valuable practice for athletes to record, in addition to workouts and signs of overtraining, body weight and the quality/quantity of sleep and other life stressors they perceive to be significant. Variance in these measures may be warning signs of infection and/or overtraining. Another preventative measure that can be taken by athletes during heavy training is the consumption of carbohydrate-containing beverages during their workout. There are preliminary reports that carbohydrate-electrolyte drinks can attenuate the relative perceived exertion as well as the release of the stress hormones cortisol and epinephrine during prolonged intense exercise (Burgess, et al, 1991; Davis et al., 1989; Deuster et al., 1992; Murray et al., 1989; Slentz et al., 1990) and limit some of the negative effects on immune function (Nieman et al., 1996). Carbohydrate feedings may also prove beneficial in avoiding the overtraining syndrome by minimizing the depletion of bodily carbohydrate stores; carbohydrate depletion during successive days of intense training may contribute to the overtraining syndrome (Costill et al., 1988; Kirwan et al., 1988).

There are also ways to directly minimize exposure to cold and flu viruses. As Eichner (1995) has pointed out, a common way in which in-

---

TABLE 7-3. *Practical Implications For Reducing the Risk of Overtraining, Immune Dysfunction, and Infection.*

- Allow for adequate recovery between days of competition or hard training.
- Maintain logs of performance and ratings of fatigue and stressful experiences; adjust training schedules accordingly to avoid the risk of overtraining.
- Keep psychological stresses to a minimum, obtain adequate sleep, do not lose weight too rapidly, eat a well-balanced diet, and "listen to your body" for abnormal symptoms.
- Back off intense training when symptoms appear.
- Do frequent dietary analyses and seek nutritional guidance to ensure optimal nutrition
- Avoid exposure to infectious agents — do not share drinking vessels, avoid sick people, wash hands frequently, etc.
- Take flu shots and consider hepatitis vaccinations for those in contact sports.
- Follow the "neck check" rule for deciding whether or not to continue training when sick.

fections are passed among teammates is through the sharing of cups, squeeze bottles, and ice. These practices should be discouraged. It may also prove beneficial, particularly in winter season sports, for athletes to receive flu shots. Those involved in contact sports may want to be immunized against hepatitis, which can be spread through direct contact.

Eichner (1995) has also provided recommendations for continued exercise once an athlete is sick. In what he calls the "neck check," the location of symptoms determines whether the athlete may continue to exercise or should rest. If the symptoms are "above the neck," such as a runny nose, sneezing, or a sore throat (i.e., symptoms of URTI), an athlete should begin the workout with 10 min at half-speed. If the athlete feels better, a normal workout can begin. If, however, symptoms are "below the neck," such as nausea, aching muscles, and a hacking cough, the athlete should avoid exercise while symptoms persist. These systemic symptoms are indicative of viral infection, and exercise should be avoided in this situation due to the known risk of viral cardiomyopathy with intense exercise (Sharp, 1989). These types of precautionary measures are particularly important for athletes who may be showing initial signs of overtraining.

Recent experimental evidence provides support for the "neck check" rule (Weidner et al., 1995). Moderately fit subjects were inoculated with rhinovirus-16, a strain of the common cold. Thirty-four of the subjects then exercised every other day for 40 min at 70% of heart-rate reserve for 10 d, while 16 subjects remained sedentary. There were no significant differences between the groups in the severity or duration of the URTI. This group of investigators has also recently reported that an upper respiratory tract infection does not limit submaximal or maximal exercise performance (Anderson et al., 1995; Cranston et al., 1995). These results provide some substantiation for the "neck check" rule in that exercise did not further exacerbate the symptoms that occurred with rhinovirus-induced URTI. It must be noted, for the purposes of this review, that this study employed moderately-intense exercise in moderately fit subjects, and the results may not necessarily apply to an overtrained population.

SUMMARY

Maximal athletic performance is not possible without heavy (stressful) training. However, there is a fine line between optimal training and overtraining that is counterproductive and unhealthy. Overtraining can lead to a complex syndrome of multiple signs and symptoms (only some of which may be present in an individual athlete), including impaired performance, exaggerated fatigue throughout the day, sore muscles, nausea, loss of appetite, mood swings, and increased susceptibility to infection.

It is logical to assume that the increased risk of infection results from exercise-induced suppression of various immune system components, especially those of the innate immune system, which serves as a first line of defense against foreign pathogens. However, it is still not clear to what extent these relatively small changes in immune function represent meaningful changes in overall host defense, and there are few data to directly link the apparent immunosuppression to increased rates of infection in athletes following intense exercise. Even less is known about the extent to which immune dysfunction may play a role in the various symptoms of overtraining.

Studies on overtraining and immune function are limited in number and study design. Little progress has been made in this area for a number of reasons, including a fundamental problem involving the diagnosis of overtraining in which there are no clearly established criteria. Indeed, there is increasing support for the position that the overtraining syndrome is not a distinct entity but a continuum of related symptoms that may have different etiologies. Nevertheless, it seems reasonable, based on the increasing evidence of immune dysfunction following acute bouts of intense exercise and the existing literature on stress immunology, that many of the symptoms of overtraining may involve alterations in immune function.

A psychoneuroimmune hypothesis was briefly outlined to help explain the etiology of various symptoms associated with overtraining and to possibly lead to prevention strategies. This hypothesis is based on exciting new discoveries in the field of psychoneuroimmunology. Good evidence now exists to link the central nervous system, endocrine system, and immune system in an elaborate network that responds to alterations in homeostasis, including both physiological and psychological stressors. Hypothalamic CRH lies at the center of this network and can respond to and control various stress hormones and cytokines whose actions may underlie many of the adverse effects of overtraining in athletes.

There are apparently no good markers of overtraining that can be used by athletes to determine when their training is going beyond that to which they are able to healthfully adapt. Prevention strategies should include ways to limit excessive metabolic, psychological, or physical stressors associated with intense training and competition, as well as to limit exposure to infectious agents. Because athletes must train very hard to achieve maximal performance, a premium should be placed on reducing extraneous stress such as inadequate recovery time, loss of sleep, rapid weight loss, and poor nutrition.

BIBLIOGRAPHY

Adams, D.O., and T.A. Hamilton (1984). Cell biology of macrophage activation. *Annu. Rev. Immunol.* 2:283–318.

Adams, F., J.R. Quesada, and J.U. Gutterman (1984). Neuropsychiatric manifestations of human leukocyte interferon therapy in patients with cancer. *J.A.M.A.* 252:38–94.

Ader, R., N. Cohen, and D.L. Felten (eds.) (1991). *Psychoneuroimmunology* (2nd ed.). San Diego: Academic Press.

Anderson, B.N., T.G. Weidner, L.A. Kaminsky, and T. Schurr (1995). The effect of an upper respiratory infection on pulmonary function and maximal exercise capacity. *Med. Sci. Sports Exerc.* 27(5): S176.

Baj, Z., J. Kantorski, E. Majewska, K. Zeman, L. Pokoca, E. Fornalczyk, H. Tchorzewski, Z. Sulowska, and R. Lewicki (1994). Immunological status of competitive cyclists before and after the training season. *Int. J. Sports Med.* 15:319–324.

Barron, J.L., T.D. Noakes, W. Levy, C. Smith, and R.P. Millar (1985). Hypothalamic dysfunction in overtrained athletes. *J. Clin. Endo. Met.* 60:803–806.

Beiger, W.P., M. Weiss, G. Michne, and H. Weicker (1980). Exercise-induced monocytosis and modulation of immune function. *Int. J. Sports Med.* 1:30–36.

Blalock, J.E. (1994). The syntax of immune-neuroendocrine communication. *Immun. Today* 15:504–511.

Bosenberg, A.T., J.G. Brock-Utne, S.L. Gaffin, M. Wells, and G. Blake (1988). Strenuous exercise causes systemic endotoxemia. *J. Appl. Physiol.* 65:106–108.

Bousquet, J., P. Chanez, J. Mercier, and C. Prefaut (1996). Monocytes, exercise, and the inflammatory response. *Exerc. Immunol. Rev.* 2:35–44.

Brenner, I.K., P.N. Shek, R.J. Shephard (1995). Heat exposure and immune function: potential contribution to the exercise response. *Exerc. Immunol. Rev.* 1:49–80.

Brenner, I.K., P.N. Shek, and R.J. Shephard (1994). Infection in athletes. *Sports Med.* 17: 86–107.

Burgess, M.L., R.J. Robertson, J.M. Davis, and J.M. Norris (1991). RPE, blood glucose, and carbohydrate oxidation during exercise: effects of glucose feedings. *Med. Sci. Sports Exerc.* 23(3): 353–359.

Cannon, J.G. (1993). Exercise and resistance to infection. *J. Appl. Physiol.* 74:973–981.

Cannon, J.G., J.L. Nerad, D.D. Poutsiaka, and C.A. Dinarello (1993). Measuring circulating cytokines. *J. Appl. Physiol.* 75:1897–1902.

Chandra, R.K., B. Au, G. Woodford, and P. Hyam (1977). Iron status, immune responses and susceptibility to infection. *CIBA Foundation Symposium* 51:249–268.

Cohen, S., D.A. Tyrell, and A.P. Smith (1991). Psychological stress and susceptibility to the common cold. *New Engl. J. Med.* 325:606–612.

Costill, D.L., and S.H. Park (1988). Effects of repeated days of intensified training on muscle glycogen and swimming performance. *Med. Sci. Sports Exerc.* 20:249–254.

Cranston, T.E., T.G. Weidner, B.N. Anderson, L.A. Kaminsky, and E.C. Dick (1995). The effect of an upper respiratory infection on submaximal physiological responses during graded exercise testing. *Med Sci. Sports Exerc.* 27(5):S176.

Dantzer, R., and K.W. Kelley (1989). Stress and immunity: an integrated view of relationships between the brain and the immune system. *Life Sci.* 44:1,995–2,008.

Davis, J.M., V.E. Cokkinides, W.A. Burgess, and W.P. Bartoli (1989). Effects of a carbohydrate-electrolyte drink or water on the stress hormone response to prolonged intense cycling: Renin, angiotensin 1, aldosterone, ACTH and cortisol. In: Z. Laron & A.D. Rogol (eds.) *Hormones and Sport,* vol. 55. Serono Symposium Publication, Raven Press, N.Y., N.Y., 10036, pp. 193–204.

Davis, J.M., M.L. Kohut, L.H. Colbert, D.A. Jackson, A. Ghaffar, and E.P. Mayer. Exercise, alveolar macrophage function, and susceptibility to respiratory infection. *J. Appl. Physiol.,* in press, 1997.

Davis, J.M., M.L. Kohut, A. Ghaffar, E.P. Mayer, L.M. Hertler, and D.A. Jackson (1994). Effect of exercise on lung tumor metastases and in vitro alveolar macrophage anti-tumor activity. *Med. Sci. Sports Exerc.* 26(suppl.):S33.

Davis, J.M., J.A. Weaver, M.L. Kohut, L.M. Hertler, A. Ghaffar, and E.P. Mayer. Immune system activation and fatigue during treadmill running: role of interferon-α /β. *Med. Sci. Sports Exerc.,* 27(suppl.):S67, 1995.

de LaFuenta, M., M.I. Martin, and E. Ortega (1990). Changes in the phagocytic function of peritoneal macrophages from old mice after strenuous physical exercise. *Comp. Innunol. Microbiol. Infect. Dis.* 13:189–198.

Deuster, P.A., A. Singh, A. Hoffman, F.M. Moses, and G.C. Chrousos (1992). Hormonal responses to ingesting water or a carbohydrate beverage during a 2h run. *Med. Sci. Sports Exerc.* 24:72–79.

Dinarello, C.A. (1984). Interleukin-1 and the pathogenesis of the acute-phase response. *New Engl. J. Med.* 311:1413–1418.

Drenth, J.P.H., S.H.M. Van Uum, M. Van Deuren, G.J. Pesman, J. Van Der Ven-Hongekrijg, and J.W.M. Van Der Meer (1995). Endurance run increases circulation IL-6 and IL -1ra, but downregulates ex vivo TNF-a and IL-1b production. *J. Appl. Physiol.* 79(5):1497–1503.

Dyment, P.G. (1993). Frustrated by chronic fatigue? Try this systematic approach. *Phys. Sports Med.* 21:47–54.

Eichner, E.R. (1995). Contagious infections in competitive sports. *Sports Sci. Exchange.* Gatorade Sports Science Institute. 8(3).

Evans, W.J., and J.G. Cannon. (1991). The metabolic effects of exercise-induced muscle damage. In: J.O. Holloszy (ed.) *Exercise and Sport Sciences Reviews.* Baltimore: Williams & Wilkins, pp. 99–126.

Fehr, H.G., H. Lotzerich, H. Michna (1989). Human macrophage function and physical exercise: phagocytic and histochemical studies. *Eur. J. Appl. Physiol.* 58:613–617.

Field, C.J., R. Gougeon, and E.B. Marliss (1991). Circulating mononuclear cell numbers and function during intense exercise and recovery. *J. Appl. Physiol.* 71:1,089–1,097.

Fitzgerald, L. (1991). Overtraining increases the susceptibility to infection. *Int. J. Sports Med.* 12(Suppl 1):S5–8.

Francesconi, R.P. (1988). Endocrinological responses to exercise in stressful environments. *Exerc. Sports Sci. Rev.* 16:255–284.

Frohlich, J., G. Simon, A. Schmidt, T. Hitschold, and M. Bierther (1987). Disposition to infections of athletes during treatment with immunoglobulins. *Int. J. Sports Med.* 8:119.

Fry, R.W., J.R. Grove, A.R. Morton, P.M. Zeroni, S. Gaudieri, and D. Keast. (1994). Psychological and immunological correlates of acute overtraining. *Br. J. Sports Med.* 28:241–246.

Fry, R.W., A.R. Morton, P. Garcia-Webb, G.P. Crawford, and D. Keast (1992). Biological responses to overload training in endurance sports. *Eur. J. Appl. Physiol.* 64:335–44.

Fry, R.W., A.R. Morton, and D. Keast (1991). Overtraining in athletes—an update. *Sports Med.* 12:32–65.

Gabriel H., L. Brechtel, A. Urhausen, and W. Kindermann (1994a). Recruitment and recirculation of leukocytes after an ultramarathon run: preferential homing of cells expressing high levels of the adhesion molecule LFA-1. *Int. J. Sports Med.* 15:S148–153.

Gabriel, H., L. Schwarz, P. Born, and W. Kindermann (1992a). Differential mobilization of leucocyte and lymphocyte subpopulations into the circulation during endurance exercise. *Eur. J. Appl. Physiol.* 65:529–534.

Gabriel, H., L. Schwarz, G. Steffens, and W. Kindermann (1992b). Immunoregulatory hormones, circulating leukocytes and lymphocyte subpopulations before and after endurance exercise of different intensities. *Int. J. Sports Med.* 13:359–366.

Gabriel, H., A. Urhausen, L. Brechtel, H.J. Muller, and W. Kinderman (1994b). Alterations of regular and mature monocytes are distinct, and dependent on intensity and duration of exercise. *Eur. J. Appl. Physiol.* 69:179–181.

Gabriel, H., A. Urhausen, and W. Kindermann (1991). Circulating leukocyte and lymphocyte subpopulations before and after intensive endurance exercise to exhaustion. *Eur. J. Appl. Physiol.* 63:449–457.

Garagiola, U., M. Buzzetti, E. Cardella, F. Confalonieri, E. Giani, V. Polini, P. Ferrante, R. Mancuso, M. Montanari, E. Grossi, and A. Pecori (1995). Immunological patterns during regular intensive training in athletes: quantification and evaluation of a preventive pharmacological approach. *J. Int. Med. Res.* 23:85–95.

Gray, A.B., R.D. Telford, M. Collins, and M.J. Weidemann (1993). The response of leukocyte subsets and plasma hormones to interval exercise. *Med. Sci. Sports Exerc.* 25:1,252–1,258.

Hack, V., G. Strobel, M. Weiss, and H. Weicker (1994). PMN cell counts and phagocytic activity of highly trained athletes depend on training period. *J. Appl. Physiol.* 77:1,731–1,735.

Hansen, J.B., L. Wilsgar, and B. Osterud (1991). Biphasic changes in leukocytes induced by strenuous exercise. *Eur. J. Appl. Physiol.* 62:157–161.

Heath, G.W., E.S. Ford, T.E. Craven, C.A. Macera, K.L. Jackson, and R.R. Pate (1991). Exercise and the incidence of upper respiratory tract infections. *Med. Sci. Sports Exerc.* 23:152–157.

Hoffman-Goetz, L., and B.K. Pedersen (1994). Exercise and the immune system: a model of the stress response? *Immunol. Today* 15:382–387.

Hooper, S.L., L.T. Mackinnon, A. Howard, R.D. Gordon, and A.W. Bachmann (1995). Markers for monitoring overtraining and recovery. *Med. Sci. Sports Exerc.* 27:106–12.

Irwin, M. (1994). Stress-induced immune suppression: role of brain corticotropin releasing hormone and autonomic nervous system mechanisms. *Adv. Neuroimmunol.* 4:29–47.

Johnson, K.J., J. Varani, and J.E. Smolen (1992). Neutrophil activation and function in health and disease. *Immunol. Ser.* 57:1–46.

Kappel, M., M. Diamant, M. Hansen, M. Klokker, and B.K. Pederson (1991a). Effects of hyperthermia in vitro on proliferative responses of individual blood mononuclear cell subsets, interferon lymphotoxin, tumor necrosis factor, interleukin 1,2, and 6. *Immunology*, 73:304–308.

Kappel, M., A. Kharazmi, H. Nielsen, A. Gyhrs, and B.K. Pedersen (1994). Modulation of the counts and functions of neutrophils and monocytes under in vivo hyperthermia conditions. *Int. J. Hyperthermia.* 10:165–173.

Kappel, M., C. Stadeager, N. Tvede, H. Galbo, and B.K. Pedersen (1991b). Effect of in vivo hyperthermia on natural killer cell activity, in vitro proliferative responses and blood mononuclear cell subpopulation. *Clin. Exp. Immunol.* 84:175–180.

Kappel, M., N. Tvede, H. Galbo, P.M. Haahr, M. Kjaer, M. Linstouw, K. Klarlund, and B.K. Pedersen (1991c). Evidence that the effect of physical exercise on natural killer cell activity is mediated by epinephrine. *J. Appl. Physiol.* 70:2,530–2,534.

Keast, D., D. Arstein, W. Harper, R.W. Fry, and A.R. Morton (1995). Depression of plasma glutamine concentration after exercise stress and its possible influence on the immune system. *Med. J. Aust.* 162:15–18.

Kent, S., R.M. Bluthe, K.W. Kelley, and R. Dantzer (1992). Sickness behavior as a new target for drug development. *Trends. Pharmacol. Sci.* 13:24–28.

Kirwin, J.P., D.L. Costill, J.B. Mitchell, J.A. Houmard, M.G. Flynn, W.J. Fink, and J.D. Beltz (1988). Carbohydrate balance in competitive runners during successive days of intense training. *J. Appl. Physiol.* 65:2,601–2,606.

Kluger, M.J., H. Ashton, J. Doshi, P.S. Hein, J.S. Newby, and R.S. Philips (1993). Letter to the Editor. *Med. Sci. Sports Exerc.* 25:303–304.

Kuipers, H., and H.A. Keizer (1988). Overtraining in elite athletes: review and future directions. *Sports Med.* 6:79–92.

Lee, D.J., R.T. Meehan, C. Robinson, T.R. Mabry, and M.L. Smith (1992). Immune responsiveness and risk of illness in U.S. Air Force Academy cadets during basic cadet training. *Aviat. Space Environ. Med.* 63:517–523.

Lehmann, M., H.H. Dickhuth, G. Gendrisch, W. Lazar, M. Thum, R. Kaminski, J.F. Aramendi, E. Peterke, W. Wieland, and J. Keul (1991). Training-overtraining. A prospective, experimental study with experienced middle- and long-distance runners. *Int. J. Sports Med.* 12:444–452.

Linde, F. (1987). Running and upper respiratory tract infections. *Scand. J. Sport Sci.* 9:21–23.

Mackinnon, L.T. (1996). Immunoglobulin, antibody, and exercise. *Exerc. Immunol.* 2:1–35.

Mackinnon, L.T., and S. Hooper (1994). Mucosal (secretory) immune system responses to exercise of varying intensity and during overtraining. *Int. J. Sports Med.* 15:S179–183.

Mackinnon, L.T., and S. Hooper (1996). Plasma glutamine and upper respiratory tract infection during intensified training in swimmers. *Med. Sci. Sports Exerc.* 28:285–290.

Mackinnon, L.T., and D.G. Jenkins (1993). Decreased salivary immunoglobulins after intense interval exercise before and after training. *Med. Sci. Sports Exerc.* 25:678–683.

Mackinnon, L.T., E.M. Ginn, and G.J. Seymour (1993). Temporal relationship between decreased salivary IgA and upper respiratory tract infection in elite athletes. *Austr. J. Sci. Med. Sport.* 25:94–99.

McDowell, S.L., K. Chalos, T.J. Housh, G.D. Tharp, and G.O. Johnson (1991). The effect of exercise intensity and duration on salivary immunoglobulin A. *Eur. J. Appl. Physiol.* 63:108–111.

Michna, H. (1988). The human macrophage system: activity and functional morphology. *Bibl. Anat.* 31:1–83.

Michna, H. (1989). Ultrastructural features of skeletal muscle in mice after physical exercise: its relation to the pathogenesis of leukocyte invasion. *Acta Anat.* 134:276–282.

Muir, A.L., Cruz, M., Martin, B.A, Thommasen, H., Belzberg, A., and J.C. Hogg (1984). Leukocyte kinetics in the human lung: role of exercise and catecholamines. *J. Appl. Physiol.* 57(3):711–719.

Muns, G. (1993). Effect of long-distance running on polymorphonuclear neutrophil phagocytic function of the upper airways. *Int. J. Sports Med.* 15(2):96–99.

Muns, G., I. Rubinstein, and P. Singer (1996). Neutrophil chemotactic activity is increased in nasal secretions of long-distance runners. *Int. J. Sports Med.* 17(1):56–59.

Muns, G., P. Singer, F. Wolf, and I. Rubinstein (1995). Impaired nasal mucociliary clearance in long-distance runners. *Int. J. Sports Med.* 16:209–213.

Murray, R., G.L. Paul, J.G. Seifert, D.E. Eddy, and G.A. Halaby (1989). The effects of glucose, fructose, and sucrose ingestion during exercise. *Med. Sci. Sports Exerc.* 21(3):275–282.

Newsholme, E.A. (1994). Biochemical mechanisms to explain immunosuppression in well-trained and overtrained athletes. *Int. J. Sports Med.* 15:S142–S147.

Nieman, D.C. (1992). Exercise, immunity, and respiratory infections. *Sports Science Exchange.* Gatorade Sports Science Institute. 4(39).

Nieman, D.C. (1994). Exercise, infection, and immunity. *Int. J. Sports Med.* 15:S131–141.

Nieman, D.C. (1996). Prolonged aerobic exercise, immune response, and risk of infection. In: L. Hoffman-Goetz. (ed.) *Exercise and The Immune Function.* Boca Raton, FL: CRC Press. pp. 143–161.

Nieman, D.C., and S.L. Nehlsen-Cannarella (1992). Exercise and infection. In: R.W. Watson and M. Eisinger (eds). *Exercise and Disease.* Boca Raton: CRC Press, pp. 121–143.

Nieman, D.C., L.M. Johanssen, J.W. Lee, and K. Arabatzis (1990). Infectious episodes in runners before and after the Los Angeles Marathon. *J. Sports Med. Phys. Fitness.* 30:316–328.

Nieman, D.C., A.R. Miller, D.A. Henson, B.J. Warren, G. Gusewitch, R.L. Johnson, J.M. Davis, D.E. Butterworth, and S.L. Nehlsen-Cannarella (1993). Effects of high- vs moderate-intensity exercise on natural killer cell activity. *Med. Sci. Sports Exerc.* 25:1,126–34.

Nieman, D.C., S. Simandle, D.A. Henson, B.J. Warren, J. Suttles, J.M. Davis, K.S. Buckley, J.C. Ahle, D.E. Butterworth, O.R. Fagoaga, and S.L. NehlsenCannarella (1995). Lymphocyte proliferative response to 2.5 hours of running. *Int. J. Sports Med.* 16:406–410.

Northoff, H., C. Weinstock, A. Berg (1994). The cytokine response to strenuous exercise. *Int. J. Sports Med.* 15:S167–171.

Ortega E. (1994). Physiology and biochemistry: influence of exercise on phagocytosis. *Int .J. Sports Med.* 15:S172–178.

Ortega, E., M.E. Collazos, C. Barriga, and M. De la Fuente (1992). Effect of physical activity stress on the phagocytic process of peritoneal macrophages from old guinea pigs. *Mech. Ageing Dev.* 65:157–165.

Parker, S., and P. Brukner (1994). Is your sportsperson suffering from chronic fatigue syndrome? *Sports Health* 12:15–17.

Parry-Billings, M., R. Budgett, Y. Koutedakis, E. Blomstrand, S. Brooks, C. Williams, P.C. Calder, S. Pilling, R. Baigrie, and E.A. Newsholme (1992). Plasma amino acid concentrations in the overtraining syndrome: possible effects on the immune system. *Med. Sci. Sports Exerc.* 24:1,353–1,358.

Pedersen, B.K., and H. Ullum (1994). NK cell response to physical activity: possible mechanisms of action. *Med. Sci. Sports Exerc.* 26:140–146.

Pedersen, B.K., M. Kappel, M. Klokker, H.B. Nielsen, and N.H. Secher (1994). The immune system during exposure to extreme physiologic conditions. *Int. J. Sports Med.* 15:S116–121.

Peters, E.M., and E.D. Bateman (1983). Ultramarathon running and upper respiratory tract infections. An epidemiological survey. *S. Afr. Med. J.* 64:582–584.

Peters, E.M., J.M. Goetzsche, B. Grobbelaar, and T.D. Noakes (1993). Vitamin C supplementation reduces the incidence of postrace symptoms of upper-respiratory-tract infection in ultramarathon runners. *Am. J. Clin. Nutr.* 57:170–174.

Pyne, D.B. (1994). Regulation of neutrophil function during exercise. *Sports Med.* 17(4):245–258.

Pyne, D.B., M.S. Baker, P.A. Fricker, W.A. McDonald, R.D. Telford, and M.J. Weidemann (1995). Effects of an intensive 12–wk training program by elite swimmers on neutrophil oxidative activity. *Med. Sci. Sports Exerc.* 27:536–542.

Raglin, J.S., and W.P. Morgan (1994). Development of a scale for use in monitoring training-induced distress in athletes. *Int J. Sports Med.* 15:84–88.

Rainwater, M.K., D.C. Nieman, and S.A. Thomas (1995). *Compendium of the exercise immunology literature*. Paderborn, Germany: International Society of Exercise and Immunology.

Rhind, S.G., P.N. Shek, and R.J. Shephard (1995). The impact of exercise on cytokines and receptor expression. *Exerc. Immunol. Rev.* 1:97–148.

Rincon, E.O. (1994). Physiology and biochemistry: influence of exercise on phagocytosis. *Int J Sports Med.*, 15:S172–S178.

Roitt, I.M., J. Brostoff, and D.K. Male (1993). In: *Immunology* (3rd ed.) London: Gower Medical Publishers pp. 1.1–1.12, 7.1–7.16.

Robertson, M.J., and J. Ritz (1990). Biology and clinical relevance of human natural killer cells. *Blood* 76:2,421–2,438.

Rohatimer, A.Z.S., P.F. Prior, A.C. Burton, A.T. Smith, F.R. Balkwill, and T.A. Lister (1983). Central nervous system toxicity of interferon. *Brit. J. Cancer* 47:419–422.

Rowbottom, D.G., D. Keast, C. Goodman, and A.R. Morton (1995). The hematological, biochemical, and immunological profile of athletes suffering from the overtraining syndrome. *Eur. J. Appl. Physiol.* 70:502–509.

Schobitz, B., E.R. deKloet, and F. Holsboer (1994). Gene expression and function of interleukin-1, interleukin-6, and tumor necrosis factor in the brain. *Prog. Neurobiol.* 44:397–432.

Selye, H. (1983). The stress concept: past, present, and future. In: *Stress Research*, C.L. Cooper (ed.) New York: Wiley, pp. 1–20.

Sharp, J.C.M. (1989). Viruses and the athlete. *Br. J. Sports Med.* 23:47.

Shephard, R.J., and P.N. Shek (1995). Heavy exercise, nutrition and immune function: is there a connection? *Int. J. Sports Med.* 8:491–497.

Sheridan, J.F., C. Dobbs, D. Brown, and B. Zwilling (1994). Psychoneuroimmunology: stress effects on pathogenesis and immunity during infection. *Clin. Microbiol. Rev.* 7:200–212.

Sherman, W.M., and E.W. Maglischo (1991). Minimizing chronic athletic fatigue among swimmers: special emphasis on nutrition. In: *Sports Science Exchange.* Gatorade Sports Science Institute. 4(35).

Shinkai, S., S. Shore, P.N. Shek, and R.J. Shephard (1992). Acute exercise and immune function. Relationship between lymphocyte activity and changes in subset counts. *Int. J. Sports Med.* 13:169–173.

Singh, A., M.L. Failla, and P.A. Deuster (1994). Exercise-induced changes in immune function: effects of zinc supplementation. *J. Appl. Physiol.* 76:2,298–2,303.

Slentz, C.A., J.M. Davis, D.L. Settles, R.R. Pate, and S.J. Settles (1990). Glucose feedings and exercise in rats: glycogen use, hormone responses, and performance. *J. Appl. Physiol.* 69(3):989–994.

Smedley, H., M. Katrak, K. Sikora, and T. Wheeler (1983). Neurological effects of recombinant human interferon. *Br. med. J.* 286:262–264.

Smith, J.A. (1995). Guidelines, standards, and perspectives in exercise immunology. *Med. Sci. Sports Exerc.* 27(4):497–506.

Smith, J.A., and M.J. Weidemann (1990). The exercise and immunity paradox: a neuro-endocrine/cytokine hypothesis. *Med. Sci. Res.* 18:749–753.

Smith, J.A., R.D. Telford, I.B. Mason, and M.J. Weidemann (1990). Exercise, training, and neutrophil microbicidal activity. *Int. J. Sports Med.* 11:179–187.

Strasner, A., J.M. Davis, M.L. Kohut, R.R. Pate, A. Ghaffar, E. Mayer (1997). Effects of exercise intensity on natural killer cell activity in women. *Int. J. Sports Med.* 18:56–62.

Tidball, J.G. (1995). Inflammatory cell response to acute muscle injury. *Med. Sci. Sports Exerc.* 27:1022–1032.

Tonnesen, E., N.J. Christensen, and M.M. Brinklov (1987). Natural killer cell activity during cortisol and epinephrine infusion in healthy volunteers. *J. Clin. Invest.* 17:497–503.

Tvede, N., C. Heilmann, J. Halkjaer-Kristensen, and B.K. Pedersen (1989). Mechanisms of B lymphocyte suppression induced by acute physical exercise. *J. Clin. Lab. Immunol.* 30:169–173.

Tvede, N., M. Kappel, K. Klarlund, S. Duhn, J. Halkjaer-Kristensen, M. Kjaer, H. Galbo, and B.K. Pedersen (1994). Evidence that the effect of bicycle exercise on blood mononuclear cell proliferative responses and subsets is mediated by epinephrine. *Int. J. Sports Med.* 15:100–104.

Tvede, N., B.K. Pedersen, F.R. Hansen, T. Bendix, L.D. Christensen, H. Galbo, and J. Halkjaer-Kristensen (1989). Effect of physical exercise on blood mononuclear cell subpopulations and in vitro proliferative responses. *Scand. J. Immunol.* 29:383–389.

Urhausen, A., H. Gabriel, and W. Kindermann (1995). Blood hormones as markers of training stress and overtraining. *Sports Med.* 20:251–276.

Verde, T., S. Thomas, and R.J. Shephard (1992). Potential markers of heavy training in highly trained distance runners. *Br. J. Sports Med.* 26:167–175.

Weidner, T.G., T.E. Cranston, L.A. Kaminsky, E.C. Dick, T.S. Schurr, and T. Sevier (1995). The effect of exercise training on the severity and duration of an upper respiratory illness. *Int. Soc. Exerc. Immunol. Conf. Proceedings.* p. 65.

Weiss, S.J. (1989). Tissue destruction by neutrophils. *N. Engl. J. Med.* 320:365–376.

Westerman, J. (1990). Lymphocyte subsets in the blood: a diagnostic window on the lymphoid system? *Immun. Today* 11:406–410.

Woods, J.A., and J.M. Davis (1995). Exercise, monocyte/ macrophage function, and cancer. *Med. Sci. Sports Exerc.* 26:147–156.

Woods, J.A., J.M. Davis, M.L. Kohut, A. Ghaffar, E.P. Mayer, and R.R. Pate (1994). Effects of exercise on the immune response to cancer. *Med. Sci. Sports Exerc.* 26:1,109–1,115.

Woods, J.A., J.M. Davis, E.P. Mayer, A. Ghaffar, and R.R. Pate (1993). Exercise increases inflammatory macrophage antitumor cytotoxicity. *J. Appl. Physiol.* 75:879–886.

DISCUSSION

NIEMAN: Mark, your review has a unique emphasis on overtraining, for which you are to be commended. The integrative model you present is excellent in many respects. I want to confirm a few points and address some areas of concern. First, there have been quite a few surveys and epidemiologic studies confirming the anecdotal reports of an increased risk of infection among athletes who are training very heavily or who have recently completed very heavy exertion such as ultra-marathons or marathons. Exercise immunologists have directed their research either a) toward finding out if chronic immunosuppression exists among athletes who are going through periods of overtraining or b) toward characterizing immune function immediately following an exercise event. There are few investigations testing the hypothesis that there is some type of chronic immunosuppression in athletes; results of these studies are inconsistent, and so far no one has come up with a measure of immune function that can predict who is going to get sick and who is not.

Some feel that the "open window" theory best fits the epidemiologic data, i.e., during the first 3–12 h following heavy exertion, the immune system is suppressed. If the athlete has been exposed to a virus before, during, or after the exertion, the virus can replicate, gain a foothold, and then lead some athletes to get sick. However, in our Los Angeles study, only 1 out of 7 athletes got sick during the week after this winter's marathon. So, although there is a risk, the majority of the athletes get through just fine. The odds are 6:1 that the athletes who are running a marathon will get sick vs. those marathon runners who don't compete in a particular race. These odds are high, but the actual percentage of runners who get sick is not very high.

DAVIS: There are two ways of looking at it. It could mean that immune suppression, probably resulting from an increase in circulating stress hormones, is not very powerful so there are only a few athletes afflicted with modest clinical outcomes. The other explanation is that the only time an athlete will get sick is upon exposure to a particular pathogen. We don't know the level of exposure in the epidemiological studies, so we don't know the exact clinical significance of a weak suppression of immune function.

NIEMAN: I agree. There have been some attempts to control the exposure and determine whether changes in immune variables predict who is going to get sick and who isn't. So far those studies have been largely unsuccessful. Perhaps I can just add that we studied these LA marathoners in March. Forty percent of the runners reported sickness during the 2 mo prior to the race, and 13% during the week after. When we studied 330 runners during the week after they ran a marathon in July, only 3% got sick. We assume that the runners in the winter were exposed to a higher dose of viruses.

DAVIS: We have inoculated mice nasally with a virus and found them to be more susceptible to respiratory infection after they have exercised exhaustively than after moderate exercise or no exercise. I think it would be instructive if a similar study were done in human beings.

NIEMAN: We have run marathoners for 2.5 h at race pace and attempted to measure how immune cells react to that level of exertion, which induces high concentrations of circulating epinephrine. Also, cortisol is elevated for 4–5 h after exercise relative to sitting controls. Meanwhile T-cell function and natural killer cell function are suppressed. Neutrophil phagocytosis is very high following heavy exertion, whereas, the oxidative burst is significantly suppressed. I think these findings agree with your model.

DAVIS: We have measured decreases in the antiviral function of macrophages after strenuous exercise, but other macrophage functions (e.g., anti-cancer functions) can be stimulated.

NIEMAN: I feel that the "Open Window" theory best explains the data. The question is, can the athlete follow certain practices to attenuate the rise in stress hormones? We have studied carbohydrate ingestion and its effect on the stress hormones and immune response. We found that T-cell function was not as suppressed in the carbohydrate-fed runners. Natural killer cells, however, were not affected. NK cells appear to be unaffected by changes in cortisol in this research condition. We also found that the neutrophil phagocyte function was much higher in the placebo group.

GISOLFI: We have recently demonstrated that with high-intensity exercise (i.e., 80% $\dot{V}O_2$max for 60 min) there is an increase in gut permeability, which presumably exposes the gut mucosa to chemotactic oligopeptides, endotoxin, and bacteria. Presumably, these factors stimulate macrophages, which in turn lead to the cytokine cascade. It is also interesting that glucose and glutamine may help to prevent this reduction in gut barrier function.

DAVIS: There is at least one report already published in the literature of endotoxemia occurring in very intense exercise.

KENNEY: Like any other emerging area of research, there is a tendency for scientific papers to over interpret and misinterpret the data somewhat. One example is the Heath study that you mentioned earlier on URTI. The take-home message often quoted from that study is that the runners who ran more than 17 mi/wk had twice the odds ratio of having an URTI than those running less than 10 mi/wk. But the higher mileage group averaged only one URTI/y, and the lower mileage group averaged 0.5 URTI/y. Furthermore, they pointed out in that paper that published data for non-exercisers shows an URTI rate of about 4/y. So while we are saying that running a lot doubles your risk, it is a very low risk, and the risk is much lower than for non-exercisers.

DAVIS: All of the studies have their weaknesses, but overall I think it is safe to say that from the epidemiological studies we can conclude with a great deal of confidence that there is a small increase in the risk for susceptibility to URTI.

KENNEY: Let me give you an example of what I consider to be an experimental misinterpretation of data. In the Muns data showing a large increase in the total PMNs after exercise, but a rather large percentage decrease in those that were functionally phagocytizing, the interpretation was that exercise decreases the function of circulating PMNs. But if you multiply the two, the large increase in number and the percentage decrease in function, you still have twice as many functional PMNs after exercise as before. You might interpret that as an improvement in immune function with exercise rather than a suppression.

DAVIS: I agree with you. It is difficult to do exact calculations, but if you factor in also the fact that each neutrophil that was functioning was not ingesting many of the bacteria, the bottom line would be a suppression in immune function, even though the total number of neutrophils increased.

KANTER: Do you have any insights into some of the nutritional effects on immune response?

DAVIS: I think nutritional deprivation or inadequate nutrition is interpreted as a physiological stress by the body. Inadequate carbohydrate, dehydration, inadequate fluids, inadequate intake of a variety of important macronutrients and micronutrients will elicit a stress response, including elevations in the stress hormones, which would result in some suppression of immune function. Adequate availability of carbohydrate, vitamins, and water is very important. I would like to see more replication of vitamin C studies. Vitamin C supplementation during long races in South Africa seemed to decrease the incidence of URTI. If the athletes were vitamin-C deficient, you might expect that supplementation with vitamin C in those circumstances makes sense, but replication of these results is needed. Also, glutamine supplementation needs to be studied more, because exercise often seems to decrease circulating glutamine, and glutamine plays an important role in immune function. Antioxidants such as vitamin E have important effects on some of the functions of the immune system. Any stress brought on by inadequate nutrition should translate into immune suppression; therefore, an athlete who tries to maintain appropriate or adequate nutrition should be better off than one who does not.

DISHMAN: It strikes me that you really describe a conundrum in the exploration of overtraining. Ethical constraints against inducing an infection or vulnerability to infection and technological constraints that require the harvesting of immune cells from lymphoid tissues dictates a fairly heavy reliance on animal models. Using an animal model brings with it an inherent confounding, perhaps necessary and rightfully so, of the exertional stress of exercise with the emotional stress of exercise because most animal training modes require forced activity. Were the mice in your model showing increased mortality accommodated to a treadmill protocol prior to the exhaustion bout?

DAVIS: They were accommodated. Rats require a very long accommodation period before they will run on a treadmill to exhaustion without shock. We do not use shock motivation for mice because they are great runners. In about 3 d of acclimation to the treadmill, mice will run to volitional fatigue. The only motivation we use is a flick on their hindquarters once in awhile to keep them running at the front of the treadmill. It is undoubtedly not emotion free for the mice, but they will run for 2–3 h before they voluntarily decide to quit.

DISHMAN: In the rat you can easily induce suppression of innate immune responses; a remarkable acute reduction in NK cytotoxicity can be induced with foot shock or with immobilization stress. We have shown in the Fisher rat that 24-h access to voluntary wheel running obliterates NK suppression, and treadmill training also attenuates NK suppression after foot shock; it cuts the NK suppression by about 50%.

Your group has done some remarkable work in rats with an intracranial self-stimulation (ICSS) model to facilitate voluntary running on the treadmill. Have you thought about trying to tease out metabolic aspects of overtraining using the ICSS model? I assume you could induce a metabolically overtrained rat using intracranial self stimulation and compare that with a traditional treadmill overtraining response.

DAVIS: It is very difficult to separate out the types of stresses. Perhaps they even operate together during very intense exercise (i.e., metabolic disturbances), pain, and exhaustion have psychological components associated with them. Unfortunately, by giving the pleasurable pulses of electrical stimulation to the animals, they will run voluntarily until they drop. The problem with that is the brain stimulation will also activate the sympathetic nervous system, so the animals get some increases in stress hormones associated with the increased motivation to run. That would be a confounding effect using that particular model.

DISHMAN: But it might not be a confounding factor with NK suppression because it does not seem as though the NK cell is particularly sensitive to cortisol. We have shown the same thing (i.e., the differences we saw in NK activity were unrelated to ACTH or cortisol or even prolactin levels).

DAVIS: But NK activity is sensitive to epinephrine.

DISHMAN: Right, but it is not sensitive to norepinephrine. There might be ways using appropriate antagonists of sympathetic nerve activity or sympathectomies permitting a controlled test of sympathetic or sympathoadrenomedullary influences on NK activity in an overtraining model.

EICHNER: I want to comment on the clinical import of the exercise-associated immune changes, which are brief, modest, and mixed. Especially after exhaustive exercise, people tend to feel cranky and sore and tired because of exhaustion and the acute-phase response. I would like to see more epidemiologic studies prove that these are URTI rather than just symptoms that laymen check off on a questionnaire. I would like proof via cultures or serology. I think some athletes confuse nonspecific symptoms with URTI.

DAVIS: That would be very difficult to achieve in epidemiological studies of hundreds of subjects. To the extent that animal models are appropriate, one can study infection rates, immune functions, manipulate the variables, standardize the dose of infection, and use different doses of exercise to address those issues.

NIEMAN: In our surveys, we have been careful to prompt the runners to only indicate infectious episodes that conform to a list of symptoms and last two or more days.

SCOTT: Randy Eichner makes an important point, and I would like to describe an example. Runners complain of increased nasal secretions with running and want some medication because they assume that the secretions are caused by an allergy; they are usually simply associated with a humidifying effect during running. Also, the extroverts that volunteer for the studies are probably a bit more neurotic than "normals" and pay attention to their bodily functions. When you use epidemiologic methods, the subjects are not blinded to treatment, they are not randomized to treatment, and the studies are usually not prospective.

NIEMAN: We do use logistic regression, which attempts to control for training variables, demographic variables, and so on. There are epidemiologic techniques to try and tease out the effect of a single variable, but I agree that the epidemiologic approach is only a beginning step.

DAVIS: It is the cumulative evidence produced from a variety of investigative approaches that is needed to gain confidence that a hypothesis is correct. We must weigh the evidence from both the epidemiologic studies and the controlled experimental studies on people and animals and make our judgements.

8

Stay in the Game: Prevention of and Recovery from Sports Injuries

JOHN R. PERRY, M.D.
THOMAS P. KNAPP, M.D.
BERT R. MANDELBAUM, M.D.

INTRODUCTION
INJURY TO THE ANTERIOR CRUCIATE LIGAMENT
    Anatomy
    Biomechanics
    Mechanisms of Injury
    Diagnosis
    Practical Implications
        Treatment Options and Decision Making
        Operative Timing
        Outpatient Reconstruction
        Prevention
        Accelerated Rehabilitation
    Directions for Future Research on Anterior Cruciate Injuries
OSTEOCHONDRAL KNEE INJURIES
    Practical Implications
        Diagnosis
        Treatment
    Directions for Future Research on Osteochondral Knee Injuries
STRESS FRACTURES
    Epidemiology
    Etiology
    Practical Implications
        Diagnosis
        Confirmatory Studies
        Treatment
        Prevention
    Directions for Future Research on Stress Fractures
ANKLE IMPINGEMENT SYNDROMES
    History
    Anatomy

Pathologic Anatomy
Practical Implications
    Diagnosis
    Treatment
    Directions for Future Research on Ankle Impingement Syndromes
SUMMARY
BIBLIOGRAPHY
DISCUSSION

INTRODUCTION

That the field of sports medicine has undergone a tremendous evolution in concept and practice is obvious from a historical perspective. Activity-related injuries and their prevention have been recorded since the Old Testament. In the *Book of Genesis* Jacob, while wrestling with a man, sustained ". . . a hallow in his thigh." The diagnosis was inexact, but the injury was recognized nonetheless. Subsequently, the Chinese, ascribing to the writings of Kung Fu, affirmed the relationship between daily exercise and quality of life. Unfortunately, most early sports injuries in the Greek civilization related to battlefield trauma, but in 762 B.C. the Greeks, in honor of the god Zeus, initiated the first Olympiad. Aristotle, with particular interest in the "marathon" run between Sparta and Athens, noted several injuries among the participants. This prompted Aristotle to declare the "uninjured victors as those who did not squander their powers by early training." In time, Greek physicians influenced by Aristotle and Hippocrates identified the principles of activity-related injuries and developed early treatment protocols. Claudius Galen, a Roman physician, was the first to characterize the relationship between the body and mind in athletics. In addition, he popularized and integrated into his clinical practice the concept that if connective tissues were protected from the stresses of physical activity, they would "waste away." For these contributions, he is often recognized as the first sports medicine physician.

At the end of the 19th century, Darling published his classic text, *"On the Effects of Training."* Paul Dudley White, often recognized as the father of American cardiology, first underscored the adaptive effects of the cardiovascular system to exercise. He described the "athletic heart" syndrome and the mechanical, structural, and physiological responses of the cardiovascular system to physical training.

In the 1960s and '70s the growth and popularity of sports exploded as the media familiarized society with the Olympic Games and a multitude of other athletic competitions. In the 1970s and '80s this interest translated into increased participation in a variety of athletic endeavors, including soccer, gymnastics, marathons, and triathlons.

Presently, with more people playing harder and longer, the sports medicine professional is increasingly confronted with diagnostic and therapeutic challenges that previously were nonexistent. At best, we have only descriptive and epidemiological data regarding the etiology and pathogenesis of these disorders. Consequently and justifiably, athletic injury diagnosis, treatment, and prevention are presently approached in a multidisciplinary fashion. Integrating the contributions of the physician, basic scientist, biomechanical engineer, trainer, physical therapist, podiatrist, chiropractor, nutritionist, and exercise physiologist has facilitated the remarkable achievements realized in sports medicine over the past 20 y. In addition, specialization has permitted sports medicine professionals to focus on specific problems of young, elder, female, and/or elite athletes.

The purpose of this chapter is to illuminate a few areas in orthopedic sports medicine that have developed significantly in the past 20 y. The four topics selected include: 1) injuries to the anterior cruciate ligament of the knee, 2) osteochondral knee injuries, 3) stress fractures, and 4) ankle impingement syndromes. As a result of more effective methods of diagnosis, therapy, rehabilitation, and prevention, athletes sidelined with these injuries are now returning to their respective sports more quickly and efficaciously.

INJURY TO THE ANTERIOR CRUCIATE LIGAMENT

Anatomy

The anterior cruciate ligament (ACL) is approximately 3.5 cm long and 1.1 cm wide. It is composed of anteromedial and posterolateral bands that originate from the posteromedial surface of the lateral femoral condyle and attach to the tibial eminence. The primary function of the ACL is the prevention of anterior displacement of the tibia on the femur. Disruption of the ACL may cause functional instability and consequent athletic disability.

Biomechanics

Muller (1983) demonstrated the close interrelationship between ligament function and articular surface congruency. The structural integrity of the ligament and the articular surface allows a normal combination of knee rolling and sliding. This precise mechanical and anatomic relationship permits the knee to function in motion and to withstand loading forces 1.3 times body weight during walking and 3-6 times body weight while running (Sobotnick, 1985).

Mechanisms of Injury

Sports commonly associated with knee injuries include skiing, basketball, soccer, football, wrestling, and softball. Athletes engaged in these sports may sustain knee injuries during deceleration, twisting, cutting, and jumping maneuvers. Knee positions associated with ACL injuries include pure valgus, valgus/external rotation, varus/internal rotation, and hyperflexion (Garrick, 1988).

Diagnosis

In most instances, diagnosing an ACL tear is possible after completing a thorough history and physical examination. The history may include a compilation of the athlete's and trainer's injury description, videotape analysis of the injury, and a re-enactment of the injury. Acutely, the physical exam reveals a swollen knee with anterior instability demonstrated by Lachman and anterior drawer maneuvers. Damage to the collateral ligament and other capsular structures may also be noted.

Plain radiographs are obtained to evaluate the bony and articular architecture, and a magnetic resonance image (MRI) is often ordered. With a high-quality MRI, the clinician can inspect the "black box" of the knee without surgery and can define associated injuries to bone, ligament, and articular and meniscal fibrocartilage. The accuracy of MRI in diagnosing ligament and meniscal tears ranges from 80–100%.

In addition to causing anterior knee instability, tears of the anterior cruciate ligament are associated with loss of articular cartilage and meniscal integrity and eventual osteoarthritis. Lomander (1991) has linked intraarticular release of stromeolysin, an enzyme that cleaves articular cartilage, with injuries to the anterior cruciate ligament. Understanding of this enzymatic process may lead to a pharmacologic treatment for inhibiting articular degeneration. Ultimately, this association between ACL injury and later cartilage degeneration may highlight the importance of reconstructing the anterior cruciate ligament to maintain long-term knee joint function and integrity.

Practical Implications

Treatment Options and Decision Making. For complete understanding of the options for operative versus nonoperative treatment of ACL injuries, ACL-deficient athletes must understand the negative biomechanical and biochemical implications of the injury. The patient's desired activity level is probably the most decisive factor concerning the appropriate treatment of an ACL tear, but other variables such as age, future goals, severity of ligament laxity, associated injuries, and rehabilitative potential must also be considered. Nonoperative treatment of acute ACL tears may be successful in patients who are not cruciate dominant (genu varus and hyperlax), have no associated injuries, and are willing to forego high-demand sports that require pivoting, jumping, and deceleration. Accepted but nonabsolute indications for operative reconstruction include symptomatic instability with activities of daily living or athletic events, functional loss in patients who cannot or are reluctant to alter their lifestyles, and failure of nonoperative management (Swenson & Fu, 1993). If surgical intervention is chosen, it should be performed, if possible, when the likelihood of reestablishing normal knee function is optimal. Operative timing is predicated on the return of full knee motion and the resolution of pain and swelling. Moreover, surgical intervention should be performed only if the athlete is deemed willing and able to comply with a rigorous and time-consuming postoperative rehabilitation program (Swenson & Fu, 1993).

In the past two decades increased understanding of the histologic, biologic, and functional significance of the menisci has established the importance of preserving damaged menisci to the greatest extent possible. Unfortunately, many surgeons still remove entire menisci, with resultant degenerative osteoarthritis in young athletes. Malcolm and Daniel (1980) showed that a complete meniscectomy can cause a 313% increase in contact stresses across the knee. Thus, restoring meniscal integrity and function through partial meniscectomy or meniscal repair, while simultaneously addressing the clinical symptoms associated with meniscal tears, is presently advocated.

Functions of the menisci include shock absorption, energy dissipation, and load transmission. They also transport lubricating fluid across the articular surfaces through their "windshield wiper" effect, increase the contact area between the femur and tibia, and improve articular congruity and knee stability (Swenson & Harner, 1995).

The incidence of meniscal tears in ACL injuries is high, ranging from 50–80%. Most meniscal tears associated with an acutely torn ACL seem to occur in the lateral meniscus (Duncan et al., 1995; Spindler et al., 1993; Swenson & Harner, 1995). Arthroscopic techniques allow facile repair of certain meniscus tears utilizing a variety of suturing techniques. Success rates of meniscal repairs range from 60% in ACL-deficient knees to 90% in ACL-reconstructed knees (Warren, 1989). Isolated meniscal tears in knees with intact anterior cruciate ligaments have been successfully repaired approximately 50–60% of the time (Cannon & Vittori, 1992; Henning et al. 1987). Furthermore, Henning et al. (1990) have shown that meniscal repairs can be enhanced with the addition of a fibrin clot, which contains many concentrated factors that promote vascular ingrowth and stimulate the healing process. In addition, the clot provides a structural scaffold that supports the ingrowth of fibrovascular tissue (Swenson & Harner, 1995).

When meniscal pathology has been appropriately addressed, arthroscopically-assisted ACL reconstruction may proceed. In recent years, arthroscopically-assisted reconstruction has undergone rapid development and become the mainstay of treatment for athletes sustaining

ACL injuries. Arthroscopically-assisted reconstruction significantly diminishes morbidity and therefore allows more predictable rehabilitation, at least initially, following surgery. Improvements in instrumentation and fixation have also refined the precision and technical quality of this procedure. Achieving isometric graft position, performing a notchplasty to create adequate space for the graft, and establishing rigid fixation with a variety of devices is easily executed with arthroscopic guidance.

Beyond the technical advancements, recent investigations have better defined when to operate, which grafts to use in specific situations, how to implement effective perioperative anesthesia, why accelerated rehabilitation speeds recovery and limits complications, and why prevention techniques need further development.

In athletes, ACL reconstruction is the treatment of choice and has had highly satisfactory results (Andersson et al., 1989; Clancy et al., 1982). Reconstruction using a central-third bone-patellar tendon-bone autograft remains the standard to which other graft materials are compared. Alternative graft choices include autogenous hamstring and quadriceps tendons as well as Achilles tendon and patellar tendon-bone allograft. Synthetic grafts, such as Gore-tex, that were utilized in the 1980s have proven ineffective in substituting for the ACL. A variety of graft materials is being employed, which attests to the fact that none of the available options should always be considered the ideal selection. Each graft type has its own merits, and proper graft selection is paramount to the evolution of ligament reconstruction surgery.

Factors that should be considered when selecting a particular graft type for reconstruction include harvest and insertion of the material, donor site morbidity, tissue stiffness and strength, tensioning and fixation of the graft, and postoperative rehabilitation.

In the landmark study by Noyes et al. (1984), various human ligament graft tissues were subjected to high strain-rate failure tests. The 14-mm wide bone-patellar tendon-bone grafts were strongest, with a mean strength of 168% of the reference ACLs. The strengths of the semitendinosus and gracilis tendons were only 70% and 49%, respectively, of the reference ACLs. These relative values, however, represent only the static strength at the time of reconstruction. Strength to failure and other mechanical properties change as implanted grafts necrose, remodel, and revascularize.

In a more recent study, Steiner et al. (1994) compared hamstring and patellar tendon graft fixation using mechanical testing to failure. Doubled semitendinosus-gracilis grafts (quadrupled) secured with soft-tissue washers demonstrated slightly greater fixation strength than did the intact ACLs. Bone-patellar tendon-bone grafts fixed with interference screws had slightly reduced fixation strength when compared to the intact ACL specimens, but this difference was not statistically significant. The authors thus concluded that the two fixation methods were equally efficacious. Although both grafts were similar in strength to the intact ACL, only the patellar tendon grafts that were secured with interference screws were comparable in stiffness to the intact ACL. The stiffness of the hamstring tendons, despite excellent fixation, was, at best, approximately 50% that of the normal ACL.

As demonstrated by Bach et al. (1995), ACL reconstruction with patellar tendon autograft reliably eliminates manual postoperative instability. Measurements with the KT-1000 arthrometer (MedMetric, Inc., San Diego, CA) on 62 patients about 2 y after surgery revealed a mean postoperative increase of only 0.3 mm in maximum manual instability. Furthermore, arthrometric parameters were statistically reduced from preoperative values. Shelbourne et al. (1990) also validated the efficacy of autogenous bone-patellar tendon-bone ACL reconstruction. At an average follow-up period of 4 y, 60 of 69 varsity athletes returned to their preinjury level of participation. Of the remaining 9 athletes, 8 chose not to participate for nonmedical reasons. After reconstruction, 131 of the 140 patients had not experienced any episodes of instability, and manual maximum KT-1000 measurements showed a mean difference of 1.3 mm between the reconstructed and uninjured knees.

In a study comparing autogenous hamstring and patellar tendon ACL reconstruction, knee stability and function were significantly better in patients with patellar tendon autografts (Specchiulli et al., 1995). In a similar comparative study by Otero and Hutcheson (1993), patients with patellar tendon autografts had significantly lower Lachman and KT-arthrometer values than did a matched group of patients who received doubled semitendinosus/gracilis autografts. Marder et al. (1991), in their prospective study comparing ACL reconstructions using patellar tendons versus semitendinosus and gracilis tendons, showed no significant difference in quadriceps strength between the two groups. However, the average hamstring peak torque was somewhat greater in the patellar tendon group.

Although the literature suggests that autogenous tissues are the most popular in ACL reconstruction, with the bone-patellar tendon-bone autograft as the current gold standard, these tissues are not without problems. Autogenous patellar graft size is limited to the width of the patellar tendon, and the presence of patella baja may preclude a suitable harvest of tendon tissue. (A clinical study by Yasuda et al. (1988) demonstrated a positive correlation between graft size and clinical stability as assessed by Lachman testing.) Furthermore, autogenous donor sites may not permit repeat reconstructions, and although rare, the patient may experience patellar tendinitis or chronic postoperative anterior knee pain.

In contrast, various allografts (Achilles tendon, bone-patellar tendon-bone) may be fashioned to sizes that provide greater mechanical strength when compared to corresponding autogenous tissues. Additionally, allogenic tissues afford an attractive alternative because of shorter operative times, more cosmetic incisions, no donor-site morbidity, superior usefulness in revisions of failed autogenous reconstructions, and perhaps less anterior knee pain (DiStefano, 1993).

The controversial issues surrounding the use of allografts focus on procurement, preparation, disease transmission, and immunogenicity. The ideal allograft is sterile, free of infectious disease, incites a low immunologic response, undergoes rapid revascularization and cellular repopulation, and ultimately attains adequate tensile strength.

Deep freezing and freeze-drying greatly reduce allograft antigenicity without significantly altering its structural properties (DiStefano, 1993). Cryopreservation, however, does not destroy viruses, and gamma irradiation is now commonly used to help sterilize allograft tissues and to inhibit the human immunodeficiency virus (HIV). The precise dose of radiation that reliably inactivates infectious agents in allografts without unduly compromising their ultimate strength has not been identified. In a study of the effects of gamma irradiation on the HIV in fresh-frozen bone-patellar tendon-bone grafts, Fideler et al. (1994) found that doses of 2–2.5 Mrad failed to destroy the viral DNA. The DNA of the HIV was not detectable, however, in the grafts treated with 3–4 Mrad of gamma radiation. This evidence notwithstanding, DiStefano (1993) discovered that 3-Mrad doses of radiation on fresh-frozen goat bone-patellar tendon-bone allografts resulted in 27% and 40% reductions in maximum force and in the ratio of strain energy to maximum force, respectively.

Olson et al. (1992) recently reported the results of 30 patients who received fresh-frozen allografts and were followed for an average of 44 mo. Seventy-four percent of patients were able to return to their preinjury level of sports activity, and 70% had less than 3 mm of increased laxity in their reconstructed knees, compared with their intact knees, with manual maximum KT-1000 testing.

In comparing functional performances, Olson et al. (1992) suspected that patients reconstructed with allografts would functionally outperform patients with autogenous ACL reconstructions strictly because of problems associated with damage to the donor sites in patients with autogenous reconstructions. Lephart et al.(1993) tested this hypothesis by comparing the functional capacity of 33 athletes 12–24 mo after surgery. Nineteen patients underwent autograft reconstructions, and 14 had allograft reconstructions. Quadriceps strength, performance testing, including the hop test, and functional capacity were statistically indistinguishable for both groups.

Making direct comparisons between these previously cited studies should be done cautiously because of differences in patient populations, indications for surgery, surgical techniques, postoperative rehabilitation protocols, patient compliance, length of follow up, and methods of follow up evaluation. The lack of a uniform, standardized system for grading and reporting results makes interpretation of the outcomes presented in these studies difficult (Swenson & Fu, 1993).

Bone-patellar tendon-bone and semitendinosus autografts, as well as allografts, have all been used successfully for ACL reconstruction. Each technique has its own pitfalls, risks, and benefits, so each method should be studied in a standardized fashion, and treatment should be individualized to match the patient's needs.

Operative Timing. Much of the debate regarding timing of ACL reconstruction centers on possible sequelae such as arthrofibrosis, worsening instability, and more frequent and severe meniscal tears and osteochondral lesions. For the early period after injury, controversy exists over the most suitable period for operative intervention (i.e., immediately after injury or after joint inflammation has resolved). Arthrofibrosis is a well recognized and disturbing complication associated with acute ACL reconstruction and may cause a greater functional deficit than the original ACL injury. The patient with arthrofibrosis is prevented from regaining full motion, particularly full extension. Shelbourne et al. (1991) performed a retrospective study of 169 young athletes following ACL reconstruction to determine the optimal time to perform acute ACL reconstruction. Patients operated on within 1 wk of injury (Group I) had a significantly higher incidence of arthrofibrosis when compared to patients who had ACL reconstruction 21 d or more after the injury (Group III). Patients operated between 8 and 21 d after injury (Group II) had a similar incidence of arthrofibrosis as Group I patients when they followed a conventional postoperative rehabilitation protocol. However, only a small number of Group II patients (4%) who followed an accelerated physical therapy program developed arthrofibrosis. Because of increased rates of arthrofibrosis, stiffness, and decreased range of motion, we consider ACL reconstruction when the acute swelling has subsided and full knee motion has returned. This typically occurs approximately 3 wk after surgery but may occur earlier. In higher level athletes, we believe early ACL reconstruction is warranted and can be performed without appreciable risk of arthrofibrosis

Outpatient Reconstruction. Because of pressure to reduce expenses, refinements in operative techniques, and improvements in perioperative anesthesia, performing ACL reconstruction as an outpatient procedure is becoming commonplace. Currently, all our ACL reconstructions are done in an outpatient setting unless otherwise dictated by insurance considerations.

For effective outpatient surgery, teamwork and patient counseling, are indispensable (Highgenboten, 1992). Our team consists of the patient, surgeon, office staff, personnel in the outpatient surgery center, and home health care agencies. Education and counseling of the patient and family and their dedication to the outpatient concept are essential prior to surgery.

Advances in perioperative anesthesia and analgesia protocols have decreased the acute recovery period and improved pain control after surgery. In our patient population, a general anesthetic (propofol; Diprivan, Stuart Pharmaceuticals, Wilmington, DE) is administered with the intent of discharge within 1–2 h after surgery. For preemptive analgesia, the knee joint is then instilled with 20 mL of bupivacaine hydrochloride (Marcaine, 0.25%) with epinephrine (1:200,000), followed by infiltration of all arthroscopy portal sites and incision margins with the same bupivacaine mixture. Arthroscopically-assisted ACL reconstruction is then performed. Approximately 30 min prior to completion of the procedure, 60 mg of ketorolac tromethamine (Toradol, Syntex Laboratories, Palo Alto, CA) is administered intramuscularly. Prior to skin closure, the incisions are infiltrated with etidocaine hydrochloride (Duranest) with epinephrine, and 20 additional mL are infused into the knee joint. A cold wrap is applied directly over the dressing.

In the recovery room, continuous passive motion is started immediately from 0–90 degrees. When fully awake, the patients begin active movements through the range of motion, isometric quadriceps exercises, and straight leg lifts. Prior to discharge, each patient performs 20 active flexion-extension exercises from 0–90 degrees. If necessary, moderate pain is managed with hydrocodone bitartrate tablets (Vicodin, Knoll Pharmaceuticals, Whippany, NJ), and severe pain is relieved with intravenous morphine sulfate.

Having returned to their homes, all patients receive intermittent home nursing care during the first 24 h after surgery. Three doses of Toradol, 30 mg, are administered intramuscularly every 6 h, and Vicodin tablets are taken as needed for pain. For its anti-inflammatory effects, naproxen (Naprosyn, Syntex, Puerto Rico), 500 mg bid, is started on postoperative day 1 and continued for 4–6 wk.

In addition to its demonstrated cost effectiveness compared to inpatient surgery (Highgenboten, 1992; Kao et al., 1995), studies have shown that very few patients require readmission for pain control, nausea, vomiting, or urinary retention (Kao et al., 1995; Tierney, 1995). Moreover, Kao et al. (1995) reported no statistically significant differences in pain relief between inpatients and outpatients, and 92% of their patients were satisfied with their outpatient experience. Obviously, outpatient surgery is an attractive and reasonable alternative for ACL reconstruction. The patient is immediately allowed to recuperate in a familiar, comfortable, and psychologically favorable setting, which undoubtedly enhances early rehabilitation.

Prevention. Most literature on ACL injuries focuses on treatment rather than on prevention. Undoubtedly, more emphasis should be placed on developing methods to reduce ACL injuries because the incidence of severe ACL sprains was once only a third the current rate (Ettlinger et al., 1995). In women athletes, especially those engaged in sports requiring jumping, cutting, and pivoting, injury rates appear to be higher than in their male counterparts. A large study by Arendt and Dick (1995) showed that women who played intercollegiate soccer and basketball had significantly higher ACL injury rates than did men engaged in the same sports. In women's soccer the ACL injury rate (0.31) was more than double that in men's soccer (0.13). Similarly, among women basketball players, the ACL injury rate (0.29) was more than four times greater than that of men basketball players (0.07).

The mechanism underlying the greater ACL injury rate among women is probably multifactorial. Possible contributing reasons may include extrinsic factors (body movement, muscular strength, shoe-surface interface, and skill level) or intrinsic factors (joint laxity, limb alignment, intercondylar notch dimensions, and ligament size). The current challenge is to explain the sex-specific factors associated with this injury and to develop preventive measures based on these findings.

Closely examining injury mechanisms may prove helpful in developing safety recommendations, effecting rule changes, or suggesting movement modifications that may reduce ACL injury rates. For example, Griffis and associates in a prospective 10–y study identified three major noncontact mechanisms associated with ACL injuries in women basketball players. When movements that alleviated ACL stretch were taught to two Division I women's basketball teams, the incidence of ACL injuries was reduced 89% after several years (Arendt & Dick, 1995). Furthermore, if ACL injuries are found to be associated with certain tactics such as slide tackles in soccer, rules limiting or restricting these maneuvers should be considered.

One study that directly addressed methods to reduce ACL injuries was reported by Ettlinger et al. (1995). Through videotape analysis of skiing accidents leading to knee sprains, the authors identified the "phantom-foot" and "boot-induced" ACL injury mechanisms as the two most common among Alpine skiers. Using this information, they developed an experimental training program for experienced ski patrollers and instructors that emphasized avoiding high-risk behavior, recognizing potentially hazardous situations, and responding quickly and appropriately when these conditions were encountered. After implementing this program, a 62% reduction in ACL sprains was noted in the patrol and ski instructor group, compared with no decrease recorded in the control group. This study is noteworthy because no other products, services, or behavior modifications that decrease ACL injuries among Alpine skiers have been identified in other studies.

Accelerated Rehabilitation. During the past 15 y, tremendous advancements in ACL reconstruction have occurred. Elegant anatomical and biomechanical studies have illustrated the importance of near-isometric graft placement and proper graft tensioning and have provided data regarding the strength of various fixation devices. Despite marked improvements in reconstruction techniques, postoperative complications remained commonplace prior to the introduction of accelerated rehabilitation. The concept of expedited rehabilitation is one of the most important advancements in ACL reconstruction during the past few years. Shelbourne and Nitz (1990) were among the first investigators to institute an accelerated rehabilitation program after correlating their patients' results with compliance to a conservative rehabilitation protocol. They discovered that patients who progressed as they desired and achieved full extension earlier than instructed (noncompliant) returned to normal function without instability sooner than patients who complied with the conservative postoperative rehabilitation protocol. In hopes of overcoming postoperative ACL complications such as prolonged knee stiffness, limitation of complete knee extension, delay in strength recovery, and anterior knee pain, they developed an aggressive rehabilitation protocol that emphasized immediate full-knee extension, weightbearing, and passive range of motion, along with early strengthening. The patients engaged in the accelerated rehabilitation protocol had earlier full-knee extension, a quicker return of quadriceps strength, fewer patellofemoral joint symptoms, and no difference in knee stability when compared to the patients involved in a slower-paced therapy regimen. Furthermore, the number of patients who required surgical management for symptomatic extensor loss was significantly less in the aggressive rehabilitation group.

In addition to illustrating the advantages of accelerated rehabilitation, such as increased patient compliance, less muscle atrophy, decreased anterior knee pain, and earlier return to fitness and athletic endeavors, this study provided impetus to directly compare the basic science and clinical rationales for accelerated rehabilitation. Based on finding slightly smaller KT-1000 tibial translation in patients rehabilitating in an accelerated fashion, Shelbourne et al. (1990) hypothesized that an increased ACL ligamentization rate would be associated with faster rehabilitation regimens.

The findings of Tipton et al. (1970) in a dog model certainly support a positive correlation between ligament strength and exercise. They demonstrated that medial collateral ligament strength and collagen fiber bundle size increase in response to exercise, whereas immobilization causes a decrease in strength. The ligaments in the exercised dogs had a significantly higher hydroxyproline content than did those in the immobilized animals, which suggested that exercise increased collagen metabolism.

In another animal study, Arnoczky et al. (1982) investigated the histologic properties and revascularization pattern of patellar tendon grafts used in ACL reconstruction. Postoperatively, the limbs were not immobilized, and the animals were allowed to exercise at will. Sixteen weeks after surgery, the grafts had hypertrophied to three times their original diameters. This increase in diameter resulted from additional deposition of collagenous tissues. Microscopically, dense, longitudinally oriented collagen bundles were observed, and revascularization of the grafts was complete by 20 wk.

During most activities of daily living, the anterior cruciate ligament is loaded to only approximately 454 newtons, which is far below the bone-patellar tendon-bone graft's initial maximum load to failure, as demonstrated by Noyes et al. (1984). In theory, an 80% safety zone exists between the most frequent forces the new graft is subjected to and its maximal load tolerance. However, all grafts undergo weakening after implantation due to tissue necrosis. For example, primate patellar grafts are weakest 6–8 wk after surgery, dropping to 15% of their preimplantation strength at that time (Noyes, et al. 1984).

Although the graft may not be able to withstand certain activities in the first few months after reconstruction, we believe it is still important to subject it to subthreshold stresses applied through normal functional activities. Because the process of collagen synthesis seems to be greater than collagen degradation in the acute healing stage of the ACL graft, applying stress to the graft tissue may promote earlier and more organized alignment of the invading host fibroblasts. In this way, the ligamentization process is accelerated.

Although several clinical studies confirm that patellar tendon (Shelbourne & Nitz, 1990; Shelbourne et al., 1990) and semitendinosus grafts (MacDonald et al., 1995) can withstand physical stresses inherent in an accelerated rehabilitation program without deleterious sequelae, certain guidelines should be followed. Aggressive rehabilitation should be done in a manner that minimizes inflammation, pain, and swelling that can reduce voluntary movements of the knee joint. Attempts at accelerated recovery with complete disregard of sound basic science and rehabilitation principles should be avoided.

Closed-chain kinetic exercises, which are performed with the foot fixed on a surface and the entire limb bearing a load, should be emphasized. During closed-chain kinetic exercises, lower shear stresses are applied to the knee joint compared to open-chain exercises because with the foot fixed, all the joints in the extremity are compressed by the load. In addition, closed-chain exercises subject the knee joint to functional stresses that are similar to normal weightbearing activities (Shelbourne & Nitz, 1990). The resultant joint compression with weightbearing and hamstrings-quadriceps cocontraction provides inherent joint stability, which may allow more rigorous strengthening workouts while avoiding the potential for graft elongation with conventional open-chain exercises. This hypothesis was experimentally confirmed in vivo by Lutz et al. (1991), who determined shear forces during isometric open- chain knee flexion, extension exercises, and closed-chain exercises at 30, 60, and 90 degrees of knee flexion. They found reduced anterior shear forces at 30 and 60 degrees of knee flexion during closed-chain exercises, compared to open-chain knee extension. Furthermore, patellofemoral joint forces are markedly decreased during closed-chain kinetic exercises compared to open-chain exercises performed in knee flexion ranges of 30–90 degrees (Shelbourne & Nitz, 1990). Based on the aforementioned rationale, closed-chain exercises should be emphasized during postoperative ACL rehabilitation. Too much reliance on open-chain exercises may cause patellofemoral irritation and inappropriate stresses across the graft. Moreover, open-chain exercises fail to simulate sports-specific activities that are necessary for return to competition.

Directions for Future Research on Anterior Cruciate Injuries

Despite numerous investigations that quantify and compare the biomechanical strength, stiffness, and elongation of various graft tissues stabilized with different fixation devices, knowing when to operate and which graft to use in various circumstances remains controversial. Further prospective, randomized, comparative studies with subjects matched for age, sex, operative timing and technique, and rehabilitation protocol are necessary to answer these questions. In addition, methods must be developed to reduce the number of ACL injuries. Future research should focus on specific injury mechanisms, movement modification, training techniques, and accessory equipment. Finally, questions regarding the timing of return to athletic endeavors need answering. Determining the functional levels and graft strength during ligamentization that must be achieved before permitting return to sports activities is imperative.

OSTEOCHONDRAL KNEE INJURIES

Human articular cartilage is composed primarily of water (60–80%) and collagen and proteoglycans (20–40%). The hyaline cartilage matrix is synthesized by chondrocytes. The articular cartilage functions in force distribution and dissipation, and its smooth surface permits knee motion with minimal friction. Generally, the articular cartilage surface in the knee is thick and firmly anchored to the subchondral bone, which helps protect the knee from shearing injuries. These properties allow functional adaptation to walking, running, and extreme knee motions. In an unstable knee, however, where larger shearing motions are allowed, chondral damage may occur. Cartilage defects may also be associated with chronic, repetitive training and wear. Once the cartilage is damaged, proteoglycans are lost from the matrix, and the chondrocytes are exposed to increased forces. In this harsh environment, the chondrocytes synthesize and release stromeolysin, which enzymatically degrades the articular surface.

Irrespective of the cause and effect, these articular lesions may lead to pain, swelling, joint dysfunction, and athletic disability. Furthermore, these lesions pose difficult treatment problems because damaged articular cartilage cannot restore its original biologic or biomechanical properties. In addition, deterioration of healthy cartilage surrounding the normal cartilage may also occur, and osteoarthritis ensues.

Practical Implications

Diagnosis. Injuries to hyaline cartilage in the knee joint are difficult to diagnose without invasive techniques. Because of the inherent inability of human articular cartilage to repair itself adequately, whether the injury is deep or superficial, there is an obvious need to detect these defects (Wojtys et al., 1987). Once diagnosed and treated either conservatively or surgically, a reliable noninvasive modality is also essential to follow the natural history of these injuries.

Anteroposterior and lateral radiographs of the knee should be obtained and may demonstrate an osteochondral defect or loose body. A supplemental tunnel or notch view may best demonstrate the location of an osteochondritis dissecans lesion. However, small defects, purely chondral fractures, or in situ osteochondritis dissecans lesions may be virtually impossible to diagnose with plain radiographs, arthrograms, or computed tomography. In such cases, MRI may assist in the diagnosis of these radiographically occult lesions. MRI, although not completely sensitive, can be utilized to detect subchondral marrow abnormalities and cartilaginous loose bodies, assess overlying cartilage integrity, and precisely determine the extent and location of these articular lesions.

Wojtys et al. (1987) in their MRI investigation of knee hyaline cartilage found the multiplane capability of MRI was excellent in detailing small (3 mm wide x 1 mm deep) defects on the femoral condyles and patellar surface. With the use of intraarticular gadolinium, chondral defects as small as 2 mm were reliably delineated on all MRI sequences (Gylys-Morin et al., 1987).

Treatment. Traditional treatment modalities for articular surface defects have demonstrated varying degrees of success. These articular resurfacing techniques include debridement, subchondral drilling, abrasion arthroplasty, and osteotomy and are intended to allow vascular ingrowth and fibroblast migration into the cartilage defect. The end result, however, is a disorganized fibrocartilage surface (Brittberg et al., 1994) that is mechanically inferior to normal articular cartilage and may not effectively withstand the forces applied by an athletic population.

Other potential treatments for focal hyaline cartilage defects include periosteal (Niedermann, et al. 1985), perichondrial (Engkvist, 1979), and osteochondral grafts and chondrocyte implantation (Peterson, et al., 1984). In animal studies, chondral tissue has successfully formed after the use of periosteal or perichondral grafts to treat focal cartilage defects. The results of both periosteal and perichondral grafts, however, are inconsistent, inconclusive, and short-term (Brittberg, et al., 1994). For example, Engkvist (1979) in his investigation of free perichondral grafts applied to patellar subchondral bone found minimal cartilage degenerative changes 8 mo after surgery. In contrast, however, cartilage degeneration was common 1 y after surgery, suggesting its inability to withstand joint forces.

Niederman et al.(1985) reported on five patients who underwent periosteal grafting for knee osteochondral defects. Four of 5 patients were free of pain and swelling 12 mo after surgery. During arthroscopic visualization, the new cartilage appeared macroscopically normal 1 y after surgery. The results of this study should be interpreted with caution because the follow up period was too short to adequately evaluate potential cartilage degenerative changes.

Perhaps a more promising treatment for athletes with localized articular knee lesions may be autologous chondrocyte implantation. In 1984, Peterson et al. reported successful treatment of focal patellar chondral defects in rabbits, using transplanted, cultured, autologous chondrocytes injected underneath a sutured periosteal flap. One year later, cartilage-like tissue typically covered the majority of each defect. This animal study spawned an autologous chondrocyte transplantation study in human subjects (Brittberg et al., 1994). In this study, 23 patients with full-thickness cartilage defects on a load-bearing surface of the femoral condyle or patellar facet and disabling symptoms were treated with autologous cartilage implantation and followed for an average of 36 mo. With cell expansion techniques, chondrocytes arthroscopically removed from the medial femoral condyle of the patient's involved knee were multiplied to approximately 12 million. Two to three weeks after the initial biopsy, open surgical techniques, as shown in Figure 8-1, were used to suture a periosteal flap over the chondral lesion. This was followed by injection of the cultured chondrocytes into the defect below the periosteal flap.

According to this report, all patients initially had resolution of knee locking, coupled with reduced pain and swelling. Fourteen of 16 patients with femoral condyle implantations had good or excellent functional results. Ensuing arthroscopic examinations revealed macroscopically normal articular cartilage in all 14 of these patients. Histologic evaluations demonstrated normal appearing cartilage in 11 of 15 patients with femoral chondral defects.

The results of cartilage implantation in the patients with patellar defects were disappointing. At a mean follow up of 36 mo, only 2 of 7 patients had good or excellent outcomes, and only one patient had a biopsy specimen exhibiting a normal hyaline appearance. More studies are necessary to better establish the relative value of cartilage implantation. In our estimation, chondrocyte implantation should be used only to repair small articular cartilage defects less than 6 cm^2.

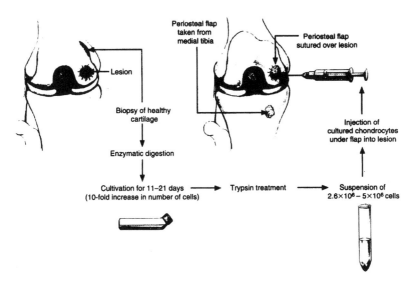

FIGURE 8–1. *Technique of implanting chondrocytes at the femoral condyle.* Adapted from Brittberg et al. (1994).

Directions For Future Research On Osteochondral Knee Injuries

Autologous cartilage implantation is in its infancy. Clearly, randomized controlled studies are necessary to corroborate the results and improve on the clinical efficacy of Brittberg et al. (1994) before cartilage implantation can become a widely accepted treatment. Further research should also focus on developing a noninvasive imaging technique that can be used to diagnose and sequentially follow nonoperatively and operatively treated cartilage lesions. In time, with continued development of autologous cartilage implantation, our ability to successfully treat focal chondral defects should improve dramatically.

STRESS FRACTURES

Stress fractures were originally described in 1855, 40 y prior to radiographic confirmation. In 1958, Devas first described stress fractures in athletes. Since then, numerous reports have followed, including descriptions of stress fractures in runners (Lombardo & Benson, 1982; Marcus et al., 1985; Noakes; 1985) and dancers (McBryde, 1975). The diagnosis of stress fractures in the athletic population has continued to increase because stress fractures in certain bony locations appear to have a degree of sports specificity. The following section will discuss the epidemiology, etiology, diagnosis, and treatment of stress fractures.

Epidemiology

Stress fractures are often discussed according to their associations with age, sex, race, skeletal location, and specific athletic endeavors. Men, with their greater lean body mass and larger overall bone structure, appear to suffer fewer stress fractures than do women. According to Markey (1987), the higher frequency of stress injuries in women runners may be ascribed to their relatively short stature. Several reports have shown that women develop up to 10 times as many stress fractures as men on the same training courses (Protzman & Griffis, 1977). Similarly, Jones et al. (1993) prospectively followed 310 military trainees participating in 8 wk of basic training and found that the women had a significantly greater incidences of time-loss injuries than did men (44.6% compared to 29.0%).

Although the assertion is frequently made, blacks and other persons with dark skin are not less likely to sustain stress injuries. In contrast, Markey (1987) found similar stress fracture incidences in a racially-mixed population of military recruits.

In most studies, the tibia is the most frequent site of stress fractures.

In an investigation of 145 males and 175 females with bone scan-positive stress fractures, Matheson et al. (1987) reported tibial and tarsal involvement in 49.1% and 25.3%, respectively. The remaining stress fracture sites, in descending order of frequency, were the metatarsals (8.8%), femur (7.2%), fibula (6.6%), pelvis (1.6%), sesamoids (0.9%), and back (0.6%). Older athletes more commonly developed femoral and tarsal stress fractures, whereas tibia and fibular stress fractures were more frequent in younger athletes.

With respect to sports-specific stress fractures, a literature review revealed a 2% incidence of stress fractures in soccer players (Matheson, et al., 1987; Orava et al., 1978). In our experience, the most common location of soccer-related stress fractures are the metatarsals, especially the fifth and second, followed by the tibia, fibula, femur, anterior iliac crest, and pars interarticularis.

Etiology

Stress fractures in collegiate and professional athletes are very common worldwide. For instance, 9 of 24 players on the U.S. National Soccer Team from 1991–94 were diagnosed with stress fractures. Currently, the most widely accepted explanation for stress fracture development is repetitive and additive subthreshold mechanical insults that together exceed the stress-bearing capacity of bone. Bone, unaccustomed to these stress levels, compensates with a rapid, focal, circumferential, periosteal resorption coupled with slower lamellar bone formation along the lines of stress. The net result is a weakened cortex susceptible to stress fracture development.

The sports medicine professional must have a working concept of connective tissue adaptation to stress. Mandelbaum (1993) has developed a hypothesis concerning connective tissue acclimatization to stresses that incorporates Wolf's Law of Transformation as well as endocrine and nutritional factors. Because connective tissue responds to external forces, bones exposed to changing conditions respond by changing their internal architecture. In essence, stress fractures result from a maladaptive response to abnormal doses of stress. By judiciously managing stress application, therefore, stress injuries are preventable.

Figure 8-2A illustrates how bone adapts to appropriate proportions of hard and easy training days, and Figure 8-2B shows how excessive training intensity coupled with inadequate rest can lead to bone injury. Assuming a normal hormonal state and adequate nutrition, training can increase bone mineral density, tensile strength, and periosteal new bone formation, thus increasing the threshold for injury to the bone. In contrast, injury to bone can occur with progressive training regimens that

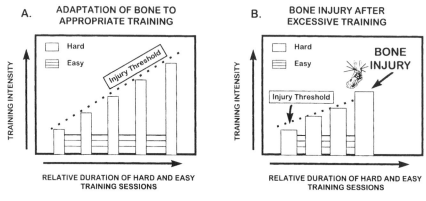

A. ADAPTATION OF BONE TO APPROPRIATE TRAINING

B. BONE INJURY AFTER EXCESSIVE TRAINING

FIGURE 8-2. *A. Adaptation of bone to appropriate cycles of hard and easy training. As training progresses, the bone becomes stronger and less subject to injury. B. Bone injury after excessive training. When the proportion of hard training days becomes excessive, the bone is unable to adapt adequately, and injury results.*

continually increase the training load beyond the bone's ability to adapt; the likelihood of injury is greater with nutritional deficits and endocrine abnormalities such as those occurring in amenorrheic women athletes.

Poorly maintained and rapidly changing field conditions and inadequate shoe design also contribute to the development of stress injuries. Certain athletes, especially younger or recreational participants, may regularly play on hard, sun-baked or soft, muddy ground with little turf. Even elite players may practice on substandard fields but play games on expertly maintained turf. Additionally, the unyielding plastic or rubber cleats of many turf shoes cannot effectively penetrate compacted soil surfaces so large ground reactive forces are transmitted through the small surface areas of the cleats, resulting in large, localized plantar pressures that can cause stress injuries.

Inadvisable training techniques and regimens also increase the risk of stress fractures. In a survey of athletes Matheson et al. (1987) found that training errors accounted for 22.4% of stress fractures. Athletes who suddenly engaged in strenuous training after a prolonged period of inactivity or who rapidly increased their training intensity, duration, and frequency are especially susceptible to stress injuries (Orava et al., 1978).

Biological factors associated with stress injuries include anatomical foot variations, such as pronated or cavus feet, metatarsus adductus, and a short first metatarsal. For example, pronated feet are the most common positional anomaly in athletes who develop stress fractures of the tibial or tarsal bones. In contrast, athletes with cavus feet most frequently sustain stress fractures of the metatarsal bones and the femoral neck (Matheson, et al., 1987).

Practical Implications

Diagnosis. It is imperative that stress fractures are diagnosed in a timely manner because a delay may increase time lost from sports participation and ultimate functional morbidity. Johansson et al. (1990) reported on stress fracture of the femoral neck in 23 subjects followed for an average of 6.5 y after injury. In these athletes (16 recreational and 7 elite) the average time to diagnosis was 14 wk after the onset of symptoms. All the elite athletes were unable to resume their careers. Thus, in the absence of prevention, early diagnosis and treatment of stress fractures are the sports medicine professional's objectives.

Athletes with stress fractures typically describe similar inciting events and symptom complexes. Predictably, each athlete has recently undergone an increased training load (e.g., by increasing training duration, intensity, or frequency). Occasionally, the provoking activity is a single event. Nevertheless, the athlete's symptoms are insidious in onset over 2–3 wk. The hallmark complaint is mild, localized pain that initially occurs toward the end of a training session and is relieved by rest. Over time, the severity of the pain increases, occurs earlier during a practice period, and persists after activity has ceased. Eventually, excruciating pain develops as soon as exercise begins and the pain forces discontinuation of training.

On physical exam, athletes with stress fractures usually have a focal area of tenderness along with variable hardening of tissue over the bone, erythema, and warmth. Percussion at a distance from the fracture may cause pain transmission from the fracture site (Markey, 1987). Additionally, anatomic anomalies, including cavus or pronated feet, pes planus, metatarsus adductus, short metatarsals, bony excrescences, and hyperkeratoses must be noted and diligently evaluated.

Other entities in the differential diagnosis, including infection, tumor (osteoid osteoma), chronic compartment syndrome, and medial tibial stress syndrome (MTSS), must be considered. In the tibia, for example, MTSS may be differentiated from a stress fracture based solely upon clinical characteristics and physical examination. Pain secondary to MTSS, as opposed to early stress fracture pain, is often present at the beginning of a workout and may last for several hours after cessation of activity. Also, the tenderness over the posteromedial distal third of the tibia in MTSS is more diffuse than the tenderness associated with stress fractures. MTSS pain is also occasionally aggravated by active ankle plantar flexion and foot inversion against resistance (Jones & James, 1987).

Differentiating tarsal navicular stress fractures from other midfoot maladies may also prove challenging. The accompanying pain is vague, and the tenderness may be an ill-defined soreness over the dorsum of the medial midfoot or along the medial aspect of the longitudinal arch. Often, swelling and palpable tissue changes are nonexistent. Associated foot abnormalities, including first metatarsal shortening and metatarsus adductus as well as decreased ankle dorsiflexion and subtalar motion, are occasionally present.

Confirmatory Studies. Although most stress fractures are recognized after a thorough history and physical exam, the diagnosis should be confirmed with radiographic studies. Plain radiographs that identify only about 50% of stress fractures may, depending upon the developmental stage of the fracture, reveal periosteal new bone formation, cortical thickening, or a lucency. Maximal periosteal bone formation occurs at 6 wk following injury.

The radiologic gold standard for diagnosing stress injuries is the technetium-99 diphosphonate, three-phase, or single-phase bone scan. The radioactive isotope, which osteoblasts incorporate in new bone formation, may allow diagnosis within 48– 72 h following clinical signs of injury (Markey, 1987), which is long before abnormalities are observed on plain radiograph films. Although the bone scan is highly sensitive for early stress fracture diagnosis, it lacks specificity. Prather et al. (1977) reported a 24% false-positive rate for scintigraphy in stress fractures. Fortunately, the sensitivity and accuracy of radioisotopic scanning can be enhanced with high-resolution views of the suspected areas and comparison scans of the uninvolved limb (Prather, et al., 1977). Also, a negative bone scan essentially excludes a stress fracture diagnosis.

Radioisotope scanning may also help differentiate stress fractures from shin splints. Table 8-1 compares the characteristic findings of each entity on bone-scan.

Because of its enhanced soft-tissue contrast resolution, MRI may also permit prompt (preradiographic) detection of stress fractures. MRI is more specific than bone scanning in stress fracture detection, but a definitive study comparing the sensitivity of MRI and scintigraphy in evaluating stress fractures has not been performed. Intuitively, MRI may have a distinct advantage in defining stress injuries in the lower leg and foot because the marrow is predominantly fatty, and MRI most readily demonstrates prefracture stress responses in regions of fatty marrow (Deutsch et al., 1992). On MRI T1– and T2–weighted sequences, stress injuries appear as globular foci of decreased signal intensity and variably increased signal intensity, respectively. Stress injuries are most effectively demonstrated on STIR (Short Tau [T1] Inversion Recovery) sequences because they highlight foci of high signal intensity against a suppressed fatty marrow background. In addition, STIR images are also

TABLE 8–1. *Bone scan appearance: stress fracture versus shin splints.*

Characteristic	Stress Fracture	Shin Splints
Bone Scan	Any phase can be positive	Only positive on delays
Intensity	Can be 1+ to 4+	Usually 1+ or 2+
Shape	Round/fusiform	Linear/vertical
Location	Anywhere in the lower leg	Mid-posterior tibia

effective in demonstrating stress fractures in bone composed primarily of hematopoietic marrow (Deutsch, et al., 1992).

Treatment. The treatment of stress fractures requires a multifaceted and multidisciplinary approach. Primary care, psychiatric, and orthopedic physicians, along with dietitians, psychologists, coaches, trainers, and parents may be involved in the therapeutic regimen.

To help prevent injury, athletes, especially young female athletes, should optimize their nutritional status. Proper nourishment includes a low-fat, high-carbohydrate diet, avoidance of phosphate-containing sodas, and calcium supplementation if necessary. Some studies suggest that excess phosphate intake and a negative calcium balance may be correlated with stress maladaptation. Women athletes require 1,000–1,500 mg of calcium per day so supplementation should be encouraged. Vitamins and trace elements should be consumed at the recommended dietary allowances.

Eating disorders such as bulimia and anorexia nervosa must always be contemplated, especially in the female athlete with multiple, recurrent stress fractures. In these cases, coaches, trainers, parents, and a psychiatrist/psychologist should be integrally involved in the athlete's treatment program.

Women athletes with secondary abnormal menstrual patterns or amenorrhea should be evaluated by a primary care physician for possible estrogen supplementation.

Concurrent with nutritional and medical evaluation, treatment following a general plan should be instituted. This plan includes rest, treatment and preventive care education, analgesics, serial radiographs, icing and physical therapy treatments, appropriate cross training to maintain cardiovascular tone, rehabilitation, and a regimented return to athletic competition (Sterling et al., 1992).

Because increasing physical activity to a level inconsistent with the ability of the bones to adapt is the most common factor associated with stress injuries, avoiding abnormal stress will allow bone repair processes to dominate over bone resorption. Six to eight weeks of rest is necessary for most fractures to heal adequately before the athlete should return to competition, but each case must be individualized. For example, fractures of the pubic rami may require 2–5 mo of healing (Markey, 1987).

Some investigators believe that bracing certain stress fractures is important for limiting unwanted motion (Markey, 1987) and expediting return to athletic participation (Whitelaw et al., 1991). For example, Whitelaw et al. (1991) provided pneumatic leg braces to 17 competitive athletes who had tibial stress fractures. They resumed intensive training an average of 3.7 wk after injury and returned to a preinjury level of competition 5.3 wk after brace application. Whitelaw theorized the brace created a venous tourniquet and hence facilitated accelerated healing. However, bracing may simultaneously transfer stress to other bony regions that may subsequently become symptomatic (Markey, 1987).

Very few stress fractures require surgical management. However, operative intervention should be considered in those bones in which a complete fracture might cause serious sequelae. The femoral neck, tibia, tarsal navicular, and fifth metatarsal are pertinent examples.

Figure 8-3 represents our treatment plan for athletes with suspected tibial stress fractures. Plain radiographs (x-rays) are obtained, even though most will be negative. They serve as reference films, however, for future x-rays. If the plain films are indeed negative, a bone scan or MRI is obtained. When a tibial stress fracture in a runner is documented, aggravating activity is avoided for 6 wk. Cardiovascular deconditioning is averted by cross training with swimming or bicycling. If asymptomatic after 6 wk, the athlete may cyclically progress through sport-specific activities. If pain persists yet plain radiographs do not show a worsening of the fracture, cyclical training progression is continued. If fracture extension is noted, however, step one is repeated for an additional 6 wk. If the pain is resolved 6 wk later, a return to sport-specific activities is allowed. If discomfort continues, a CT scan is performed (if x-rays are equivocal). If the CT scan demonstrates a large lucency or definite fracture line without signs of healing, reamed intramedullary rodding of the tibia is performed. Thereafter, the player may return to athletic competition, using cyclical progression.

Figure 8-4 outlines the treatment plan we follow in managing metatarsal stress fractures. The concepts and treatment sequence are similar to those for injuries to the tibia, except operative intervention involves cancellous screw fixation and possible bone grafting.

Figure 8-5 is the treatment protocol developed by Torg (1987) for tarsal navicular stress fracture. Incomplete and complete but nondisplaced navicular fractures should be immobilized for 6–8 wk in a short leg cast with no weightbearing. Weightbearing and a gradual return to athletic endeavors are guided by the patient's symptomatology and radiographic evidence of union. Complete displaced fractures can be treated as just noted with non-weightbearing cast immobilization or

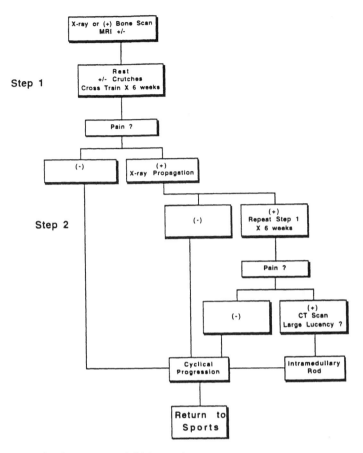

FIGURE 8-3. *Plan for treatment of tibial stress fractures.*

with open reduction and internal fixation coupled with cast immobilization and no weight bearing for 6 wk. Navicular fractures complicated by delayed or failed union should be treated with medullary curettage and bone grafting, along with internal fixation if the fracture fragments are mobile. If a fibrous union is encountered, no attempts should be made to reduce the fragments after bone grafting. Again, surgery is followed by 6–8 wk of cast immobilization. Solid healing may not occur for 3–6 mo in fractures requiring bone grafting.

Prevention. To avoid exercise-induced injuries to bones, severe exercise stress should be alternated with light exercise and adequate rest periods. Ultimately, the biologic status of the athlete, including nutritional and hormonal factors, determines the amount of rest required and the training load that can be tolerated.

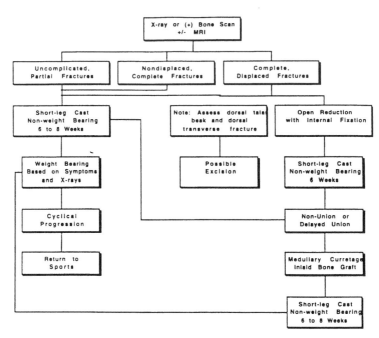

```
                    ┌─────────────────────┐
                    │ X-ray or (+) Bone Scan │
                    │      +/-  MRI         │
                    └─────────────────────┘
        ┌───────────────────┬─────────────────┬─────────────────┐
 ┌──────────────┐    ┌──────────────┐    ┌──────────────┐
 │ Uncomplicated,│    │ Nondisplaced,│    │  Complete,   │
 │Partial Fractures│  │Complete Fractures│  │Displaced Fractures│
 └──────────────┘    └──────────────┘    └──────────────┘
```

FIGURE 8-4. *Plan for treatment of metatarsal stress fractures.*

We have developed the following stress fracture prevention guidelines for the athletes, coaches, and trainers we serve.

1) To minimize injuries associated with habitual exposure to a particular pair of athletic shoes, practice and game shoes must be
   different

2) Training must progress in a cyclical fashion that allows.proper
   musculoskeletal adaptation. The quality of training should be
   emphasized over quantity, and both training loads and rest periods should be carefully monitored.

3) Training programs should be individualized according to the
   athletes' biologic status and abilities.

4) Year-round training programs should be monitored especially
   carefully because the greatest incidences of stress fractures are in
   temperate climates such as California and Florida.

5) If the number of stress fractures seems inordinately high, yet
   training methods are proper, consider altering the playing conditions (e.g., shoes, cleats, and fields).

6) Women athletes who have delayed menarche or abnormal menstrual cycles should be promptly identified and appropriately
   treated.

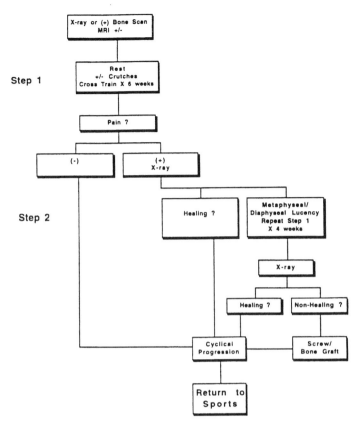

FIGURE 8-5. *Plan for treatment of tarsal navicular stress fractures.* Adapted from Torg et al. (1987).

7) Because the child is not a small adult, training programs for youths should be individualized by puberty stage, not by age.

8) Athletes, especially those with multiple stress fractures, should be observed closely to detect possible eating disorders.

Directions For Future Research on Stress Fractures

Recently, sports medicine specialists have better defined the complex response of the musculoskeletal system to exercise. Further investigations that define the biomechanical and hormonal parameters and nutritional needs of the athlete and their relationship to training regimens and stress fracture prevention are needed. For example, pertinent research might include biomechanical evaluations of athletic equipment such as cleated shoes in soccer and football. Further studies are also needed to examine various training techniques in order to reach a more optimal balance between quality and quantity of training without sacrificing performance. Finally, studies should better address the role of nutrition in the etiology of stress fractures and stress fracture prevention.

ANKLE IMPINGEMENT SYNDROMES

Ankle sprains represent 85% of all ankle injuries and are the most common injury sustained by athletes (Attarian et al., 1985). Among soccer players, ankle sprains are also the most frequent injury, accounting for 31% of all injuries (Ekstrand & Tropp, 1990). In recent years, the acute care of ankle sprains has focused on diminution of swelling and inflammation, functional taping or bracing, increasing the effective range of motion, strengthening the muscles around the ankle joint, and using proprioceptive rehabilitation techniques.

Despite proper treatment and rehabilitation techniques, a subgroup of athletes with ankle sprains develops residual problems. These sequelae include chronic, recalcitrant pain, functional instability, gross instability, weakness, proprioceptive loss, and consequent athletic disability. Smith and Reischl (1986), in their investigation of young basketball players with ankle sprains, reported that 50% had lingering symptoms. Moreover, 15% of these players developed symptoms that hindered their performance.

Assuredly, chronic ankle problems encompass a spectrum of pathological changes in anatomy and movement patterns with resultant overlapping clinical signs and symptoms, including instability, pain, and impingement. Both chronic ankle instability and ankle impingement, the latter being the focus of this section, lie within this spectrum of chronic ankle pathology. Some patients may develop a combination of instability and impingement that poses a difficult diagnostic and therapeutic challenge to the sports medicine specialist. Clinicians must become skilled in discerning these various chronic ankle problems and implementing appropriate treatment. Recent advances in diagnostic and therapeutic techniques, including ankle arthroscopy, MRI, and innovative rehabilitation protocols, have improved these patients' overall care and prognosis.

History

Wolin et al. (1950) were the first to describe "chronic ankle sprains" in nine patients. These patients all developed intractable anterolateral ankle pain and swelling following inversion ankle sprains. Instability, however, was not noted. Because of chronic symptoms, all patients underwent arthrotomy and exploration. A dense mass of hyalinized connective tissue originating from the anteroinferior portion of the talofibular ligament and extending into the joint was observed. The authors labeled this tissue "meniscoid" because it resembled a torn meniscus in the knee, and they thought the disability experienced by these patients was secondary to entrapment of the tissue between the fibula and talus.

More recently, McCarroll et al. (1987) described a similarly placed band of fibrous, meniscus-like tissue during arthroscopic examination of four collegiate soccer players who had suffered repeated inversion ankle sprains accompanied by persistent pain, swelling, and trapping. This "meniscoid" lesion is shown in Figure 8-6.

Anatomy

Thoroughly understanding the normal anatomy of the lateral gutter of the ankle joint will enable the sports medicine professional to better appreciate pathologic changes in this region. The lateral gutter, as demonstrated in Figure 8-7, is bordered by the fibula laterally, the talus medially, and the tibia with the tibiofibular ligament superiorly. The anterior talofibular, calcaneofibular, and anterior inferior tibiofibular ligaments constitute the anterior border. The posterior border is comprised of the posterior talofibular, calcaneofibular, and posterior inferior tibiofibular ligaments. In cross section, the lateral gutter extends from anterior to posterior between the fibula and talus, as shown in Figure 8-8.

Pathologic Anatomy

Inversion ankle sprains result in a pathoanatomic spectrum of injury involving ligament, capsule, cartilage, and bone. Consequently, the clinician often has difficulty assessing the degree of anatomic injury

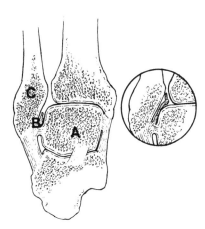

FIGURE 8-6. *"Meniscoid" lesion in the anterolateral aspect of an ankle joint.* From McCarroll et al. (1987).

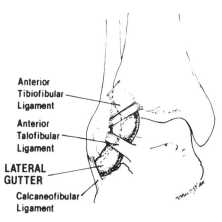

FIGURE 8-7. *Anterior borders of lateral gutter.* From Ferkel et al. (1991).

solely from the patient history, the physical exam and the radiologic studies. Typically, the pathologic entity found in anterolateral ankle impingement is a dense mass of hypertrophic scar tissue extending from the anterolateral capsule posteriorly into the lateral gutter. Histologic specimens in the report by Wolin and colleagues (1950) revealed a combination of fibrous, fibrocartilaginous, and inflammatory tissue as well as hypertrophic synovium. Subsequent studies reported similar histologic findings (Bartolozzi et al., 1987; Bassett, et al., 1990; Ferkel et al., 1991), although the hypertrophied mass is typically synovial in origin (Jacobson & Liu, 1992; Martin et al., 1989; Meislin et al., 1993).

Ferkel et al. (1991) believe anterolateral impingement develops following an inversion ankle sprain. With repetitive motion, the ends of the incompletely healed ligament become inflamed with resultant synovitis and scar formation. As this scar tissue grows, a cyclical inflammatory

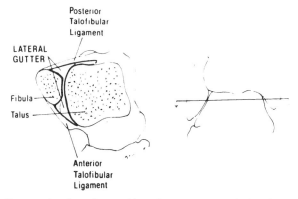

FIGURE 8-8. *Cross-section through area of lateral gutter.* From Ferkel et al. (1991).

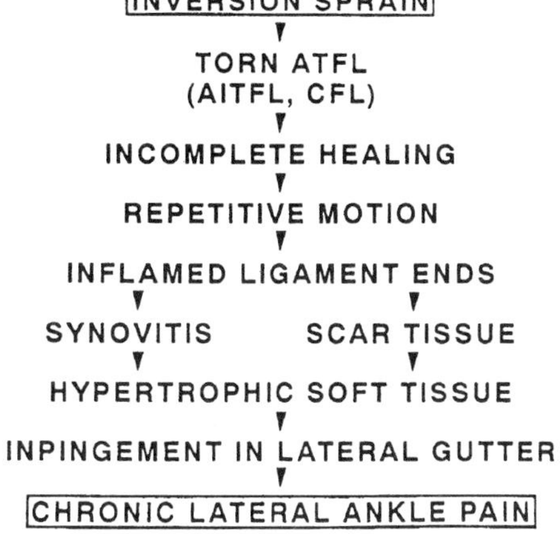

```
                    ┌─────────────────┐
                    │ INVERSION SPRAIN │
                    └─────────────────┘
                             ▼
                        TORN ATFL
                       (AITFL, CFL)
                             ▼
                    INCOMPLETE HEALING
                             ▼
                     REPETITIVE MOTION
                             ▼
                   INFLAMED LIGAMENT ENDS
                      ▼               ▼
                  SYNOVITIS        SCAR TISSUE
                      ▼               ▼
                   HYPERTROPHIC SOFT TISSUE
                             ▼
                INPINGEMENT IN LATERAL GUTTER
                             ▼
              ┌─────────────────────────────┐
              │ CHRONIC LATERAL ANKLE PAIN   │
              └─────────────────────────────┘
```

FIGURE 8-9. *Sequence of development of chronic lateral ankle pain.* ATFL, anterior talofibular ligament; AITFL, anterior inferior tibiofibular ligament; CFL, calcaneofibular ligament. From Ferkel et al. (1991).

process ensues as the mass causes irritation and impinges on the space between the talus, tibia, and fibula. This pathologic process is depicted in Figure 8-9.

In 1990, Bassett et al. described a separate distal fascicle of the anterior inferior tibiofibular ligament. This distinct fascicle running parallel and distal to the anterior inferior tibiofibular ligament was present in 10 of 11 cadaver specimens. In the same study, they reported on seven patients with chronic anterior ankle pain who were found to have a thickened "Bassett's" ligament that impinged on the anterolateral talus during ankle dorsiflexion. The distal fascicle was resected in all seven patients, with subsequent pain relief and without loss of stability. These authors theorized that the anterolateral talar dome in an ankle with increased lateral laxity may extrude anteriorly with ankle dorsiflexion and impinge against this distal fascicle, with resultant anterior ankle pain. In some situations, then, ankle impingement may embody an amalgam of pathologic soft tissue formation and occult kinematic instability.

Practical Implications

Diagnosis. To accurately diagnose ankle impingement, the sports medicine specialist must employ a systematic approach and maintain a high level of suspicion. In short, an ankle sprain may be more than "just a sprain." Ankle impingement should be suspected in an athlete who has a history of repetitive ankle sprains, chronic and persistent anterolateral ankle pain when performing activities such as pivoting and pushing off, and sensations of weakness and "giving way" in the ankle joint. Often, these subjective symptoms are absent before or after activity. Physical examination usually reveals localized tenderness in the anterolateral gutter. Occasionally bogginess, erythema, and diffuse swelling are present. Ankle motion is usually normal or slightly limited in dorsiflexion. Excessive foot pronation, pes planus, or posterior tibialis tendinitis may aggravate the impingement (Jacobson & Liu, 1992). Increased lateral laxity with anterior drawer or varus stress tests is not present in pure impingement. Plain radiographs and stress views are obtained to help rule out other differential diagnostic entities, including pathologic lateral ligamentous laxity. Subjective functional instability may be present secondary to pain, but chronic lateral ankle instability is not seen in the classical anterolateral soft-tissue impingement syndrome. Secondary imaging techniques (e.g., CT, MRI) can also facilitate a correct diagnosis and exclude other sources of pathology. As reported by Meyers et al. (1988), 13 of 31 consecutive patients with chronic residual ankle pain had avulsed intra- or juxta-articular fragments of traumatic origin that were detected by CT scanning but were not readily apparent on standard radiographs. Sagittal MRI slices usually demonstrate excessive soft tissue with low signal intensity in the lateral gutter, although MRI has been associated with false-negative results in some patients (Ferkel et al., 1991).

Many other entities besides impingement can cause anterolateral ankle pain, including those listed in Table 8-2. The sports medicine professional must encompass these in his differential diagnosis.

Distinguishing lateral gutter ankle pain from pain in the sinus tarsi can be particularly difficult. If an injection of local anesthetic into the sinus tarsi alleviates the symptoms, the diagnosis is not anterolateral impingement (Ferkel et al., 1991).

Bartolozzi et al. (1987) proposed a classification for athletes with impingement syndrome (Table 8-3). The classification incorporates not only pathologic soft tissue changes but also the possibility of concomitant "patholaxity."

Treatment. When the diagnosis of impingement syndrome has been made, all patients should undergo a systematic conservative therapy

---

TABLE 8–2. *Differential diagnosis of ankle impingement pain.*

1. Osteochondral fractures of the talus
2. Calcific densities beneath the medial or lateral malleoli
3. Peroneal subluxation or dislocation
4. Tarsal coalition
5. Subtalar joint dysfunction
6. Degenerative joint disease
7. Chronic lateral ligament laxity
8. Sinus tarsi syndrome
9. Syndesmotic ligament injury

TABLE 8-3. *Classification of ankle impingement syndrome.*

Grade I:	Normal X-rays, anterolateral capsular thickening seen on MRI and verified arthroscopically
Grade II:	Extra-articular or intra-articular osteophytes with articular surfaces entirely normal
Grade III:	Bony abnormalities involving articular surface (i.e. osteochondritis dissecans)
Grade IV:	Previous intra-articular fracture

program combining physical therapy, nonsteroidal anti-inflammatory medication, bracing, and possible steroid injection. A systematic approach to diagnosis and appropriate therapeutic intervention for chronic recurrent ankle sprains is presented in Figure 8-10. We have used a rehabilitation program that requires a baseline range-of-motion assessment and isokinetic testing. The rehabilitation protocol includes the application of ice, phonophoresis, electrical stimulation, exercise and strengthening (isometric, isokinetic, and isotonic), range-of-motion activities (stretching, joint mobilization), and cross training. Functional progression with multidirectional exercises, proprioceptive training, and sport simulation are gradually incorporated into the rehabilitation regimen.

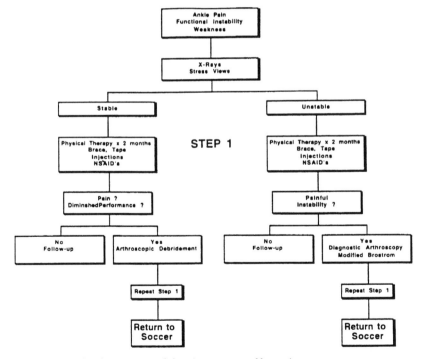

FIGURE 8–10. *Plan for treatment of chronic recurrent ankle sprains.*

Arthroscopic intervention is indicated when a patient with an otherwise negative work up and a history of recurrent ankle sprains develops subsequent chronic ankle pain and tenderness in the lateral gutter that does not respond to conventional treatments. Arthroscopic intervention includes initial joint inspection, debridement of the impingement mass, removal of distal tibia and talar dome osteophytes, and chondroplasty of the tibia and talus when indicated. Fifty-one percent of the patients in the study by Ferkel et al. (1991) had chondromalacia of the anterolateral talar dome. During debridement of the pathologic mass, care must be taken not to excise the anterior talofibular ligament.

In the subgroup of athletes with impingement who fail to adequately respond to an aggressive rehabilitation program, diagnostic and therapeutic arthroscopy has proven to be an effective and efficient treatment. Bartolozzi and Mandelbaum(1987) reported 77% "good" or "excellent" results. In similar studies, all with follow up periods exceeding 2 y (Ferkel et al., 1991; Liu et al., 1994; Meislin et al., 1993), good or excellent results were reported in 84%, 87%, and 90% of patients, respectively.

Directions for Future Research on Ankle Impingement Syndromes

Chronic ankle impingement, although suspected clinically, is ultimately diagnosed and treated arthroscopically. The exact incidence of anterolateral impingement following an ankle sprain is unknown because there is no clinical test that reliably identifies soft-tissue impingement. Many patients with impingement undoubtedly improve with conservative therapy, thus avoiding diagnostic arthroscopy. We hope that future investigations will enable us to more precisely define the incidence of ankle impingement. By developing different coils and imaging planes, MRI and cine-MRI may eventually better define the pathoanatomical and pathomechanical aspects of these lesions. In addition to allowing us to determine the number of patients with impingement who require surgery, this improved diagnostic capability might also reveal a correlation between the incidence and size of the impingement mass and sprain severity.

SUMMARY

Sports medicine has undergone exponential development since the 1970s. This evolving growth perhaps can be primarily attributed to sports medicine specialists responding to the expanding needs and rising expectations of an athletic population. Consequently, athletes are now treated in a multidisciplinary fashion. The efforts of physicians, basic scientists, biomechanical engineers, trainers, physical therapists, podiatrists, chiropractors, nutritionists, and exercise physiologists have spawned an amazingly healthy, synergistic relationship, with their combined achievements outpacing their individual contributions. In each of the athletic injuries discussed previously, this cooperation has markedly improved the care of our athletic population with respect to diagnosis, treatment, performance enhancement, and prevention. Accordingly, the athlete has been allowed to stay in the game at a maximally functional level.

BIBLIOGRAPHY

Andersson, C., M. Odensten, L. Good, and J. Gillquist (1989). Surgical or non-surgical treatment of acute rupture of the anterior cruciate ligament. *J. Bone Joint Surg.* 71A:965–974.

Arendt, E., and R. Dick (1995). Knee injury patterns among men and women in collegiate basketball and soccer: NCAA data and review of literature. *Am. J. Sports Med.* 23:694–701.

Arnoczky, S.P., G.B. Tarvin, and J.L. Marshall (1982). Anterior cruciate ligament replacement using patellar tendon. *J. Bone Joint Surg.* 64A:217–224.

Attarian, D.E., H.J. McCrackin, D.P. DeVito, J.H. McElhaney, and W.E. Garrett Jr., (1985). A biomechanical study of human lateral ankle ligaments and autogenous reconstructive grafts. *Am. J. Sports Med.* 13:377–381.

Bach, B.R. Jr., G.T. Jones, C.A. Hager, F.A. Sweet, and S. Luergans (1995). Arthrometric results of arthroscopically assisted anterior cruciate ligament reconstruction using autograft patellar tendon substitution. *Am. J. Sports Med.* 23:179–185.

Bartolozzi, A.R., B.R. Mandelbaum, G.A.M. Finerman, J.E. Zachazewski, P. Padilla, and M. Meyerson (1987). The anterior capsular impingement syndrome of the ankle. Presented at 13th Annual Meeting of the American Orthopaedic Society for Sports Medicine, Orlando, FL.

Bassett, F.H. III, H.S. Gates, J. B. Billys, H.B. Morris, and P.K. Nikolaou (1990). Talar impingement by the anteroinferior tibiofibular ligament. *J. Bone Joint Surg.* 72A:55–59.

Brittberg, M., A. Lindahl, A. Nilsson, C. Ohlsson, O. Isaksson, and L. Peterson (1994). Treatment of deep cartilage defects in the knee with autologous chondrocyte tranplantation. *N. Eng. J. Med.* 331:889–895.

Cannon, W.D. Jr., and J.M. Vittori (1992). The incidence of healing in arthroscopic meniscal tears in anterior cruciate ligament reconstructed knees versus stable knees. *Am. J. Sports Med.* 20:176–181.

Chen, Y.C. (1985). Arthroscopy of the ankle joint. In: M. Watanabe (ed.) *Arthroscopy of Small Joints.* New York: Igaku-Shoin, pp. 116.

Clancy, W.G. Jr., D.A. Nelson, B. Reider, and R. Narechania (1982). Anterior cruciate ligament reconstruction using one-third of the patellar ligament, augmented by extraarticular tendon transfers. *J. Bone Joint Surg.* 64A:352–359.

Deutsch, A.L. (1992). Traumatic injuries of bone and osteonecrosis. In: A.L. Deutsch, J. Mink, and R. Kerr (eds.) *MRI of the Foot and Ankle.* New York: Raven Press, pp. 75–109.

Devas, M.B. (1958). Stress fractures of the tibia in athletes or "shin soreness." *J. Bone Joint Surg.* 40B:227–239.

DiStefano, V. (1993). Anterior cruciate ligament reconstruction: Autograft or Allograft? *Clin. Sports Med.* 12:1–11.

Duncan, J.B., R. Hunter, M. Purnell, and J. Freeman (1995). Meniscal injuries associated with acute anterior cruciate ligament tears in Alpine skiers. *Am. J. Sports Med.* 23:170–172.

Ekstrand, J., and H. Tropp (1990). The incidence of ankle sprains in soccer. *Foot & Ankle* 11:41–44.

Engkvist, O. (1979). Reconstruction of patellar articular cartilage with free autologous perichondral grafts. *Scand. J. Plast. Reconst. Surg.* 13:361–369.

Ettlinger, C.F., R.J. Johnson, and J.E. Shealy (1995). A method to help reduce the risk of serious knee sprains incurred in Alpine skiing. *Am. J. Sports Med.* 23:531–537.

Ferkel, R.D., R.P. Karzel, W. Del Pizzo, M.J. Friedman, and S.P. Fischer (1991). Arthroscopic treatment of anterolateral impingement of the ankle. *Am. J. Sports Med.* 19:440–446.

Fideler, B.M., C.T. Vangsness Jr., T. Moore, Z. Li, and S. Rasheed (1994). Effects of gamma irradiation on the human immunodeficiency virus. *J. Bone Joint Surg.* 76:1032–1035.

Garrick, J.G. (1988). Epidemiology of the ACL. In: J.A. Feagin Jr. (ed.) *The Crucial Ligaments.* New York: Churchill Livingstone, pp. 173–176.

Gylys-Morin, V.M., P.C. Hajek, D.J. Sartoris, and D. Resnick (1987). Articular cartilage defects: Detectability in cadaver knees with MR. *Am J. Radiol.* 148:1153–1157.

Henning, C.E., M.A. Lynch, K.M. Yearout, S.W. Vequist, R.J. Stallbaumer, and K.A. Decker (1990). Arthroscopic meniscal repair using a fibrin clot. *Clin. Orthop.* 252:64–72.

Henning, et al. (1987).

Highgenboten, C.L. (1992). Outpatient anterior cruciate ligament reconstruction and patient-controlled analgesia. *JAMA* 268:3,432.

Jacobson, K.E., and S.H. Liu (1992). Anterolateral impingement of the ankle. *J. Med. Assoc. Georgia* 81:297–299.

Johansson, C., I. Ekenman, H. Tornkvist, E. Eriksson (1990). Stress fractures of the femoral neck in athletes: The consequences of a delay in diagnosis. *Am. J. Sports Med.* 18:524–528.

Jones, B.H., M.W. Bovee, J.M. Harris III., and D.N. Cowan (1993). Intrinsic risk factors for exercise-related injuries among male and female army trainees. *Am. J. Sports Med.* 21: 705–710.

Jones, D.C., and S.L. James (1987). Overuse injuries of the lower extremity: Shin splints, iliotibial band friction syndrome, and exertional compartment syndromes. *Clin. Sports Med.* 6:273–290.

Kao, J.T., C.E. Giangarra, G. Singer, and S. Martin (1995). A comparison of outpatient and inpatient anterior cruciate ligament reconstruction surgery. *Arthroscopy* 11:151–156.

Lephart, S.M., M.S. Kocher, C.D. Harner, and F.H. Fu (1993). Quadriceps strength and functional capacity after anterior cruciate ligament reconstruction: Patellar tendon autograft versus allograft. *Am. J. Sports Med.* 21:738–743.

Liu, S.H., A. Raskin, L. Osti, C. Baker, K. Jacobson, and G. Finerman (1994). Arthroscopic treatment of anterolateral ankle impingement. *Arthroscopy* 10:215–218.

Lomander, L.S. (1991). Markers of cartilage metabolism and arthrosis: A review. *Acta Orthop. Scand.* 62:623–632.

Lombardo, S.J., and D.W. Benson (1982). Stress fractures of the femur in runners. *Am. J. Sports Med.* 10: 219–227.

Lutz, G.E., R.A. Palmitier, K.N. An, and E.Y.S. Chao (1991). Comparison of tibiofemoral joint forces during open kinetic chain and closed kinetic chain exercises. Presented at the 58th annual conference of the American Academy of Orthopaedic Surgeons, Anaheim, CA.

MacDonald, P.B., D. Hedden, O. Pacin, and D. Huebert (1995). Effects of an accelerated rehabilitation program after anterior cruciate ligament reconstruction with combined semitendinosus-gracilis autograft and a ligament augmentation device. *Am. J. Sports Med.* 23:588–592.

Malcolm, L.L., and D. Daniel (1980). The biomechanical rationale for partial meniscectomy. Presented at the International Arthroscopy Association Meeting, Philadelphia, PA.

Mandelbaum, B.R. (1993). Intensive training in the young athlete: Pathoanatomic change. In: B.R. Cahill and A.J. Pearl (eds.) *Intensive Participation in Children's Sports.* Champaign, IL: Human Kinetics Publ. pp. 217–233.

Marcus R., C. Cann, P. Madvig, J. Minkoff, M. Goddard, M. Bayer, M. Martin, L. Gaudiani, W. Haskell, and H. Genant (1985). Menstrual function and bone mass in elite women distance runners: Endocrine and metabolic features. *Annals Int. Med.* 102:158–163.

Marder, R.A., J.R. Raskind, and M. Carroll (1991). Prospective evaluation of arthroscopically assisted anterior cruciate ligament reconstruction: Patellar tendon versus semitendinosus and gracilis tendons. *Am. J. Sports Med.* 19:478–484.

Markey, K.L. (1987). Stress fractures. *Clin. Sports Med.* 6:405–425.

Martin, D.F., W.W. Curl, and C.L. Baker (1989). Arthroscopic treatment of chronic synovitis of the ankle. *Arthroscopy* 5:110–114.

Matheson, G.O., D.B. Clement, D.C. McKenzie, J.E. Taunton, D.R. Lloyd-Smith, and J.G. MacIntyre (1987). Stress fractures in athletes: A study of 320 cases. *Am. J. Sports Med.* 15: 46–58.

McBryde, A.M. Jr. (1976). Stress fractures in athletes. *J. Sports Med.* 3:212–217.

McCarroll, J.R., J.W. Schrader, K.D. Shelbourne, A.C. Rettig, and M.A. Bisesi (1987). Meniscoid lesions of the ankle in soccer players. *Am. J. Sports Med.* 15:255–257.

Meislin, R.J., D.J. Rose, J.S. Parisien, and S. Springer (1993). Arthroscopic treatment of synovial impingement of the ankle. *Am. J. Sports Med.* 21:186–189.

Meyer, J.M., P. Hoffmeyer, and X. Savoy (1988). High resolution computed tomography in the chronically painful ankle sprain. *Foot & Ankle* 8:291–296.

Muller, W. (1983). Kinematics of the rolling-gliding principle. In W. Muller (ed.) *The Knee: Form, Function, and Ligament Reconstruction.* New York: Springer-Verlag. pp. 8–13.

Niedermann, B., S. Boe, J. Lauritzen, and J.M. Rubak (1985). Glued periosteal grafts in the knee. *Acta Orthop. Scand.* 56:457–460.

Noakes, T.D., J.A. Smith, G. Lindenberg, C.E. Wills (1985). Pelvic stress fractures in long-distance runners. *Am.J. Sports Med.* 13:120–123.

Noyes, F.R., D.L. Butler, E.S. Grood, R.F. Zernicke, and M.S. Hefzy (1984). Biomechanical analysis of human ligament grafts used in knee-ligament repairs and reconstructions. *J.Bone Joint Surg.* 66A:344–352.

Olson, E.J., C.D. Harner, F.H. Fu, and M.B. Silbey (1992). Clinical use of fresh, frozen soft-tissue allografts. *Orthopedics* 15:1225–1232.

Orava, S., J. Puranen, and L. Ala-Ketola (1978). Stress fractures caused by physical exercise. *Acta Orthop. Scand.* 49:19–27.

Otero, A.R., and L. Hutcheson (1993). A comparison of the doubled semitendinosus/gracilis and central third of the patellar tendon autografts in arthroscopic anterior cruciate ligament resconstruction. *Arthroscopy* 9:143–148.

Peterson, L., D. Menche, and D. Grande (1984). Chondrocyte transplantation—an experimental model in the rabbit. In: *Transactions from the 30th Annual Orthopedic Research Society, Atlanta, GA, February 7–9*. Palatine, Ill.: Orthopedic Research Society. pp. 218 (Abstract).

Prather, J.L., M.L. Nusynowitz, H.A. Snowdy, A.D. Hughes, W.H. McCartney, and R.J. Bragg (1977). Scintigraphic findings in stress fractures. *J. Bone Joint Surg.* 59A:869–873.

Protzman, R.R., and C.G. Griffis (1977). Stress fractures in men and women undergoing military training. *J.Bone Joint Surg.* 59A:825.

Shelbourne, K.D., and P. Nitz (1990). Accelerated rehabilitation after anterior cruciate ligament reconstruction. *Am. J. Sports Med.* 18:292–299.

Shelbourne, K.D., H.J. Whitaker, J.R. McCarroll, A.C. Rettig, and L.d. Hirschman (1990). Anterior cruciate ligament injury: Evaluation of intraarticular reconstruction of acute tears without repairs: Two to seven year followup of 155 athletes. *Am. J. Sports Med.* 18:484–489.

Shelbourne, K.D., J.H. Wilckens, A. Mollabashy, and M. DeCarlor (1991). Arthrofibrosis in acute anterior cruciate ligament reconstruction: The effect of timing of reconstruction and rehabilitation. *Am. J. Sports Med.* 19:332–336.

Smith, R.W., and S.F. Reischl (1986). Treatment of ankle sprains in young athletes. *Am. J. Sports Med.* 14:465–471.

Sobotnick, S.I. (1985). The biomechanics of running: Implications for the prevention of foot injuries. *Sports Med.* 2:144–153.

Specchiulli, F., R. Laforgia, A. Mocci, L. Miolla, L. Scialpi, and G. Solarino Jr. (1995). Anterior cruciate ligament reconstruction: A comparison of two techniques. *Clin. Orthop.* 311:142–147.

Spindler, K.P., J.P. Schils, J.A. Bergfeld, J.T. Andrish, G.G. Weiker, T.G. Anderson, D.W. Piraino, B.J. Richmond, and S.V. Medendorp (1993). Prospective study of osseous, articular and meniscal lesions in recent anterior cruciate ligament tears by magnetic resonance imaging and arthroscopy. *Am. J. Sports Med.* 21:551–557.

Steiner et al. (1994).

Sterling, J.C., D.W. Edelstein, R.C. Calvo, and R. Webb II (1992). Stress fractures in the athlete: Diagnosis and management. *Sports Med.* 14:336–346.

Swenson, T.M., and F.H. Fu (1993). Anterior cruciate ligament reconstruction: long term results using autograft tissue. *Clin. Sports Med.* 12:709–722.

Swenson, T.M., and C.D. Harner (1995). Knee ligament and meniscal injuries: Current concepts. *Orthop. Clin. N. Am.* 26:529–546.

Tierney, G.S., R.W. Wright, J.P. Smith, and D.A. Fischer (1995). Anterior cruciate ligament reconstruction as an outpatient procedure. *Am. J. Sports Med.* 23:755–756.

Tipton, C.M., S.L. James, W. Mergner, and T. Tcheng (1970). Influence of exercise on strength of medial collateral knee ligaments of dogs. *Am. J. Physiol.* 218:894–902.

Torg J.S., H.Pavlov, and E. Torg (1987). Overuse injuries in sport: the foot. *Clin. Sports Med.* 6:291–320.

Warren, R.F. (1989). Meniscectomy and repair in the anterior cruciate ligament-deficient patient. *Clin. Orthop. Rel. Res* 252:55–63.

Whitelaw, G.P., M.J. Wetzler, A.S. Levy, D. Segal, and K. Bissonnette (1991). A pneumatic leg brace for the treatment of tibial stress fractures. *Clin. Orthop.* 270:301–305.

Wojtys, E., M. Wilson, K. Buckwalter, E. Braunstein, W. Martel (1987). Magnetic resonance imaging of knee hyaline cartilage and intraarticular pathology. *Am. J. Sports Med.* 15:455–463.

Wolin, I., F. Glassman, S. Sideman, and D.H. Levinthal (1950). Internal derangement of the talofibular component of the ankle. *Surg. Gynecol. Obstet.* 91:193–200.

Yasuda, K., Y. Tomiyama, Y. Ohkoshi, and K. Kaneda (1988). Arthroscopic observations of autogeneic quadriceps and patellar tendon grafts after anterior cruciate ligament reconstruction of the knee. *Clin. Orthop.* 246:217–224.

DISCUSSION

HOUGH: Many decisions using high-technology interventions depends on how much access the physician has to the technology and the willingness of managed-care organizations or health insurers to pay for expensive procedures that might lead to a definitive diagnosis. In particular, when do you think it is best to order an MRI, and under what circumstance does the MRI result actually change the way that the physician treats a knee injury involving the ACL or a meniscal tear?

MANDELBAUM: There are two populations for which use of the MRI technique is indicated. The first is elite athletes, especially professional athletes, because time away from competition is a critical variable. If there is a positive MRI result, the physician and athlete can be confident in deciding to initiate a surgical intervention quickly, whereas with a negative MRI result, the physician can be about 95% confident that there is no serious pathology. The second population is patients who have defined knee injuries with pain and swelling but who want no surgical intervention. In these patients, a negative MRI result can be very useful in making the decision to avoid surgery.

HOUGH: In our geographic area there seems to be great variability among the radiologists reading or interpreting MRIs. Much of this variability is related to the fact that upwards of 20% of lateral meniscal tears may be misread on an MRI. What are your recommendations for dealing with suspected meniscal tears when the MRI is negative?

MANDELBAUM: If the clinical picture strongly suggests a meniscal tear, but the MRI doesn't reveal it, the physician must make a decision based on clinical experience; if the knee fails to respond to less invasive techniques, arthroscopic surgery is indicated. In such cases, the MRI is not especially helpful.

HOUGH: Under what circumstances would you do an ACL reconstruction? How do you factor in patient age and level of activity that the patient wishes to pursue? In our practice we have a lot of patients 50–80 years old that want to be extremely active and do not want to be limited by problems of an ACL-deficient knee. How do you deal with these issues?

MANDELBAUM: If you had injured an ACL in 1985, you would have had a large incision, would have spent 4 d in the hospital, would have worn a cast for 2 mo, and the probability for success was 50%. Today, the surgery is an out-patient procedure, you would have a range of motion of about 100 degrees in the recovery room, you would probably be done with the rehabilitation program after about 6 mo, and the probability for success is 90–95%. So the nature of what we can accomplish and the indications for surgery have changed dramatically in the last 10 y or so. If a patient simply wants to jog every morning and does participate in any pivoting sports, I would be inclined to avoid surgery with that individual unless the knee was very instable. On the other hand, if a competitive tennis player, squash player, or volleyball player has moderate instability, ACL reconstruction may well be indicated. Also, the results of ACL reconstruction for those older than 40 y, both men and women, are no different than those for younger people. I had a 68–year-old retiree who skied 60 d/y and tore his ACL. He said, "Doc, I retired to ski. You can't tell me that I am too old to fix my ligament. Fix it." I did, and he got to ski 50 d during the following year. In another 10 y, the preferred treatment is probably going to be entirely different; the molecular biologists will help evolve new techniques to make injury care much more effective than it is even now.

BARTON: Would you comment on your ideas of when to brace, and when not to brace? I don't think there is a great deal of agreement on this topic among sports practitioners today.

MANDELBAUM: In the days when we couldn't stabilize joints very well, even with an operation, the brace had a greater impact, but we now know that braces have little impact on the ACL-reconstructed knee. There is some evidence that during the early months of rehabilitation, as the ligament is getting stronger, there may be some benefit of bracing. We are getting away from the use of braces in athletic participation, but use postoperative braces in case there is a traumatic injury while the ligament is going through its biological ligamentization process and getting stronger. So I believe we should be gradually moving away from using braces during sport participation after full recovery from ACL reconstruction in most athletes. On the other hand, there is some evidence that reconstructed knees that continue to have excessive instability and laxity may benefit somewhat from bracing.

BARTON: You mentioned that ankles that stay swollen for an extended period of time are much more likely to experience ankle-impingement syndrome, but many of our high-level athletes participate daily on swollen ankles. How strong a relationship is there between continual play throughout a season on swollen ankles and the likelihood of having impingement syndrome?

MANDELBAUM: The ankle sprain involves an entire spectrum of injuries to ligaments, bones, or cartilages. So a small ligament sprain has no consequences, but an osteochondral injury in association with a ligamentous injury has much greater potential for developing into an impingement syndrome. To illustrate, if we do an MRI on a sprained ankle, and it shows an osteochondral bruise, we know that this is likely to be a 6–wk injury. If the athlete resumes practice the next week, the athlete is going to limp. The physician must say, "You are not going to be able to play for 6 wk." When both the athlete and the coach understand this and allow the injury to heal adequately, a greater problem in the future can be prevented. As we better understand the relationships between pain, relative instability of the ankle, and impingement, we will be able to not only treat these problems, but to prevent them.

SCOTT: I think the physician must differentiate between intra-articular swelling and extra-articular swelling. In the high school and college athletes who sustain inversion sprains, the lateral ligaments sometimes pull on the distal fibula and cause a periosteal swelling. After a couple of weeks you can see that the ankle joint is not swollen, but the bottom of the lateral malleolus is still swollen. The physical exam will reveal that this is bony swelling instead of intra-articular swelling. I find that they can play with this bony swelling without causing further problems. Persistent intra-articular swelling of the ankle is an indication that there is something wrong, and that should be a good tip-off to investigate further.

TERJUNG: You described in the chapter how an affected athlete can look back and see the development of a stress fracture from a mild, localized onset of pain that occurs toward the end of an exercise bout, to a greater pain starting earlier in the exercise with continued volume of exercise until finally a fairly severe exercise-induced pain that becomes devastating. The athlete, in fact, may not recover. Obviously, the best treatment is prevention. Can't this well-described progression be used to preempt the severity of stress fracture injury?

MANDELBAUM: Most definitely. What we try to do is help the athletic trainers and athletes understand that progression, that red flag, so that the problem is stopped somewhere between a stress reaction and stress fracture.

TERJUNG: So a lot has to do with the education of the athletes?

MANDELBAUM: Certainly.

KOTO: Will you expand on the difference between becoming more aggressive with functional activities in the rehab program and early return to sports activities? The idea that athletes should quickly return to full practice and competition puts pressure on the practitioner, especially the orthopaedists, the physical therapists, and the athletic trainers, to get the patient back to participation as soon as possible, and that may be unrealistic. When dealing with elite athletes, ski racers, elite soccer players, or highly-paid professional athletes, there are a lot of incentives to getting an individual ready to play in 4–6 mo vs. 9–12 mo. Is there any way to minimize this "rush to return?"

MANDELBAUM: I think it is realistic that many athletes, professional, elite, and recreational, can get back to their sports in 4–5 mo after serious ACL injury.

SCOTT: I think patients who push doctors or trainers to get them better faster after an ACL reconstruction may be the wrong persons to be operating on because ACL reconstructions require tremendous patient responsibility. The way to get around being "put on the spot" is to show patients the entire protocol, emphasizing every step that they have to go through successfully before the next step is attempted.

KOTO: Could you expand on practical techniques that might be used to minimize knee injuries in female athletes, whose musculature may not be as strong as that in males?

MANDELBAUM: The question of why ACL tears in women are on the increase is a fascinating one. Chuck Henning identified an increase in the incidence of ACL tears in female high school basketball players and modified the players movement patterns to decrease ACL injuries. That is a good example of how laboratory or clinical findings can be translated into coaching techniques that can help prevent injuries. We are collecting data on ACL injuries in soccer players and plan to evaluate with biomechanical analyses how the ACL tears occur and perhaps teach the players how to alter their movements to minimize the risk of injury or how to avoid situations that are likely to lead to injury.

KOTO: There is a lot of confusion among athletic trainers on how to differentiate between stress fractures at the base of the 5th metatarsal and Jones fractures of that bone. The first would probably require decreased activity with some weight bearing, and the second would require immobilization, perhaps no weight bearing, and even surgical intervention. Can you clarify this?

MANDELBAUM: As you know, the Jones fracture is in the zone of transition between the metaphysis and the diaphysis, where there is a poor blood supply; the Jones fracture does not heal as quickly as the more proximal fractures at the base of the bone do. To treat Jones fractures, especially in soccer athletes, the physician should operate early by putting in a screw and/or bone graft.

KOTO: Have you had any success with orthotic devices to put the rear foot and the forefoot in more of a neutral position to decrease ankle impingement?

MANDELBAUM: I don't think there is much evidence that orthotics can prevent the incidence of impingement syndromes, but I think orthotics can minimize certain anatomic variations; they can be used as an adjunct therapy.

MURRAY: How is the function and integrity of ligaments and cartilage influenced by the dehydration that is so common during training and competition?

MANDELBAUM: With dehydration comes fatigue, and with fatigue comes a higher incidence of variety of injuries late in the game. We know that the more exhausted athlete in the last 30 min of a soccer game or in the last part of a distance run will have a greater incidence of stress injuries or acute injuries.

MURRAY: But do we know anything about the direct effect of dehydration on the function, the morphology, or the integrity of connective tissue?

MANDELBAUM: I don't know that there is any information to answer that question.

CLARKSON: You provided an overview of the relationship between nutrition, particularly insufficient calcium intake, and stress fractures in female athletes and stated that women athletes with secondary abnormal menstrual function or amenorrhea should be evaluated by a primary care physician for possible estrogen supplementation. Because amenorrhea and abnormal menstrual cycles may be the result of insufficient caloric intake, I suggest that the athletes should first be seen by a nutritionist for a nutritional evaluation and that nutritional intervention should be tried before considering estrogen supplementation.

Also, a particular problem that I have noticed with classical ballet dancers who have insufficient caloric intake is that not only do they have recurrent stress fractures, their stress fractures heal very slowly or not at all.

MANDELBAUM: Your point is well taken.

SCOTT: With repeated stress fractures, you have to look at the psyche of the patient. There was a female member of the United States Olympic rowing team who was also a medical student, and had 11 stress fractures of the ribs. That person knew the physiology but ignored the bodily signs. There may be an underlying eating disorder affecting any athlete who has repetitive stress fractures. Such persons may be using their exercise as something other than just fun or competition. I think you have to look at their psyches.

EICHNER: Why are there so many stress fractures in your male soccer players? Is it just "too much too fast?" Is your ability to diagnose stress fractures improving with the use of MRIs? Is there possibly a nutritional aspect, such as low dietary calcium?

MANDELBAUM: The answer is probably, "Yes," to each of those questions. There are many factors involved in soccer injuries, including the type of shoe worn by the player, the nature of the playing field, the training progressions, and the dietary factors.

ARROYO: What can be done to prevent soccer players from getting stress fractures?

MANDELBAUM: Preventing stress fractures through improved education of coaches, athletes, and sports health professionals is critical.

ARROYO: When you perform an MRI procedure and the radiologist finds nothing wrong with the ACL, but clinically you are convinced that it is injured, will the insurance companies allow you to perform the arthroscopic procedures?

MANDELBAUM: That is variable. Even in California, which is a very restricted managed-care environment, I would say that 95% of the time the clinical judgment is respected, especially if there is some objective evidence of injury (e.g., if a knee has a 2+ Lachman test result and a 2+ pivot shift), usually it is not a problem.

WENZEL: I would like to reemphasize the tremendous pressure to which athletic trainers are subjected to get athletes back on the playing field quickly with accelerated rehabilitation of ACL injuries. How can a football coach or an athletic trainer effectively communicate with the doctor the notion that it is too early for an athlete to return to action, even though all the data for strength, flexibility, power, and endurance indicate that no adverse effects of returning to action are likely? As a trainer of professional athletes who make $25,000 a night only when playing, I feel enormous pressure to put the athlete back in action, and when that occurs, I am sitting there on the bench saying, "God, I hope he doesn't tear his ACL again." If that happens, the team may not renew the athlete's contract for six-million dollars, and I may lose my job because the player's health and well being is my responsibility. How can I effectively communicate with the doctor to make a decision on whether an athlete should return to play 4 mo after surgery as opposed to 6 or 7 mo?

MANDELBAUM: I don't think I have any great advice to offer on this issue. Obviously, we need to develop better criteria for judging when an athlete should be allowed to return to play.

BEHNKE: Track athletes often develop tibial periostitis, which is commonly called shin splints. Particularly at the high school level, coaches may expect the athlete to "run through" this problem, and invariably we see stress fractures develop. Is there any solid information that shows that continued training with shin splints is likely to lead to stress fractures.

MANDELBAUM: Unfortunately, I don't know of any substantial published data on this issue.

Index

Accuracy, exercise testing, 68–70
ACL (anterior cruciate ligament), 319–330; accelerated rehabilitation, 328 330; anatomy, 319; biomechanics, 319; decision making, 320–325; diagnosis, 320; future research, 330; injury mechanisms, 319–320; outpatient reconstruction, 325–326; practical implications, 320–330; prevention, 327 328; reconstruction timing, 325; treatment options, 320–325
ACTH (adreno-corticotropin), 272
Acute phase response, cytokines, 276–277
Adaptive immune system, 273
Adaptive immunity, lymphocyte function, 285–287
Aerobic exercise, caffeine performance effects, 219
Ambient temperature, exercise performance effects, 144–145
Anaerobic energy production, measurement, 79–80
Anaerobic threshold; Conconi-test, 77–78; non-invasive measurement, 76–78; plasma lactate, 74–75
Animal studies, immune system, 289
Ankle impingement syndromes; anatomy, 345; future research, 350; history, 344 345; pathologic anatomy, 345–347; practical implications, 347–350
Anomalous coronaries, 257
Anomalous coronary arteries, sudden death of athletes, 241
Anxiety, relaxation-induced, 8–11
Aortic stenosis, sudden death of athletes, 241
Applied sport psychology, 5–6; goal-setting hypotheses, 14
Arrhythmias, 257–258
Athlete's heart, 244–246
Athletes; following through a competitive season, 293–294; health problem detection, 239–268; sudden death impact, 240–241

B cells (B lymphocytes), immune system, 275–276
Badminton, field tests, 82
Basketball; ACL (anterior cruciate ligament) injury, 319; field tests, 82
Blunt chest trauma, sudden death of athletes, 242

Body carbohydrate stores, sport performance fuel, 98
Body fat stores, sport performance fuel, 97–98
Body temperature, exercise performance manipulations, 143–144
Burnout, 270

Caffeine; diuretic effect, 222; dosage, 220–221; early research, 211–212; endurance performance studies, 213–217; ergogenicity theories, 211; ethical considerations, 222; exercise performance study complications, 212–213; field studies, 220; future research, 228; habitual consumption, 221–222; improved endurance mechanisms, 217–218; intense aerobic exercise, 219; metabolism effect study complications, 212–213; practical implications, 220–222; response variability, 221; shorter-term exercise performance effects, 218 220; short-term intense exercise effects, 219–220; urinary doping levels, 221
Carbohydrate; exercise ingestion rate, 114; exercise ingestion timing, 113 114; exercise ingestion types, 113; feeding during exercise, 110–115; ingestion rates following exercise, 116–117; metabolic responses, 115–116; muscle glycogen resynthesis ingestion types, 117–118; necessity due to muscle's fat oxidation limitations, 103–104; preexercise nutrition, 120–123
Carbohydrate stores, sport performance fuel, 98
Cardiovascular problems; chest pain, 247; echocardiography screening, 249 250; heart murmurs, 248–249; laboratory testing, 250–251; medical history, 247–248; needle-in-haystack dilemma, 246; physical exam, 248; practical alternative, 246; screening, 246–251; syncope, 248
Carnitine; exercise effects, 205–206; exercise supplement effects, 208–210; function, 202–204; future research, 227; macronutrient diet effects on muscles, 205–206; metabolism effects, 208–210; performance effects, 208–210; practical implications, 210; resting metabolism, 205; supplemental effects on plasma and muscle levels, 207; theoretical basis for ergogenic effect, 202 204

Chest pain, cardiovascular problems, 248
Chronic fatigue, 270
Cognitive strategy, 22–38; dissociative, 33–34; elite distance runners, 28 32; lunggom, 24–28; marathon runners, 23–38; non-elite distance runners, 32 38; predominant, 33–34; pre-elite distance runners, 32–38; RSQ (Running Style Questionnaire), 34–35; tumo, 24–25
Competition, immune system relationship, 287–290
Competitive sport, hydration optimization, 139–184
Conconi test, anaerobic threshold, 77–78
Consent procedures, sports psychology, 21–22
Consumers; described, 44; sports psychology concerns, 48–49
Cortisol, 272
CPT (carnitine palmitoyltransferase activity), 103
Creatine; additional supplementation effects, 199–201; ergogenicity theoretical basis, 188–189; exercise performance following supplementation, 192–199; function, 188–189; future research, 227; metabolism, 189–190; practical implications, 201; supplementation effects on muscle content, 190–192
Cycling, field tests, 81
Cytokines, immune system, 276–278, 285

Diagnosis; ACL (anterior cruciate ligament) injury, 320–325; osteochondral knee injuries, 331–332; stress fractures, 337–338
Dietary fat, glycogen resynthesis influences, 118
Diets, high fat/low carbohydrate, 105–106
Dissociative cognitive strategy, 33–34
Distance runners, cognitive strategy, 28–38

Echocardiography, cardiovascular screening role, 249–250
Elite distance runners, cognitive strategy, 28–32
Endurance capacity; energy cost as efficiency measurement, 71–72; indices, 70 79; maximal oxygen uptake (VO2max), 70–71; non-invasive anaerobic threshold measurement, 76–78; plasma lactate response to exercise, 74–78; power output or running velocity at VO2max, 72–74; simulated time trials, 78–79; ventilatory threshold, 77
Endurance performance; caffeine mechanisms, 217–218; caffeine studies, 213 217
Endurance training; fat oxidation increase, 107–109; plasma free fatty acid mobilization, 108–109
Epidemiological studies, immune system, 288–289
Epinephrine, 272

Ergogenic aids, 185–238; caffeine, 210–227; carnitine, 201–210; creatine, 187 201; erythropoietin, 222–226; introduction, 186–187
Erythropoietin, 222–226; ergogenic potential, 223–224; future research, 228; hematological response to rhEPO administration, 224–225; practical implications, 226; recombinant human, 223; rhEPO administration detection, 225–226; safety concerns, 223–224
Exercise; aerobic, 219; ambient temperature performance effects, 144–145; body temperature manipulation during performance, 143–144; caffeine performance effect study complications, 212–213; carbohydrate feeding, 110 115; carbohydrate ingestion timing, 118; carnitine supplement effects, 208 210; fat supplementation methods, 104–105; fatty acid availability, 102–103; fluid ingestion performance effects, 147–149; gastrointestinal function effects, 159–160; graded tests of caffeine effects, 218; heat tolerance mechanisms, 149–151; high-intensity carbohydrate ingestion, 114–115; high intensity fuel use, 101–102; hydration status performance effects, 145–147; infection relationship, 287–288; innate immunity, 279; intense exercise and immune function, 278–287; low-intensity fuel use, 99; moderate-intensity carbohydrate ingestion, 110–113; moderate-intensity fuel use, 99–101; muscle glycogen resynthesis, 116–120; plasma lactate response, 74–78; postexercise rehydration, 161–166; preexercise carbohydrate feedings, 120–123; preexercise hydration, 160–161; rhEPO administration responses, 224–225; shorter-term caffeine performance effects, 218–220; short-term intense caffeine effects, 219–220; temperature regulation, 141–143
Excessive training, 270; immune system relationship, 287–290
Exercise testing; accuracy and variability, 68–70; development, 64; specificity and validity, 67
Exertional sudden death, 240–241
External validity, sport psychology, 16–17

Fat stores, sport performance fuel, 97–98
FFA (free fatty acids); CPT (carnitine palmitoyltransferase activity), 103; exercise intensity availability 102–103; sport performance fuel, 96
Field tests, sport performance, 81–83
Fluid loss, exercise determinations, 142–143
Fluids; exercise ingestion performance effects, 147–149; gastric emptying, 151–156; intestinal absorption, 157–158; rehydration, 166–170; replacement limitations, 151–160; tracer methods, 159; water and

carbohydrate provision balancing,
166–169; water overload and hyponatremia, 169–170
Football, ACL (anterior cruciate ligament)
injury, 319
Fuels, sport performance, 95–138

Gastric emptying, fluids, 151–156
Gastrointestinal function, exercise effects,
159–160
Glutamine, 294–296

HCM (hypertrophic cardiomyopathy), sudden death of athletes, 240–241
Health problems; anomalous coronaries,
257; anomalous coronary arteries, 241;
aortic stenosis, 241; arrhythmias, 257–258;
athlete's heart, 244–246; blunt chest
trauma, 242; cardiovascular screening,
246–251; detection in athletes, 239–268;
epidemiological information on sudden
deaths, 241–244; future research, 259; gender differences, 243; HCM (hypertrophic
cardiomyopathy), 240–241; hypertension,
256; hypertrophic cardiomyopathy,
251–253; introduction, 240; Marfan syndrome, 241, 253–254; mitral valve prolapse, 254 256; myocarditis, 241; practical
implications, 258–259; sudden deaths of
athletes, 240–241
Heart murmurs, 248–249
Heart-rate monitors, sports training, 83
High fat/low carbohydrate diets, 105–106
High-intensity exercise; carbohydrate ingestion during, 114–115; sport performance
fuel use, 101–102
Hydration optimization; ambient temperature performance effects, 144–145; body
temperature performance manipulation,
143–144; exercise performance effects,
145–147; fluid ingestion performance effects, 147–149; fluid replacement limitations, 151–160; heat tolerance mechanisms, 149–151; hydration status exercise
performance effect, 145–147; introduction,
139–141; postexercise rehydration,
161–166; practical implications, 170–172;
preexercise, 160–161; rehydration fluid
formulation, 166–170; temperature regulation, 141–143; thermoregulation and
fluid balance, 141–151
Hypertension, 256
Hypertrophic cardiomyopathy; continuing
competition, 251–252; defining problems,
252; molecular discoveries, 252–253; sudden death of athletes, 251 253; symptoms,
251
Hyponatremia, 169–170

Ice hockey, carbohydrate ingestion during,
114–115

Ideographic modeling, sport psychology, 6,
39
Immune system, 269–316; adaptive immunity, 227–273, 285–287; animal studies,
289; B cells (B lymphocytes), 275–276; cytokines, 276–278, 285; epidemiological
studies, 288–289; exercise training,
287–290; exercise/infection relationship,
287–288; following athletes through a
competitive season, 293–294; glutamine
focus, 294–296; immune function, 290 296;
infection, 290–296; innate immunity,
272–273; intense exercise and immune
function, 278–287; introduction, 270–272;
macrophages, 274–275;
monocyte/macrophage function,
283–285; monocytes, 274–275; natural
killer cells, 275; neutrophils, 273–274;
overtraining, 290–303; practical implications, 303–305; psychological stress study,
289–291; stress hormones, 272; T cells (T
lymphocytes), 275–276
Immunomodulators, overtraining, 298–300
Indices, endurance capacity, 70–79
Induced overtraining, 291–293
Infection; exercise relationship, 287–288; immune system, 290–296
Inflammatory cytokines, 276
Injuries; ACL (anterior cruciate ligament),
319–330; ankle impingement syndromes,
344–350; diagnosis history, 318–319; introduction, 318–319; osteochondral knee
injuries, 331–334; stress fractures, 334–344
Innate immune system, 272–273
Innate immunity, exercise, 279
Intestinal absorption, fluids, 157–158
Intravenous infusions, plasma FFA exercise
ingestion methods, 104–105
IZOF (individual zone of optimal function
modeling), sport psychology, 7–8

L-carnitine, 201–210
Long-QT syndrome, sudden death of athletes, 257–258
Low-intensity exercise, sport performance
fuel use, 99
Lung-gom (swiftness of foot) cognitive
strategy, 24–28
Lymphocyte function, adaptive immunity,
285–287

Macrophage function, immune system,
283–285
Macrophages, immune system, 274–275
Mahetangs, lung-gom cognitive strategy,
24–28
Marathon runners; cognitive strategy,
23–38; field tests, 81
Marfan syndrome; diagnosis, 254; features,
253–254; management, 254; sudden death
of athletes, 241
Maximal aerobic power (VO2max), 22–23

Maximal oxygen uptake (VO2max), endurance capacity indice, 70–71
MaxLASS (Maximal lactate steady state), 75
MCT (Medium chain triglycerides), exercise ingestion methods, 105
Mental practice, motor skills, 11–13
Mitral valve prolapse, 254–256; additional testing, 255; clinical features, 255; complications, 255; diagnosis, 254–255; disqualifiers, 256; management tips, 255–256; pathogenesis, 255
Moderate-intensity exercise; carbohydrate feeding, 110–113; sport performance fuel use, 99–101
Monocyte function, immune system, 283–285
Monocytes, immune system, 274–275
Mood states, performance effects, 38–40
Motor skills, mental practice, 11–13
MTTS (medial tibial stress syndrome), 337
Muscle glycogen; carbohydrate ingestion timing, 118; carbohydrate resynthesis rates, 116–117; carbohydrate types, 117–118; dietary fat/protein resynthesis influence, 118; maximizing prior to competition, 119–120; resynthesis following exercise, 116–120
Muscles; carnitine exercise effects, 205–206; creatine supplementation effects on total creatine content, 190–193; creatine supplementation exercise performance, effects, 193–199; macronutrient diet exercise effects, 205–206; supplemental carnitine effects, 207
Muscular strength, described, 80–81
Myocarditis, sudden death of athletes, 241

Neutrophils, immune system, 273–274
NK cells (natural killer cells) immune system function, 275, 279–283
Nomothetic modeling, sport psychology, 6, 39
Non-elite distance runners, cognitive strategy, 32–38
Nutrition, prexercise, 120–123

Observers, described, 44
Osteochondral knee injuries; diagnosis, 331–332; future research, 334; practical implications, 331–333; treatment, 332–333
Overexertion, 270
Overreaching, 270
Overtraining, 270; following athletes through a competitive season, 293–294; glutamine focus, 294–296; immune function, 290–296; immunomodulators, 298 300; induced, 291–293; integrated psychoneuroimmune hypothesis, 301–303; mechanisms, 297–303; studies, 290

Physical exam, cardiovascular problems, 248

Plasma FFA; endurance training mobilization, 108–109; intravenous infusions during exercise, 104–105
Plasma, supplemental carnitine effects, 207
Plasma lactate; anaerobic threshold, 74–75; exercise response, 74–78; factors, 75–76; maximal lactate steady state, 75; non-invasive anaerobic threshold measurement, 76–78
Postexercise rehydration, 161–166
Predominant cognitive strategy, 33–34
Pre-elite distance runners, cognitive strategy, 32–38
Preexercise hydration, 160–161
Prevention; ACL (anterior cruciate ligament) injury, 327–328; stress fractures, 341–343
Prexercise nutrition, carbohydrate feedings, 120–123
Protein, glycogen resynthesis influences, 118
Providers, described, 44
Psychological stress, immune system relationship, 289–291
Psychologists, applied sport, 5–6
Psychoneuroimmune hypothesis, overtraining, 301–303
Publications; American Psychological Association Observer, 16; Ethical Principles of Psychologists and Code of Conduct, 18–19; Inner Tennis, 3; Keep on Running: The Science of Training and Performance, 3; On the Effects of Training, 318; RSQ (Running Style Questionnaire), 34; Self-Efficacy: A Predictor But Not a Cause of Behavior, 15; Sport Psychologist (The), 21; Supernature, 24

Recombinant human erythropoietin, 223
Rehydration fluids; formulation, 166–170; water and carbohydrate provision, 166–169; water overload and hyponatremia, 169–170
Relaxation; ideographic research modeling, 6; IZOF (individual zone of optimal function modeling), 7–8; mental practice, 11–13; nomothetic research modeling, 6; procedures, 7–8; relaxation-induced anxiety, 8–11; ZOF (zone of optimal function modeling), 7–8
Relaxation-induced anxiety, sport psychology, 8–11
Resting metabolism, carnitine, 205
Rowers, relaxation-induced anxiety, 9–10
RSQ (Running Style Questionnaire), cognitive strategy, 34–35
Runners; cognitive strategy, 28–38; field tests, 81

Self-efficacy research, sport psychology, 14–16
Short-term intense exercise, caffeine effects, 219–220

Simulated time trials, endurance capacity, 78–79
Skiing, ACL (anterior cruciate ligament) injury, 319
Soccer; ACL (anterior cruciate ligament) injury, 319; carbohydrate ingestion during, 114–115; field tests, 82
Softball, ACL (anterior cruciate ligament) injury, 319
Specificity, exercise testing, 67
Speed, described, 81
Speed indices, sports training, 80–81
Sport performance, field tests, 81–83
Sport performance fuels, 95–138; active people applications, 123–124; body carbohydrate stores, 98; body fat stores, 97–98; carbohydrate feeding during exercise, 110–115; dietary carbohydrate influences, 109–110; dietary carbohydrate metabolic responses, 115–116; fat oxidation endurance training increase, 107–109; fat supplementation during exercise, 104–105; FFA (free fatty acid), 96; future research, 124; high fat/low carbohydrate diets, 105 106; introduction, 96; muscle glycogen resynthesis, 116–120; practical considerations, 119; prexercise nutrition, 120–123; substrate use during exercise, 98–104
Sport psychology, 1–62; 4–min-mile barrier, 3–4; applied, 5–6; cognitive strategies, 22–38; consent procedures, 21–22; consumer concerns, 48–49; earlier reviews, 41–44; early work focus, 2–3; ethical principles and training, 18–22; external validity, 16–17; future practice, 46; future research, 46; goal-setting, 13–14; historical anecdotes, 3–5; ideographic research models, 6, 39; intuitive versus natural science/empirical models, 2; lawfulness of behavior, 20–22; mind game interventions, 17–18; nomothetic research models, 6, 39; performance and mood states, 38–40; practical implications, 44–45; qualitative survey data, 23–24; relaxation, 6–18; relaxation-induced anxiety, 8–11; self-efficacy research, 14–16; VMBR (visuo motor behavior rehearsal), 3
Sports injuries, prevention/recovery, 317–359
Sports training, 63–94; anaerobic energy production measurement, 79–80; described, 64; endurance capacity indices, 70–79; exercise testing, 67–70; exercise testing development, 64; field tests, 81–83; future research, 85–86; heart-rate monitors, 83; plasma lactate response to exercise, 74–78; practical implications, 84–85; speed indices, 80–81; strength indices, 80–81; volume performance effects, 65–66
Sprinting, field tests, 81
Squash, field tests, 82
Staleness, 270
Strength indices, sports training, 80–81
Stress fractures, 334–344; confirmatory studies, 338–339; diagnosis, 337–338; epidemiology, 334–335; etiology, 335–336; future research, 343–344; MTTS (medial tibial stress syndrome), 337; practical implications, 337–343; prevention, 341–343; treatment, 339–341
Stress hormones, 272
Syncope, cardiovascular problems, 248

T cells (T lymphocytes), immune system, 275–276
Team physicians; health problem conflicts, 258; hypertrophic cardiomyopathy help, 253
Temperature regulation; exercise, 141–143; fluid loss determinations, 142 143; sweat loss determinations, 142; sweat rates, 142
Tracer methods, fluids, 159
Training; described, 64; exercise/infection relationship, 287–288; mental practice, 11–13; relaxation, 6–11
Treatment; ACL (anterior cruciate ligament) injury, 320–325; osteochondral knee injuries, 332–333; stress fractures, 339–341
Triathletes, field tests, 81
Triglycerides; exercise ingestion methods, 104; medium chain, 105
Tumo, cognitive strategy, 24–25

Validity, exercise testing, 67
Variability, exercise testing, 68–70
Ventilatory threshold, described, 77
Ventricular preexcitation, sudden death of athletes, 257
VMBR (visuo-motor behavior rehearsal), 3
Volleyball, field tests, 82

Water overload, 169–170
Wrestling, ACL (anterior cruciate ligament) injury, 319

ZOF (zone of optimal function modeling), sport psychology, 7–8